Amphetamine Misuse

Amphetamine Misuse

International Perspectives on Current Trends

Edited by

Hilary Klee
Manchester Metropolitan University, UK

hoap **harwood academic publishers**
Australia • Canada • China • France • Germany • India • Japan
Luxembourg • Malaysia • The Netherlands • Russia • Singapore
Switzerland • Thailand • United Kingdom

Amsteldijk 166
1st Floor
1079 LH Amsterdam
The Netherlands

British Library Cataloguing in Publication Data

Amphetamine misuse : international perspectives on current
   trends
   1. Amphetamine abuse — Cross-cultural studies
   I. Klee, Hilary
   362.2'99

   ISBN 90-5702-081-5 (Softcover)

Contents

Preface

The idea for this book arose from a sense of frustration in the early 1990s that amphetamine misuse, a chronic and growing problem in the United Kingdom, was being overlooked – by government and researchers alike. Drug workers and other health professionals were uncertain of how to provide appropriate care – their services were not designed for stimulant users, they were under-resourced and there was no research to guide them. It took some time for their voice to be heard in official circles. Amphetamine misuse has gradually climbed up the agenda of drug policy makers since then, no doubt helped by international concern about the use of amphetamine-type stimulants by young people on the 'rave' scene and the corresponding increase in trafficking, and also the HIV risk to health revealed by studies of injection and sexual practices. It now seems to be acknowledged that the neglect needs to be remedied.

This book is published at a time when there are signs of a shift in emphasis in the international drug markets away from heroin and cocaine and towards cheaper synthetic drugs, particularly the amphetamines. The United Nations Drug Control Programme, the World Health Organization and the Council of Europe are taking initatives that are designed to improve and increase the data-base on these drugs and encourage international co-operation that will limit trafficking. The de-stabilization of Eastern European states and their drive towards modernization, the opening of borders in the European Union, the emergence of China and the rapid economic development of some Southeast Asian states, all contribute to a high level of uncertainty that impedes the establishment of effective mechanisms that will facilitate inter-state control and the sharing of drug intelligence.

The ease of production of amphetamines, the technical and business expertise of the manufacturers and drug traffickers and the exceptionally high profits to be made, mean that law enforcement is no longer simply a matter of national concern. Market growth is heavily influenced by international agreements concerning drug control and legislation, and also the contagiousness of trends to new populations. Thus in each nation, the nature of drug misuse is the result of forces within its boundaries and some that are external to them, over which they have less control. To quote Dorothy Black (1991) ... "the nature and size of a drug problem can be affected by a host of factors within a country and by the effects of legal, social and economic change in other countries. The Opium Wars of the nineteenth century demonstrated all too clearly how the trade and economic policy of one country (the United Kingdom) had adverse consequences for the social and economic life of India and China".

These chapters address the phenomenon of amphetamine misuse from the perspectives of seven countries. Some have a historical problem of heavy use, some have a recurring cycle of use and others a growing problem with MDMA (Ecstasy) on the 'rave' scene. The emphasis in this book is on the amphetamines, but the relationship with MDMA is explored in several chapters. We start wtih an overview by Tokuo Yoshida from the World Health Organization that establishes terminology, summarizes developments in international law, and describes the world history of licit and illicit use of amphetamines. The final section attempts to summarize critical factors of universal relevance that have influenced the growth and decline of amphetamine misuse at both national and international levels. Between the first and the final observations, authors from the United Kingdom, Australia, the United States, Japan, Sweden, Germany and The Netherlands provide us with insights into the diversity of amphetamine misuse in different cultures, how governments have reacted to it and what the future may hold in store. They reveal many similar experiences in the use of drugs and the individual and social consequences of that use, but greatly dissimilar attitudes and ways of dealing with them. Internationally there is a wealth of knowledge that could be shared, there are nations not represented in this book that have their own stories to tell but a research base too small to be able to substantiate the observations. If predictions about market growth in amphetamines are accurate, a strategy that takes account of the difficulties and ambitions of undeveloped nations will be needed to contain it and one that will accept some compromise on fundamental issues that affect the mechanisms of control.

Black, D. (1991) The recent history of British drugs policy. In: *Drug Misuse in Local Communities: Perspectives Across Europe*, T. Bennett (ed.), p. 31. London: The Police Federation.

Acknowledgements

There are many people who have contributed directly or indirectly to this book. I am grateful for research grants from the Economic and Social Research Council, the Department of Health, the Home Office Drugs Prevention Initiative, the Higher Education Funding Council and the British Council, that have supported my interest in the misuse of amphetamines at a time when this was not a popular research area. I would also like to thank Mildred Blaxter and Liza Catan for their continuing encouragement over several years. Many researchers collected data with dedication and enthusiasm under difficult field conditions – Paul Reid has been a particularly valuable and reliable source of support. Some colleagues have readily provided help and information – notably Julie Morris, John Witton, Mike Donmall and Tim Millar. Other colleagues have shared my interest in the topic and this has been an incentive to keep pursuing it – Tom Carnwath, John Merrill, Neil Hunt, Richard Pates and Philip Fleming. Drug workers in the Northwest of England have been generous with their time to help recruit volunteers for the research. I thank my authors for their hard work towards this personal goal of mine. Some of them may have suffered rather than enjoyed my editorship at times but did not complain and I hope they now feel it was worth it.

Finally there were two main players in the production of this book:– David Legge, who has read my own contributions painstakingly and often several times, providing constructive, objective criticism and unfailing support; and Gail Meaden without whose cheerful, efficient and diligent work the book would never have reached the publisher.

Contributors

RACHEL ANDERSON
Rachel Anderson is a research associate at the University of California, Davis, Infection and Immunologic Diseases (Division of General Medicine). Currently a member of the board of directors of Harm Reduction Services she is also an administrator of the Sacramento area Needle Exchange. Her research interests include HIV/AIDS prevention work among injecting drug users and the efficacy of treatment services, particularly with respect to gender issues.

JEROME E. BECK
Jerome Beck has extensive experience in the substance abuse field. As a drug information specialist and instructor at the University of Oregan, he was able to closely monitor the long-standing popularity of methamphetamine among student and blue collar populations there. His research interest continued in the San Francisco Bay Area, eventually culminating in his role as co-principal investigator for the federally-funded sociological study of *Ice and Other Methamphetamine Use*. More recently, he served as principal investigator and investigator, respectively, on two other federally-funded studies: an ethnographic exploration of *LSD, MDMA and Other Psychedelics* and an *Epidemiological Study of Marijuana and Health* assessing long-term outcomes among a large healthcare-based cohort of users and non-users.

NEIL FLYNN

Neil Flynn is professor of clinical medicine at the University of California Davis School of Medicine, in the Department of Internal Medicine, where he is a specialist in infectious diseases. His research interests focus on the study of the epidemiology and public health impact of HIV transmission. Since 1987 he has undertaken several studies of HIV among injecting drug users in the Sacramento area and participates in the medical care of approximately 1,500 HIV-infected people in Sacramento. He is a supporter of the harm reduction model of injection drug use.

SUSUMU FUKUI

Division of Drug Dependence, National Institute of Mental Health, National Center for Neurology and Psychiatry, Chiba, Japan.

WAYNE HALL

Wayne Hall is currently chair of drug and alcoholic studies and director of the National Drug and Alcohol Research Centre (NDARC) at the University of New South Wales, Australia. His principal areas of interest are research design and data analysis in the drug and alcohol field. More widely his interests include: patterns of cannabis use and the health and psychological consequences, aboriginal alcohol use, the evaluation of methadone maintenance treatment, and patterns of psychostimulant and heroin use.

JULIE HANDO

Julie Hando is a senior research officer at the National Drug and Alcohol Research Centre, Sydney, Australia where she has been working since 1990. She is currently completing her doctorate on Australian patterns of psychostimulant use and correlates of harm. Other research interests include: drug use among detained youths, developing treatment and prevention interventions to reduce harm among psychostimulant users, and monitoring trends in illicit drug use.

WOLFGANG HECKMANN

Wolfgang Heckmann started his research in the field of addiction in 1976, and has also served as a drug commissioner (planning and administration) for West Berlin. His particular interest over the past ten years has been research on HIV/AIDS and he was, until 1993, director of the Social Research Department of the AIDS Research Center at the German Federal Institute of Health. As professor at FH Magdeburg he also teaches social psychology and he has edited texts and journals in the field of drugs and AIDS research.

KAREN A. JOE-LAIDLER

Karen Joe-Laidler is assistant professor of sociology at the University of Hawaii, Manoa and has been involved in criminal justice and drug research for the last fourteen years. She has worked on a number of areas including adult felony sentencing policy, prison classification, and the impact of juvenile court intervention. In the last six years, her writings have centred on drug use patterns among women and Asian Americans, drugs and violence among youth gangs in the US, and runaways and the juvenile justice system.

KERSTIN KÄLL

Kerstin Käll, is a clinical psychiatrist and researcher at the Karolinska Institute in Stockholm. Amphetamine is the main drug injected by Swedish drug injectors and she has interviewed many hundreds of amphetamine users over the years. Since 1987 she has conducted an ongoing epidemiological study of HIV seroprevalence and risk behaviour among injecting drug users at the Remand Prison in Stockholm. Her PhD thesis, based on this study, focused on the sexual behaviour of a subpopulation of heavy drug injectors. She is presently involved in a study of HIV in prison sponsored by the European Commission. Her main clinical interest is in the psychopathology of the abuse of various substances, including cannabis.

HILARY KLEE

Hilary Klee is research professor of psychology and director of the Centre for Social Research on Health and Substance Abuse (SRHSA) at the Manchester Metropolitan University, Manchester, UK. Her research has covered a wide range of drug misuse and health concerns – for example: polydrug use and the misuse of prescribed pharmaceuticals; HIV-related risk behaviour; peer-group leaders and prevention; pregnancy, motherhood and drugs; homelessness and drug misuse. She has a special interest in amphetamine misuse and drug service provision for amphetamine users.

KYOHEI KONUMA

Since 1988 Kyohei Konuma has been director of the Drug Dependence Treatment and Research Department at the National Psychiatric Institute of Shimohusa, Chiba-ken in Japan. Prior to that he was deputy director of the Narcotic Division of the Pharmaceutical Affairs Bureau for the Ministry of Health and Welfare. His speciality is in the treatment and clinical research of drug dependence.

MARISSA A. MILLER

Marissa Miller is a medical epidemiologist in the United States Public Health Service currently positioned within the United States Food and Drug Administration (USFDA). She holds adjunct professor status at the Uniformed Services University of the Health Sciences, teaching epidemiology to medical students. Dr Miller's expertise is in epidemiology and disease surveillance. She has conducted outbreak investigations and field studies, as well as designed drug abuse surveillance systems targeted to minority populations, while with the National Institute on Drug Abuse, now part of the National Institutes of Health. Presently Dr Miller is involved in implementing a national antimicrobial susceptibility monitoring system and directing associated activities and analytic research studies, with the Center for Veterinary Medicine, part of the USFDA.

PATRICIA MORGAN
Pat Morgan is associate professor of public health at the University of California, Berkeley, USA. Her publications derive from 20 years of cross-cultural comparative research in the alcohol and drug field and many focus on policy, political economy, social control and gender, race and class comparisons. The recipient of a Fulbright Fellowship, and a Pacific Rim Fellowship, Dr Morgan has directed two national research studies, and served as co-investigator on three more.

JUDITH MYLES
Judy Myles is consultant psychiatrist in Drug Dependence and Specialty Director of the Avon Drug Problem Team (Bristol, England), an area of the United Kingdom with a particularly pronounced amphetamine misuse problem. She is a member of the Royal College of Psychiatrists and of the Society for the Study of Addiction. Her research interests focus on opiate detoxification, including the use of α-2 agonists and buprenorphine, and the efficacy of substitute amphetamine prescribing in a clinical setting.

THOMAS PIETSCHMANN
Thomas Pietschmann after graduation worked in the Regional and Country Studies Branch of the United Nations Industrial Development Organisation (UNIDO) and then in the Asia Section of the United Nations Drug Control Programme (UNDCP). He now works in the newly established Research Section of UNDCP's Technical Services Branch. As part of the research team he has been actively involved in the preparation of a number of UNDCP research papers, including the Social and Economic Consequences of Drug Abuse and Illicit Trafficking, the Status of Knowledge on the Global Illicit Drug Industry (to be published in 1996) and on a Global review of Amphetamine-type Stimulants (to be published in 1996). His main area of research interest is in the interface of economics, shadow economies, illicit markets and drugs.

INGE P. SPRUIT
Inge Spruit is a medical anthropologist and epidemiologist and at the time of co-authoring a chapter in this book, is head of the department of Information and Research of The Netherlands Institute on Alcohol and Drugs. In 1996 this institute will merge with The Netherlands Institute for Mental Health

Care and will be known as the Division of Substance Use and Addictions. A core programme will be the epidemiology and monitoring of the use and abuse of alcohol and illegal drugs. Special attention goes to youth in general, and pupils in school surveys. Another core programme is the Dutch Alcohol and Drugs Report. The focus here is on societal developments and a series of coherent multidisciplinary XTC studies will be co-ordinated from within and outside the institute. Applied research and monitoring, policy evaluation, identification of information gaps and dispersion of information are intricately interwoven in this programme.

HIROSHI SUWAKI

Hiroshi Suwaki is presently professor and head of the Department of Neuropsychiatry at the Kagawa Medical School in Kagawa, Japan. His main interests of research are within addiction psychiatry – epidemiologic and clinical research on alcohol, volatile solvents and methamphetamine dependencies. He is a member of the WHO Expert Advisory Panel on Drug Dependence and Alcohol Problems, on the Board of Directors of ICAA (International Council on Alcohol and Addictions), on the International Advisory Board for 'Addiction' and Editorial Advisory Board of 'Alcohol and Alcoholism'.

MARGRIET W. van LAAR

Margriet van Laar is a bio-psychologist specializing in the field of human psychopharmacology. She has been involved in research on the therapeutic, cognitive and physiological effects of legal and illegal psychoactive drugs in target populations at the University of Utrecht. Drugs of primary interest are the recently developed serotonergic compounds that (may) have promising applications in a variety of disorders, such as anxiety, depression and substance abuse disorders. Currently she is a 'Focal Point' staff member at The Netherlands Institute on Alcohol and Drugs (NIAD). The NIAD has been designated by the Ministry of Health as facilities organization ('Focal Point') within the structure of the European Monitoring Centre for Drugs and Drugs Addiction (EMCDDA) in Lisbon, established by the Council of the European Union. Primary tasks of the Focal Point are to collect and process existing information concerning drugs and drug related problems, to improve data-comparison methods, and to disseminate information to relevant organizations in The Netherlands, to the EMCDDA and to Focal Points in other EU Member States.

TOKUO YOSHIDA

A pharmacist by education and a 'technical bureaucrat' by profession Tokuo Yoshida has worked in the field of drug control since 1966. While in the health ministry in Tokyo, he served as the first secretary to the Japanese

Expert Committee on Dependence-Producing Drugs during the late 1960s as Deputy Director, Narcotics Division, and in the Pharmaceuticals and Chemicals Safety Division during the 1970s and 1980s. International experience includes a four year assignment at the United Nations narcotics laboratory. Currently, he is chief of the Regulatory Control Unit, Division of Mental Health and Prevention of Substance Abuse at the WHO Headquarters in Geneva, Switzerland.

1

Use and Misuse of Amphetamines:
An International Overview

TOKUO YOSHIDA

Amphetamines are potent stimulants of the central nervous system (CNS) with some sympathomimetic activity. They were placed on the market before World War II and used extensively for a wide range of therapeutic indications and for nonmedical purposes as 'pep pills' during the war and post-war reconstruction periods. As their use became widespread, their habit-forming properties came to light, and their misuse gradually emerged as a public health problem. Discussions on the misuse of amphetamines led to an international consensus, in 1971, to place amphetamines under strict control measures similar to those applied to narcotic drugs.

Today, the medical use of amphetamines is limited in terms of both quantity and scope of therapeutic indication, but the illicit traffic in, and misuse of, amphetamines are prevalent throughout the world. Furthermore, the problem of amphetamine misuse has become even more complex with the emergence of many amphetamine-like substances. This chapter first discusses terminology which often creates confusion, and provides an overview of the history of use and misuse of amphetamines from an international point of view.

TERMINOLOGY

In discussing problems associated with the misuse of drugs, there has been some confusion arising from the use of many similar and closely-related terms. Since different authors may use a variety of terms to describe the various aspects of use and misuse of amphetamines in the subsequent chapters of this book, it will be useful to review commonly used terms first.

Terms Related to Drug Identity

Amphetamine, in the singular form, properly applies to the racemate of 2-amino-1-phenylpropane. The molecule of amphetamine has one asymmetric carbon, yielding two optical isomers. The spelling of its English INN (International Nonproprietary Name) is *amfetamine* (WHO, 1992a). The INNs are a standard drug nomenclature consisting of generic names of pharmaceutical substances determined by WHO (the World Health Organization) in order to help avoid confusion with regard to the identity of pharmaceutical substances. INNs are indicated in parentheses the first time they appear in this chapter in order to facilitate cross-referencing.

Dexamphetamine (INN: *dexamfetamine*) is the dextro rotatory or (+)-isomer of amphetamine. Since the (+)-form is known to be significantly more potent than the *levo*-form, amphetamine, which is the mixture of the same quantity of *dextro*- and *levo*-forms, is less potent than dexamphetamine.

Methamphetamine (INN: *metamfetamine*) is the *N*-methyl derivative of amphetamine. Unlike *amfetamine* (INN) which corresponds to the racemic mixture, *metamfetamine* (INN) refers to the *dextro*-isomer of 1-phenyl-2-methylaminopropane. Methamphetamine is more potent than dexamphetamine.

Amphetamines, in the plural form, usually applies at least to the above three substances. In this chapter, the term amphetamines will be used in this sense. Some people include, in addition, *levamfetamine* (INN), the *l*-form of amphetamine, as well as levomethamphetamine and methamphetamine racemate or, in other words, all stereoisomers of both 2-amino-1-phenylpropane and 2-methylamino-1-phenylpropane. In its broadest context, however, the term can even embrace a large number of structurally and pharmacologically related substances. In this chapter, some of these amphetamine analogues are briefly mentioned under amphetamine-like substances.

Amphetamines have a primary or secondary amino group in their molecules and form stable and crystalline water-soluble salts by reacting with several inorganic acids. Because of these advantages amphetamines are used in salt forms. Of these salts, amphetamine sulphate and methamphetamine hydrochloride are the commonest.

Terms Related to Patterns and Consequences of Use

Misuse is a term employed in the national drug control legislation of the United Kingdom (Misuse of Drugs Act, 1971) and other countries having similar drug control systems. Without prejudice to legal definitions that may exist in these countries, misuse is used in this chapter as a general term to mean 'bad use' or a use which is medically and/or socially unacceptable.

Abuse is another term used in a similar way, also quite widely. For example, the international drug control treaties use the term abuse rather than misuse.

Except in legal discussions where subtle differences in meaning may have practical implications, misuse and abuse may be used interchangeably. *Recreational use* and *nonmedical use* are also similar but they are more neutral because they do not necessarily imply bad use. In the early days when amphetamines were not controlled drugs, taking amphetamines to stay awake at night was seen as nonmedical use but not as misuse or abuse. However, the use of the same quantities of amphetamines for the same purpose may be considered today as misuse or abuse, because such use is no longer considered as appropriate by society. In several Islamic countries, recreational use of alcohol may be considered as misuse or abuse regardless of the quantity drunk, but in other countries, drinking may be considered as alcohol abuse only when it becomes "excessive". As social and/or medical norms change, so will change what most people call misuse or abuse of drugs.

As a diagnostic term not influenced by social norms, WHO's ICD-10 (International Classification of Diseases, 10th revision) guidelines (WHO, 1992b) employs the term *harmful use*, which refers to a pattern of psychoactive substance use that is causing damage to health. Harmful use commonly, but not invariably, has adverse social consequences. Social consequences in themselves, however, are not sufficient to justify a diagnosis of harmful use.

Misuse of drugs usually begins with *experimental use*, out of curiosity or in response to an offer from drug-using friends. It may stop afterwards, if the user does not feel good at all. The use can also continue occasionally as opportunities permit — a mode of use often called *casual use*. The user may be enjoying the effect of the drug, but can stop using it if highly motivated, without too much difficulty. The user may continue using the drug further, to feel good or to avoid feeling bad, until it becomes difficult to stop using the drug. Having to continue taking the drug is a state of being dependent on the drug and the type of drug use at this phase is referred to as dependent use (WHO, 1974).

Since drug dependence is one of the most serious health problems associated with the misuse of amphetamines, let us examine its meaning in more detail.

Drug Dependence

Drug addiction and *drug habituation* were the terms used widely by experts up until the 1960s, and by many people including medical doctors even today. During the 1960s, the WHO Expert Committee on Drug Dependence (which will be referred to as "the Expert Committee", whose name has changed several times since its first meeting in 1949) made serious attempts to clarify the difference between the two, only to abandon this effort and to propose instead the use of drug dependence as a term to replace both addiction and habituation (WHO, 1964).

The Expert Committee made a distinction between *psychic dependence* and *physical dependence* and described these in its meeting report in 1974 as follows: "psychic dependence is a condition in which a drug produces a feeling of satisfaction and a psychic drive that require periodic or continuous administration of the drug to produce pleasure or to avoid discomfort, whereas physical dependence refers to an adaptive state that manifests itself by intense physical disturbances when the administration of the drug is suspended" (WHO, 1974). These disturbances, i.e., withdrawal (or abstinence) syndromes, are a group of symptoms of variable clustering and severity occurring on absolute or relative withdrawal of a substance after repeated, and usually prolonged and/or high dose use of that substance. Onset and course of the withdrawal syndrome are time-limited and are related to the type of substance and the dose being used immediately before abstinence. Withdrawal syndrome does not exclude "rebound" phenomena.

Both "physical dependence" and "psychic dependence" are commonly used even today. However, the ICD-10 guidelines do not make a distinction between the two. Speaking of only one dependence, the guidelines describe dependence syndrome as follows.

> *"Dependence syndrome — A mental and behavioural disorder due to psychoactive substance use, described in ICD-10 as a cluster of physiological, behavioural, and cognitive phenomena in which the use of a substance or substances takes on a much higher priority for a given individual than other behaviours that once had greater value. A central descriptive characteristic of the dependence syndrome is the desire (often strong, sometimes overpowering) to take psychoactive drugs (which may or may not have been medically prescribed), alcohol, or tobacco. There may be evidence that return to substance use after a period of abstinence leads to a more rapid reappearance of other features of the syndrome than occurs with non-dependent individuals."*

The non-distinction of physical dependence from psychic dependence was endorsed subsequently by the Expert Committee, which felt that the term physical dependence might lead to confusion with the general term drug dependence (WHO, 1993). Such confusion actually occurred because clinicians often interpreted the manifestation of withdrawal syndromes as evidence of physical dependence, and, based on the notion that physical dependence is a type of drug dependence, they would diagnose the person as drug dependent. This is not correct since, if the withdrawal syndromes are not so severe and are well tolerated, they will not make it difficult for the user to come off the drug, and the user who can come off the drug without much difficulty is not dependent on the drug by definition. Furthermore, the distinction is not consistent with the modern view that all drug effects on the individual are potentially understandable in biological terms. It is in fact difficult to differentiate between psychic reactions and physical symptoms as they often occur simultaneously and are closely interrelated.

In summary, the essential component of drug dependence is a strong desire or a sense of compulsion (craving) to take the drug as manifested by drug-seeking behaviour which is difficult to control. Withdrawal syndrome and tolerance (a reduction in the sensitivity to a drug following its repeated administration) are both considered merely as consequences of drug exposure which, alone, are not sufficient evidence for a positive diagnosis of drug dependence.

In pharmacology, when a drug is a reinforcer, it makes the desire for the drug stronger as the subject continues using the drug. Therefore, repeated use of drugs having marked reinforcing efficacy can easily lead to a state of dependence.

The definition of dependence does not explicitly exclude dependence on the therapeutic effect of a drug. Psychological "dependence" can develop on the therapeutic effect of a drug when the drug is effective in alleviating severe suffering of the user, particularly when the suffering is of a chronic nature. Such a condition, for example, may occur with psychoactive as well as non-psychoactive drugs. This state, however, is not considered as real drug dependence. For example, a strong desire for amphetamines in patients suffering from narcolepsy does not necessarily represent dependence on amphetamines. If the craving for amphetamines persists even after the disease has been cured, it could then be regarded as a sign of drug dependence.

THERAPEUTIC USE OF AMPHETAMINES

Originally, amphetamine was introduced as a nasal astringent presented in inhaler form sold over-the-counter in the early 1930s. During this decade, the CNS stimulant effects were discovered in the USA, as well as therapeutic effects of amphetamine for the treatment of narcolepsy. The marketing of oral preparations of amphetamine sulphate began in the USA and the United Kingdom, followed by Germany and other countries. Soon after the marketing of amphetamine sulphate in the USA, methamphetamine hydrochloride was placed on the market in Germany towards the end of the 1930s. During the following decade, both amphetamine and methamphetamine were sold under a variety of brand names in many countries.

Numerous studies and reports have been published on the effects, use and misuse of amphetamines. Amphetamines have a marked CNS stimulant effect and some sympathomimetic effects with adrenergic agonist activity. Subjective mood-elevating effects of amphetamines are due to the CNS stimulation. Cocaine is chemically different, but pharmacologically similar to amphetamines except that it is shorter-acting. At moderate doses, amphetamines cause wakefulness and euphoria, increase motor activity and performance, reduce appetite and food and water intake. At higher doses, symptoms of CNS overstimulation appear such as insomnia, nervousness, restlessness, anxiety, irritability, and aggression. Even when the initial effects are a pleasant mood elevation and euphoria, there are often dysphoria, depression and feelings of fatigue afterwards. Blood pressure and pulse rate are generally, but not always, increased due to stimulation of the sympathetic nervous system.

After oral administration, amphetamines are absorbed through the gastrointestinal system, reaching a peak plasma level in 2–3 hours and remaining relatively close to this level at 5 hours post administration. However, the subjective effects of mood elevation do not necessarily correspond to the blood level of the drug; they tend to reach a peak before the drug level does and wane earlier than the drug does from the blood. Much of the orally administered amphetamines are excreted in the urine within the first 24 hours. The rate of urinary excretion increases as the urine becomes acidic. Metabolic changes include ring-hydroxylation, oxidative demethylation (in the case of methamphetamine), beta-hydroxylation and deamination.

Tolerance develops as a result of the repeated use of amphetamines with respect to subjective mood-elevating effects as well as anorectic effects. Other than the difference in potency, there is no difference in pharmacological profile between amphetamine and methamphetamine.

Initially, amphetamines were indicated for a wide range of conditions, including asthma, enuresis, epilepsy, motion sickness, myasthenia gravis, obesity, overdose of hypnotics and narcotic analgesics, schizophrenia, narcolepsy and hyperactivity disorders in children. A number of pharmaceutical preparations, e.g., inhalers and oral dosage forms, were sold, sometimes without requiring a physician's prescription. Today, their therapeutic use is very limited, both in scope and quantity, for rare cases of narcolepsy and as an adjunct to psychological and educational treatment for attention-deficit hyperactive children. Use as anorectic agents, once widespread, is strongly discouraged. Changing medical views on amphetamine misuse and psychotoxicity, as well as the development of safer alternative drugs, have contributed to this change in prescribing practices.

MISUSE OF AMPHETAMINES AND THEIR INTERNATIONAL CONTROL

As the use of amphetamines for a broad range of therapeutic purposes became widespread during the late 1930s and early 1940s, iatrogenic amphetamine dependence came to be recognized as a problem. Patients who were prescribed amphetamines on a chronic basis to reduce appetite, for example, complained of depression or inability to work when the drug was reduced or discontinued. Furthermore, non-medical use of amphetamines became common in some countries where these drugs were used by the military for night operations, by factory workers on a night shift, by truck drivers on extended duties and even by students preparing for examinations. By today's standards, all such non-medical uses and most of the above therapeutic uses would be regarded as misuse or abuse of amphetamines. In those days, however, there was no clear notion of what might constitute a misuse of amphetamines.

WHO became aware of the misuse of amphetamines in the early 1950s. The Expert Committee that met in 1952 was concerned about the misuse of amphetamines by opiate abusers when opiates were not available to them, and it recommended a close watch on the use of amphetamines (WHO, 1952). The Expert Committee discussed the issue again the following year and recommended that governments should take measures to strengthen the control of amphetamines on the national level. As control measures, the committee specifically suggested that: preparations of amphetamines should be dispensed only on prescription; each prescription should specify the number of times it may be refilled; and a careful record should be kept of each prescription (WHO, 1953). In 1955, this Expert Committee examined the misuse of amphetamines for the third time, focusing on the extent of the problem and countermeasures taken in Japan (WHO, 1956).

Misuse of amphetamines was recognized as a hazard to public health in Japan, where amphetamines were placed on the market in 1941 (Study Group on Dependence-Producing Drugs, 1988). When World War II ended in 1945, stocks of amphetamines previously held by the military were sold on the black market. Pharmaceutical companies also promoted the marketing of their products containing amphetamines, with a claim that amphetamines removed sleepiness and fatigue. Under these circumstances, the use and misuse of amphetamines increased rapidly. The tightening of distribution controls under pharmaceutical regulations, such as prescription requirements introduced in 1950, failed to turn around the increasing trend of amphetamine misuse, and the government was forced to enact the stringent Stimulant Control Law in 1951. Despite strict enforcement of this law, misuse of amphetamines still continued to increase for a few more years until 1954, when the number of current users was estimated to be over half a million. Users found it difficult to give up the drug when the licit supply was cut off, and obtained illicit methamphetamine manufactured in clandestine laboratories. The dependence-producing property of amphetamines was thus quite apparent. As the police crackdown on the illicit market proceeded successfully, Japan's first amphetamine epidemic quickly subsided after 1955.

Though not so explosive as the epidemic in Japan, the misuse of inhaler preparations of amphetamines became a significant problem in the USA during the 1940s, leading to the withdrawal of these preparations from the market.

During the 1950s, amphetamines became generally recognized as dependence-producing drugs liable to be misused. However, misuse of amphetamines was considered as a local problem and not one for international action (WHO, 1956). This perception changed during the following decade as an increasing number of countries including Australia, Sweden, and the United Kingdom, began to face similar problems. Misuse of CNS depressants such as barbiturates and hallucinogenic drugs such as *lysergide* (INN; commonly known as LSD) also emerged and became an international concern.

The spreading misuse of CNS stimulants, depressants and hallucinogens led to the discussions on the desirability of setting up an international control system for psychotropic substances at the United Nations Commission on Narcotic Drugs during the 1960s. At that time, such an international control system existed only for narcotic drugs based on the Single Convention on Narcotic Drugs, 1961, an international drug control treaty which covered opium, opiates and synthetic opioids as well as coca leaves, cannabis and their products.

The Expert Committee held in 1969 actively contributed to this discussion by presenting a draft protocol on psychotropic substances together with proposed lists of CNS stimulants, depressants and hallucinogens to be placed under control (WHO, 1970). Most of these proposals were accepted by the United Nations and were incorporated into the Convention on Psychotropic Substances (United Nations, 1977) adopted in 1971. The list of 32 psychotropic substances placed under international control included amphetamines and amphetamine-like CNS stimulants, CNS depressants such as hypnotics, sedatives and anxiolytics, as well as hallucinogens. Under this Convention, amphetamines are subject to a set of control measures similar to those applicable to narcotic drugs such as morphine and pethidine. Since the time the Convention came into effect in 1976, the number of controlled psychotropic substances has increased from 32 to 105 (as of February 1995). The procedures for modifying the list of controlled substances involve a medical and scientific assessment of individual substances by WHO and decision by the United Nations.

PROBLEMS ASSOCIATED WITH AMPHETAMINE MISUSE

Known patterns of amphetamine misuse include quasi-therapeutic use of nasal inhalant and oral preparations, oral ingestion and intravenous injection of illicit amphetamines, as well as inhalation of the sublimate of illicit methamphetamine upon heating. Alternating or concomitant use of other drugs and alcohol is not uncommon. The purity and the quantity of the drug ingested fluctuate, particularly when illicit amphetamines are taken. Individual variations are known to be significant in human reactions to psychoactive substances. The seriousness of health consequences of misuse varies considerably, depending on such factors and conditions of use.

Chronic Effects of Amphetamines

Past outbreaks of amphetamine misuse have clearly indicated that drug dependence is one of the major problems associated with the chronic use of amphetamines. The strong dependence liability of amphetamines has been confirmed also by laboratory tests. Like cocaine, amphetamines are potent reinforcers in experimental animals, including monkeys. Animals allowed to self-administer amphetamines continue taking the drug, until they become exhausted due to increased motor activity and reduced food intake. Compared with oral use, dependence develops more rapidly with intravenous injection because of quicker onset of action and more intensive euphoric effects. Dose escalation is not uncommon.

The Expert Committee once considered that the lack of physical dependence was one of the characteristic features of amphetamine-type drug dependence (WHO, 1974). The basis for this view was the absence of amphetamine-specific withdrawal symptoms. At that time, depression and sense of fatigue commonly experienced during the withdrawal state may have been considered merely as psychic rebound phenomena. However, there is no agreement among researchers that the definition of withdrawal symptoms should exclude psychic rebound phenomena. Furthermore, the differentiation between physical and psychic dependence is no longer considered useful, as discussed earlier. It would therefore be appropriate not to mention physical dependence, and note instead depression, apathy and fatigue as common withdrawal symptoms.

According to the ICD-10 guidelines, a definite diagnosis of dependence should usually be made only if three or more of the following have been experienced or exhibited at some time during the previous year:

(a) a strong desire or sense of compulsion to take the substance;

(b) difficulties in controlling substance-taking behaviour in terms of its onset, termination, or levels of use;

(c) a physiological withdrawal state when substance use has ceased or been reduced, as evidenced by: the characteristic withdrawal syndrome for the substance: or use of the same (or a closely related) substance with the intention of relieving or avoiding withdrawal symptoms;

(d)   evidence of tolerance, such that increased doses of the psychoactive substance are required in order to achieve effects originally produced by lower doses (clear examples of this are found in alcohol- and opiate-dependent individuals who may take daily doses sufficient to incapacitate or kill non-tolerant users);

(e)   progressive neglect of alternative pleasures or interests because of psychoactive substance use, increased amount of time necessary to obtain or take the substance or to recover from its effects;

(f)   persisting with substance use despite clear evidence of overtly harmful consequences, such as harm to the liver through excessive drinking, depressive mood states consequent to periods of heavy substance use, or drug-related impairment of cognitive functioning; efforts should be made to determine that the user was actually, or could be expected to be, aware of the nature and extent of the harm.

Another serious consequence of chronic use is what is generally known as amphetamine psychosis. This psychotic disorder is characterized by schizophrenia-like hallucinations and paranoid delusions without disorientation or confusion. The onset of the initial psychotic disorder varies considerably among the individuals misusing amphetamines, depending, in part, on the route of administration and dosage, ranging from 2–4 weeks of use up to several years of use. During the methamphetamine epidemic in Japan, it was observed that the initial psychotic disorder developed in approximately two-thirds of the chronic users within three years of misuse (Study Group on Dependence-Producing Drugs, 1988). The hallucinations are mainly visual and auditory, and the paranoid reactions can lead to sudden aggressive behaviour, including homicide. It should be pointed out that, in users who have already experienced this psychosis once, it can recur more easily after a short period of reuse, even when there has been a long period of abstinence. In some users, even a single dose of amphetamines can trigger the recurrence of the psychosis.

Hallucinations and paranoid delusions usually disappear within a month after discontinuation of the drug use. However, cases of residual psychotic disorder, lasting for more than half a year, as well as 'flashbacks' triggered by other psychoactive substance use or even by non-specific stimuli, are also known to occur.

Long-term misuse of amphetamines has been suspected of bringing about personality changes characterized by increased apathy and irritability. Such personality changes are not specific to amphetamines.

Toxicity

Amphetamines are not safe drugs in terms of acute toxicity. Although fatal cases are rare, acute intoxication can occur in misusers who repeatedly inject the drug at short intervals in an attempt to maintain the euphoric effect, or who unknowingly use illicit amphetamines of higher purity.

Symptoms of acute intoxication include nervousness, anxiety, hypersensitivity to light and sound stimuli, irritability, and aggressiveness. Acute psychotic reactions, including stereotyped behaviour such as shoe-shining or nail polishing lasting for hours, hallucinations, paranoid reactions, confusion and delirium, may occur. In some cases, anxiety and motor unrest, pale skin, nausea, vomiting, tremor, convulsions and coma may develop and lead to cardiovascular shock, with a fall in blood pressure. In other cases, elevated blood pressure may cause cerebral haemorrhages. Dry mouth, sweating, anorexia and mydriasis (pupil dilation) are often observed.

There is some similarity between psychotic reactions of acute intoxication and psychotic disorder due to chronic use. The two may be distinguished by the absence of acute effects such as mydriasis and sweating in the latter.

General Health and Social Problems

In addition to the health problems caused directly by the pharmacological effects of amphetamines, amphetamine misuse leads to general health and social problems commonly associated with the misuse of illicit drugs, such as cocaine and heroin. They include the transmission of HIV/AIDS due to the sharing of contaminated injecting equipment, unsafe sexual behaviour, accidents, family disruption, violence, criminality and productivity loss.

AMPHETAMINE-LIKE SUBSTANCES

There are a large number of other CNS stimulants and stimulants with hallucinogenic effects having varying degrees of similarity in chemical structure to amphetamines. Of these, without counting the three stereo-isomers of amphetamines mentioned earlier, 29 substances are placed under international control as of February 1995. Furthermore, the addition to the list of three amphetamine-like substances (aminorex, methcathinone and mesocarb; all INNs) is being proposed by WHO.

Five of the 29 amphetamine-like substances were in the original list of controlled substances and 24 were subsequently added to it. Pharmacologically, 17 of them (Table 1) are CNS stimulants similar to or less potent than amphetamines. Many of them have a therapeutic use as anorectic drugs. The second group (Table 2) consists of 12 substances which are chemically related to amphetamines, but have a varying degree of hallucinogenic activity mixed with CNS stimulation. They have no recognized therapeutic use.

Many of the substances in the second group were produced by chemists in clandestine laboratories through a minor modification to the chemical structure of a known controlled substance. Analogues of controlled substances produced this way are often referred to as 'designer drugs' since

Table 1   (* = non-INN)

amfepramone (diethylpropion*)
benzfetamine
cathine
cathinone
etilamfetamine
fencamfamin
fenetylline
fenproporex
mazindol
mefenorex
4-methylaminorex*
methylphenidate
pemoline
phendimetrazine
phenmetrazine
phentermine
pyrovalerone

Table 2   (* = INN)

2,5-dimethoxyamphetamine (or DMA)
2,5-dimethoxy-4-bromoamphetamine (or DOB, brolamfetamine*)
2,5-dimethoxy-4-ethylamphetamine (or DOET)
mescaline (3,4,5-trimethoxyphenethylamine)
4-methoxyamphetamine (or PMA)
5-methoxy-3,4-methylenedioxyamphetamine (or MMDA, 5- methoxytenamfetamine)
3,4-methylenedioxyamphetamine (or MDA, tenamfetamine*)
3,4-methylenedioxymethamphetamine (or MDMA, Ecstasy)
N-ethylmethylenedioxyamphetamine (or MDEA, MDE, *N*-ethyltenamfetamine)
N-hydroxymethylenedioxyamphetamine (or *N*-OH MDA, *N*- hydroxytenamfetamine)
STP (or DOM, 2-amino-1-(2,5-dimethoxy-4-methyl)phenylpropane)
3,4,5-trimethoxyamphetamine (or TMA)

their chemical structures are 'designed' by clandestine chemists in an attempt to circumvent the drug control regulations.

For example, MDMA, commonly known as Ecstasy, is a derivative of methamphetamine. MDMA, a CNS stimulant with some hallucinogenic activity, was misused first in North America and was placed under international control in 1985. Its misuse by young people, often at dance parties, is spreading to Western Europe and Australia. Serious symptoms of acute MDMA intoxication include confusional state with a high temperature, dilated pupils, tachycardia, muscle rigidity and intravascular coagulation resulting in low platelet count.

CURRENT TRENDS IN USE AND MISUSE OF AMPHETAMINES

Extent of Therapeutic Use

According to the statistics compiled by the International Narcotics Control Board (INCB), the levels of medical use of amphetamines was the highest in the following countries on a per capita basis for the years 1991 to 1993. As expressed in the number of standard daily doses (DDD = defined daily dose) consumed by 1,000 inhabitants per day, only two countries, the USA and Spain, consumed more than 0.5 daily doses. Belgium, Chile, the United Kingdom, Israel and Australia consumed between 0.1 and 0.5, followed by Canada and Sweden which consumed approximately 0.1 daily doses. Other nations consumed less or did not consume amphetamines at all (United Nations, 1995).

In the case of the highest consumer, the USA, a 0.77 daily dose of amphetamines was consumed by 1,000 inhabitants per day. This figure could represent a situation where one out of 1,300 inhabitants have used one standard daily dose of amphetamines every day, or all the inhabitants have used one dose only once in three and half years, or anywhere between these two extreme situations. Whatever the case, the figures show low levels of use in comparison with some other psychotropic drugs. For example, benzodiazepine hypnotics are used almost 100 times more in the highest consumer country.

The INCB data also illustrate significant variations in per capita medical consumption of amphetamines between countries. This, however, is not surprising since such a striking difference in drug consumption between countries is not unique to amphetamines. For instance, even within the relatively homogeneous European Union, Denmark's per capita medical consumption of morphine was 33 times higher than Italy's during the years 1986 to 1990 (United Nations, 1991a).

It is known that many factors influence physicians' prescribing practices. To mention a few, medical education and training; perceptions of the prescriber, patient and general public about the efficacy and safety of the drug in question; drug cost, who pays for it and how payment is made; sales promotion by the drug company; indications approved by the health authorities; regulatory control on distribution; availability of alternative drugs — these all affect the extent of use of a particular drug product.

Of these, regulations on distribution and use can play a significant role in the case of controlled drugs such as amphetamines. Although drug control regulations do not intend to restrict therapeutic use *per se*, cumbersome procedural requirements, such as record-keeping and reporting obligations, often discourage physicians from prescribing controlled drugs.

Many of these factors vary considerably from one country to another. Even when the difference is rather small on each factor, the combined effect can be very significant.

Current Trends in Misuse of Amphetamines

Information from various sources indicates that misuse of amphetamines, alone or in combination with other drugs, is widespread throughout the world. Along with the global escalation of misuse of illicit drugs during the last few decades, misuse of amphetamines is persisting, spreading to previously unaffected countries, and revived even in countries where it was once brought under control, such as Japan.

Of all the illicit drugs, cannabis, cocaine and heroin are the three most widely misused drugs, probably in that order. Globally, amphetamines seem to follow. According to the INCB (United Nations, 1993), methamphetamine is the most commonly misused drug in Japan and the Republic of Korea, and amphetamines come in second position after cannabis in Australia. In Thailand, a random testing in 1993 revealed that one third of bus drivers in Bangkok were taking amphetamines. Clandestine laboratories were detected in Australia, China and Thailand. In the USA, more than 100 clandestine methamphetamine laboratories were seized in the first six months of 1993, and many South American countries reported misuse of amphetamines. In Europe, clandestine laboratories in the Netherlands, which used to supply most of the illicit amphetamine in Europe, are facing the challenge of large-scale production in eastern and central Europe, above all Poland.

Amphetamine is more frequently encountered than methamphetamine in illicit traffic in Europe whereas methamphetamine is predominant in Asia and north America. The choice of manufacturing methods by clandestine laboratories, rather than a difference in the taste of consumers, is considered to be the reason for this difference.

The abuse of amphetamine-like substances is also a problem, such as fenetylline in West Asia, pemoline in eastern Africa, methylenedioxymethamphetamine (MDMA) in Australia, Europe and USA, and methcathinone in the Commonwealth of Independent States. In addition, the illicit manufacture of MDA and MDEA were also reported in Europe. Furthermore, there are signs suggesting that the traditional use of Khat, a plant containing cathinone and cathine, is spreading slowly from North Africa to Australia, Europe and North America.

In an effort to counter the escalating misuse of illicit drugs, the international community agreed to step up concerted action against illicit traffic in drugs. A new convention adopted in 1988 by the United Nations calls for international cooperation in applying intensified control measures, such as the control of money laundering, confiscation of illicit proceeds and control of precursors and essential chemicals used for clandestine manufacturing of drugs (United Nations, 1991b).

As a result, precursors and chemicals frequently used in the illicit manufacture of amphetamines, such as ephedrine, became subject to diversion control measures in a number of countries. There are encouraging reports indicating that these measures led to shortages of precursors for methamphetamine in the USA (United Nations, 1993b). The same INCB report, however, states that there has been an increase in the smuggling of the necessary chemicals across the northern and southern borders of the USA.

It is surprising that, despite decades of concerted national and international efforts against the misuse of amphetamines, and despite considerable progress in the rationalization of their medical use, the problem of amphetamine misuse has always persisted, and now presents an even more complex picture with the addition of an array of amphetamine-like substances.

Why is this so? In trying to answer this question, we need to recognize the fact that laws and regulations are effective only to the extent that they are enforced. In this connection, we have seen people respond to regulations in two contrasting ways. While ordinary citizens are generally responsive to regulatory requirements, professional criminals, unless overpowered, tend to disregard them. Regulating drugs may thus have significant effects on the distribution and use of licit drugs which are handled by generally law-abiding licensees, but will have little impact on the availability of illicit drugs which are supplied by criminal organizations. The fight against illicit drugs has little chance of success unless enforcement capabilities are strengthened, and effective measures to reduce non-medical use of drugs are launched at the same time.

REFERENCES

Study Group on Dependence-Producing Drugs [Amphetamines] (1988) Japan: *Dependence-Producing Drug Information Monograph Series*, No. 2.

United Nations (1977) Report: *Convention on Psychotropic Substances, 1971*. New York: UN.

United Nations (1991a) *Narcotic Drugs — Estimated world requirements for 1992, statistics for 1990*. New York: UN.

United Nations (1991b) *United Nations Convention against Illicit Traffic in Narcotic Drugs and Psychotropic Substances, 1988*. New York: UN.

United Nations (1993) *Report of the International Narcotics Control Board for 1993*. New York: UN.

United Nations (1995) *Psychotropic Substances — Statistics for 1993*. New York: UN.

WHO (1952) WHO Expert Committee on Drugs Liable to Produce Addiction: Third report. *WHO Technical Report Series, No. 57*. Geneva: WHO.

WHO (1953) WHO Expert Committee on Drugs Liable to Produce Addiction: Fourth report. *WHO Technical Report Series, No. 76*. Geneva: WHO.

WHO (1956) WHO Expert Committee on Drugs Liable to Produce Addiction: Sixth report. *WHO Technical Report Series, No. 102*. Geneva: WHO.

WHO (1964) WHO Expert Committee on Addiction-Producing Drugs: Thirteenth report. *WHO Technical Report Series, No. 273*. Geneva: WHO.

WHO (1970) WHO Expert Committee on Drug Dependence: Seventeenth report. *WHO Technical Report Series, No. 437*. Geneva: WHO.

WHO (1974) WHO Expert Committee on Drug Dependence: Twentieth report. *WHO Technical Report Series, No. 551.* Geneva: WHO.

WHO (1992a) International Nonproprietary Names (INN) for Pharmaceutical Substances. Cumulative List No. 8. Geneva: WHO.

WHO (1992b) The ICD-10 Classification of Mental and Behavioural Disorders. Clinical descriptions and diagnostic guidelines. Geneva: WHO.

WHO (1993) WHO Expert Committee on Drug Dependence. Twenty-eighth report. *WHO Technical Report Series, No. 836.* Geneva: WHO.

Introduction to Section 1 — United Kingdom and Australia

There are reasons for putting the United Kingdom and Australia in the same section. They are very similar in many ways. Most notably they both have a serious amphetamine problem that is getting worse — in both countries the drug is second in popularity to cannabis and there is an ethos of harm reduction on the part of the authorities rather than the criminalization of the drug. Having become aware of a bias in focusing fairly exclusively on heroin and cocaine as potential threats to health and social order, the Australian government is now taking amphetamine more seriously and allocating resources to its control and prevention. The UK lags behind and is still at a stage of enquiry that precedes decisions about policy.

It is acknowledged that in Europe and elsewhere in the world amphetamine misuse has been overshadowed by other drugs. The reasons for this are explored with reference to the UK in the first chapter. This is followed by a typology of amphetamine users based on UK samples which can be compared with the American typology in section 2. Treatment in the UK is included here because it is a problem area full of controversy. It is an issue that is being addressed in the UK in the context of an examination of service delivery to all drug misusers. The perception of amphetamine as a relatively harmless, controllable drug that does not have the stigma of 'hard' drugs is fairly universal and there has been little demand for treatment. In the UK this is partly because services have been developed largely with heroin in mind. Substitute drug prescribing, following the example of using methadone for heroin dependence, has been tried in the past in Sweden and the UK and failed fairly traumatically. There is understandable resistance in both countries, and elsewhere in the world, to trying it again. However, the arguments for well-controlled, highly limited prescribing for problem users is made by Myles in Chapter 4 and it would be wise to consider these arguments dispassionately, taking account of the current social context rather than the past. If control and preventive interventions fail and the problem grows it would be better to be prepared with a treatment strategy.

2

Amphetamine Misusers in Contemporary Britain: The Emergence of a Hidden Population

HILARY KLEE

The escalation in drug misuse in the United Kingdom over the last two decades has been characterized by a trend towards an ever increasing repertoire of drugs and a wide range of both illicit and prescribed drugs can be bought on the streets. However, the attention that any particular drug receives from the media, or even government, seems to have little to do with the extent of its use. Channelled by the media, public anxiety has been focused selectively on heroin and its associated stereotype of the 'dope fiend', on an expected influx of crack-cocaine and its reputation for provoking violence, and on the use of MDMA (Ecstasy) by young 'ravers'. Amphetamine, to modify a common phrase, has not been noticeable by its absence. Its absence, until very recently, has not been noticed at all.

EARLY HISTORY

Following the synthesis of amphetamine in 1887 in Germany, its significance was not recognized until 1927, when it was suggested by a chemist working in Los Angeles that it would be a cheap substitute for ephedrine (for a more extended account see McKim, 1986). Ephedrine, isolated from a herb traditionally used in China, was used widely to treat asthma, but there were fears that supplies would soon be exhausted. A cheap synthetic drug with known and controllable composition, not vulnerable to the variable quality and

19

availability of a natural herb was a major step forward. A number of therapeutic uses were identified in the 1930s, notably to treat hyperactivity in children, obesity, depression, narcolepsy and nasal congestion. In particular, the over-the-counter sales of nasal inhalers became very popular and began to be marketed extensively in the United States and United Kingdom. The absence of pharmaceutical remedies in the treatment of depression, particularly in the economically depressed '30s, made amphetamines very attractive to the medical profession and were increasingly prescribed to patients. The Second World War contributed to its acceptance as a valuable and legally endorsed drug when UK troops, along with most other nations involved, were supplied with amphetamine to delay fatigue and enhance alertness.

Post-War Developments

After the war the liberal prescribing of amphetamines such as Drinamyl (a combination of amphetamine and a barbiturate — known on the streets as 'purple hearts') and Dexedrine (dexamphetamine sulphate), and the sale of non-prescribed preparations continued. Following reports of their potential for inducing psychotic episodes they were made available only on prescription from 1957. There was also increasing concern that amphetamines could induce dependence. A similar picture developed subsequently in the UK as in the US, with widespread use of amphetamine products diverted from legitimate sources and used recreationally or for occupational reasons, mostly to keep awake or for sustained energy. In the UK it assumed epidemic proportions among the young in the boom time of the 1960s, and was a part of the 'Swinging Sixties' social scene of pop-groups, Hollywood films and a new generation of young people with spending power and greater freedom from parental economic control. Different groups could be identified at around that time — 'mods' and 'rockers' (associated with different types of music and fashion), and 'bikers' who developed a subculture that still persists in many European countries and the United States. Whereas opiates, also initially widely used and not controlled, had been used across a broad spectrum of society since the nineteenth century (Berridge, 1989), the amphetamines were mainly associated with youth, gangs and deviance. To parents in the sixties, who were the products of a socialization process based on family dependence and control, the trend was threatening. It was considered to be a short step away from the induction of their children into serious use of 'hard' drugs, that is, heroin. In fact amphetamines ('pep-pills') were largely used recreationally and tended to be confined to weekend socializing.

The Context of an Opiate Oriented Society

The response of the establishment was heavily influenced by a model of drug use based on opium and, subsequently, heroin, and the 'British System' of treatment set up by the Rolleston Committtee in the 1920s. The committee comprised eminent physicians, addiction was regarded primarily as a medical problem and treatment was left to the clinical judgement of practitioners. Compulsory treatment and the official notification of addicts were both resisted. The Dangerous Drugs Act of 1920 in Britain differed from its counterpart, the American Harrison Act of 1914 in allowing medical practitioners considerable freedom in dealing with drug misuse. In the US, by contrast, the addict was criminalized (Berridge, 1989). In these early days most heroin users were mature individuals from all socio-economic classes and there were relatively few young people among those dependent on it. The pattern changed in the 1960s. In 1959 no heroin addict under the age of 20 years was recorded by the Home Office but in 1968 the figure was 709 (Teff, 1975). The steady rise in heroin use and the epidemic of recreational amphetamine misuse among young people indicated the need for changes in legislation.

Measures to Counteract Increasing Drug Use

A series of amendments to drugs legislation in 1964 and 1967 criminalized the possession, supply and importation of amphetamine. At the same time a system of registration of opiate addicts (but not amphetamine users) with the Home Office was instituted, and a nation-wide network of regional treatment centres set up. The emphasis in providing health care for drug users was on heroin. This was the drug associated with the most serious health and social problems and treatment included the substitute prescribing of opioids.

By 1972 the number of centres had reached 25, with the greatest concentration in London. A Department of Health memorandum in 1967 identified one aim of these centres as containing the spread of heroin addiction. According to Teff (1975, op cit.) the effect was to "widen the already artificial distinction between heroin addiction and other forms of drug dependence by disregarding the prevalence of multiple drug abuse…. It is easy to elevate the heroin problem out of all proportion to its overall significance" (page 93). The terms of reference of the treatment centres effectively precluded them from dealing with non-opiate users, including those with amphetamine related problems. However cocaine use was considered to be a sufficiently threatening problem and treatment was part of the services provided, despite the very low use of cocaine anywhere outside London.

By 1971 and the passing of the Misuse of Drugs Act the amphetamines had been classified according to a system that orders drugs with respect to the severity of penalties imposed for their possession, supply or trafficking. Allocated to Class B for non-injectable forms and Class A if injected, the potential punishments were, apparently, having little effect since there had developed in the late sixties a group of more dedicated users in London who had turned to injecting methamphetamine. Overprescribing to cocaine addicts by doctors was identified as responsible for the glut of metham-phetamine on the black market. An attempt was made to determine whether these users could be encouraged away from this practice by offering them a period of treatment with injectable methamphetamine (Mitcheson *et al.*, 1976). The extent of the trial was limited to 20 patients, 12 were prescribed injectable methamphetamine, and the rest were offered counselling, six of whom were given a variety of oral amphetamine substitutes. The majority were described as polydrug users with occasional use of heroin and other substances. After an average of eight weeks in treatment the outcomes were assessed and no particular benefit was observed among those prescribed substitutes. This single, small scale study has had a lasting effect on all subsequent dialogues about treatment for problem amphetamine users and is usually cited as evidence against amphetamine prescribing whenever the issue is raised.

The voluntary banning of prescribing all products containing amphet-amine by doctors in one town in the UK in 1969 had a more positive outcome in virtually eliminating all abuse of tablet forms within a year. Called the 'Ipswich Experiment' the move was supported by educational campaigns in schools, provision of more recreational facilities and was also helped by a negotiated reduction in the manufacture of amphetamine based products (Wells, 1980). However, it seems that this worthy effort was limited in real value since there were reports of the arrival of amphetamine sulphate, presumably of uncertain purity and hence potentially more dangerous, on the illicit market.

The use of amphetamines in the UK in the 1970s tends to be shrouded in mystery although a scan of the medical literature shows widespread reporting of abuse. In one of the rare social surveys, Hartnoll and Mitcheson (1973) found that amphetamine was the most used drug among a sample of British school children, apart from cannabis users who disapproved of it. Greaves (1980) suggests that one reason for the lack of social research at this time was because of the overemphasis on heroin use. Heroin was regarded as a major social ill despite its comparatively limited use and therefore deserving of more attention. However, there may have been a genuine decrease in the use of amphetamine with the arrival of cheap heroin on the market. If amphetamine users switched allegiances easily, this challenges observations (Klee, 1992) that there can be significant differences between those who are attracted to these two drugs, and that many people have distinct preferences for 'uppers' or 'downers'. However, for polydrug users with both stimulants and opiates in their repertoires, cheap heroin would have been attractive and perhaps induced more frequent use.

For young primary amphetamine users there could have been other factors that may have brought about a decline in the numbers. The effect of the earlier media coverage in the 1960s is likely to have popularized amphet-amine (Power, 1989). Illicit drug use was added to the symbols of youth empowerment, and part of the growing confrontation with establishment values and control. It could be that the battle was won in the late sixties, teenage rebellion became rather pointless, recreational drugs lost their symbolic value and they may simply have become less fashionable.

It is often proposed (see Hando and Hall, Chapter 5; Suwaki, Chapter 10) that the misuse of amphetamine is epidemic in nature. While the initial outbreak in the UK may have been traceable to factors such as social change, the public acceptability arising from the previously legal status of amphetamine based products, and overprescribing, a convincing explanation of why amphetamine misuse should decline and then recur is difficult without research-based data. The apparent decrease in the popularity of amphetamines in the UK in the 1970s may have been due to a temporary abeyance while a generation of young people grew out of it and the next generation were seeking an alternative style. It is difficult to know the extent of its decline and whether amphetamine use became hidden rather than absent. The media had turned to heroin as a cause celebre and it could be that the continued use of amphetamine went unnoticed.

THE 1980s

The early 1980s became a time of preoccupation with heroin (Hartnoll *et al.*, 1984; MacGregor, 1989; Pearson, 1987) by the media and government as the black market became flooded with supplies from South West Asia, the price went down and levels of crime and demands for treatment went up. (For a discussion of the international context of this development see Hartnoll, 1989.) How to meet treatment demands appropriately was a concern of the Advisory Council on the Misuse of Drugs (ACMD), an independent statutory body set up under the Misuse of Drugs Act of 1971 to advise Government on drug issues. Their report in 1982 on Treatment and Rehabilitation suggested a definition of the "problem drug taker" as a person who "experiences social, psychological, physical or legal problems related to intoxication and/or regular excessive consumption and/or dependence as a consequence of his own use of drugs or other chemical substances". It was recommended that services for drug users should focus on problem use rather than restricting the availability of treatment to those dependent on particular substances.

The development of services was hampered however by inadequate funding (MacGregor, 1989) and the major customers continued to be problem opiate users to whom oral methadone (a heroin substitute) could be offered. Despite the acknowledgement of other needy populations of drug users it is interesting to read references to treatment provision in the literature even now since it is immediately apparent that most writers were predominantly concerned with opiate addiction. The five examples of potential clients of services given at the beginning of the chapter on treatment in Drug Scenes (Chapter 11, Royal College of Psychiatrists, 1987) are more eclectic — problem users of heroin, cannabis, tobacco, alcohol, and a polydrug user. There is no mention of stimulants, in particular, amphetamines. It goes on to explain that the focus of the chapter on problems associated with opiate misuse is justified by the needs of the group and the need to examine issues relevant to the expansion of services. The needs of other unnamed groups are acknowledged however.

The emphasis on heroin is understandable since the services provided by Drug Dependence Units since their inception in the UK in 1968 had been aimed at heroin users. Subsequent developments were much influenced by the ACMD report on treatment and characterized by a shift towards a flexible system that could tailor a treatment programme to individual needs. A diversity of resources would be needed from other agencies — GPs, voluntary agencies, social services and self-help groups. Initiated by John Strang in the Northwest of England (see Strang, 1989 for a full account) the drug agencies, renamed Community Drug Teams in that region, were developed in the Northwest from 1983. The success of such developments has been restricted by the decline in resources as other groups requiring health care compete for limited funds. With high methadone costs, waiting lists and staff shortages, the development of services for non-opiate users has tended to take a back seat.

The government drugs campaigns were also focused on heroin at this time. Multi-media advertising aimed at the young, along the lines of 'Heroin screws you up' were initiated and claimed to be successful in raising awareness and increasing negative evaluations although there have been criticisms (Marsh, 1986). There is, perhaps a more sinister consequence of a campaign targeted in this way: problem users of other drugs are able to disassociate themselves from the warnings.

Along with heroin there was a new scare from increasingly dramatic publicity about the American drug scene. There is a general consensus in the UK that many trends in the US, including commercial and industrial innovations, economic health and even the weather, soon find their way to the shores of the UK. Thus it was only a matter of time before British cities would see organized crime and crack-related violence too. It is suggested that the over-reaction by public, press and police was largely in response to the implications for social order (MacGregor, 1989, op cit.). The glamour of cocaine was enhanced by news items and films about drugs 'barons' (an interesting choice of a term associated with the aristocracy) and casualties or repented transgressors among musicians and sports stars. Although the problem use of cocaine was almost unknown outside London and its prevalence was small in comparison to other drugs, it was viewed with some foreboding.

The 1980s ended with drug workers and government pre-occupied with potentially disastrous world trends that threatened health and social order. Concerns focused on the possibility of outbreaks of HIV not only among injecting drug users but also, and in particular, their partners; the deterioration in control over illicit drug use; the large numbers of young people using stimulants recreationally; increasing injecting, and increasing drug-related violence. Stimulants were becoming important, though it was Ecstasy and crack-cocaine that stole the headlines. This was noted by Davies and Ditton (1990) who, in asking whether the 1990s would be the decade of the stimulants, noted the high-profile role of the media in stimulating interest in certain drugs. However, the nature of the relationship between media coverage and drug trends remains largely unexplored.

AMPHETAMINE — AN UNSUITABLE CASE FOR TREATMENT

It is interesting to speculate on why amphetamine use has been neglected by policy makers and the media in the UK. There might be good reasons why it should not be taken seriously, and hence justify the delay in addressing any health and social order issues that may be associated with it. In particular the extent of concern may be determined by an evaluation of its status in giving rise to 'problem use' in terms of health and social order. A recreational drug that is reasonably well controlled and produces few casualties perhaps takes lower priority unless public pressure against it is set into motion. When resources for treatment are already stretched, the initiation of proactive measures aimed at devising ways of dealing with a population that may not want or need treatment seems ill-advised.

In this section the delay among policy makers in the United Kingdom in recognizing the extent and danger of amphetamine misuse will be examined. Was it a product of studied disregard or excusable ignorance? Looking at the emergence into the light of a hidden drugs problem is revealing — of the inadequacies of processes of detection, of obstructions to effective communication, of predilictions in key players and their evaluation of dangers to health and social order, and of the part played by purely fortuitous events.

Sources of Information

In the UK drug scene, non-opiate users, along with women and ethnic minorities have been described as 'hidden' populations, that is, sub-groups of drug users who are 'hard-to-reach' by the authorities and about whom little is known. There could be several reasons why the characteristics of hidden drugs populations stay hidden. One could be that there is insufficient intelligence about them, another is that the information is known but not communicated effectively to people with an investment in rendering them visible and yet another is that the information is known but not acted upon. Standard ways of gathering information such as surveys, law enforcement statistics, data on health treatment may be insufficient to reveal much about the characteristics of such groups.

Notifications

There are several routes of information about drug misuse to Government in the UK. One of the most influential is through notifications to the Home Office of people considered or suspected of being addicted to any of the 14 controlled drugs. Doctors are required by law to send details of such patients to the Chief Medical Officer and subsequently have to renotify annually if they are still receiving treatment. The drugs are all opiates apart from cocaine. Amphetamine misuse, however problematic, is not notifiable.

Inevitably the picture of drug prevalence that emerges from official notifications is highly distorted and is recognized as such. The potential for dependence of a drug corresponds partly but not completely with the legal sanctions against its use. All Class A drugs are controlled drugs which carry the most severe penalties. This also includes LSD and MDMA. Amphetamines are regarded as Class B drugs (along with cannabis) if not injected, carrying a custodial sentence from three months to five years for possession and a heavy fine. Their status is Class A if injected and has more serious penalties. Class C includes pharmaceutical preparations such as benzodiazepines and analgesics.

Research

Most of the information from independent research has, until quite recently, been similarly biased towards opiates and acquired from samples taken from treatment agency clients — typically older, white, male opiate users. They are easier to access and more compliant. These characteristics render them unsuitable for generalizing results to populations that are not in treatment. They reveal little about amphetamine misuse except as a minor component in a polydrug repertoire. However, commissioned research on the general population such as the British Crime Survey (Mott and Mirlees-Black, 1995) and The Four Cities Survey (Leitner *et al.*, 1993) both confirmed the currently high prevalence of amphetamine. Only very recently have research studies been mounted with the expressed aim to inform about the majority of non-agency drug users about whom little is known. Social research among such drug users is difficult, needs persistence, is getting more dangerous, and progress is slow. It is not an attractive option for social scientists.

Drug seizures

Another primary source of information about drug misuse is through the drug seizures made by police and officials of HM Customs and Excise.

Cannabis has traditionally been top of the list, but if the number of seizures is taken as an index of popularity, then amphetamine sulphate would be second in line and rising. As an index of prevalence the data are flawed by fluctuations in policies, often at a local level, that govern apprehension and arrest. The statistics on seizures and arrests over recent years have all supported the increasing and widespread popularity of street amphetamine. The number of police seizures of amphetamine tripled between 1989 and 1992 (Home Office, 1992, 1993). Seizures of amphetamine imports showed a similar trend as local suppliers failed to keep up with demand. At the same time, the quality declined to about 5% purity, a level that has been fairly constant since the late 1980s, and a possible indication that the limited supplies have been stretched by adding substances at various levels of dealing to increase bulk (ISDD, 1994).

Drug misuse data bases

A more sophisticated and comprehensive system of reporting on the drug scene, although still limited to drug users presenting to services, was developed by Donmall (1990) and is now used by the majority of health authority regions in England and Wales. Local intelligence is gathered by doctors, drug agencies and needle-exchanges, stored in a data base within each region, and summary information is fed back regularly to the Department of Health. The anonymized data include information about the range of drugs used, how they are used, as well as social and treatment profiles, and this is an important step forward in tracking drugs such as amphetamine and the benzodiazepines and detecting patterns of use over time.

Information Deficit and Uptake

The intelligence on current amphetamine misuse in the UK is improving but is still seriously deficient. A telling estimate of the information on amphetamine that is in the public domain is through the publications held by the UK's main library resource for those interested in drug misuse at the Institute for the Study of Drug Dependence (ISDD) in London. The total number of publications held by the Library in February 1995 was 58,000. The distribution between popular illicit drugs is interesting. Heroin was the main focus for 14,000 of these, 8,700 were about cannabis, 6,000 about cocaine and those on amphetamine numbered 3,300, (John Witton; personal communication). This is not unexpected, but it is a graphic indication of the status of this drug when compared with the ISDD summary of the drug scene in 1992: "Heroin dependence is increasing, but probably limited to no more than 100,000 people, mainly young men. Cocaine retains its role as a 'fashionable accessory'. Between cannabis and heroin it is a 'fuzzy' area heavily influenced by contemporary youth culture. One constant however is the central role of amphetamine — boosted by the 'rave' scene", (ISDD, 1992).

As a complete explanation for not noticing the increase in amphetamine misuse, inadequate intelligence will not do. It seems that the signs were read by some people and not others. In the Home Office Report of the Drugs Branch Inspectorate of 1987 it was reported that all branches had noted increases in amphetamine misuse and a high rate of injecting. This was not their first warning — "The perception of the amphetamine problem, which the Inspectorate has been signalling for some years, has clearly changed within enforcement, treatment and prevention agencies. Since the drug presents, on the one hand, the worst manifestations of heroin misuse because it is injected, and on the other an established stimulant market ready made for the promotion of cocaine, it is now widely acknowledged that it occupies a central position". This was a somewhat optimistic evaluation of the extent to which amphetamine was regarded as a serious problem. In the same year the Royal College of Psychiatrists published *Drug Scenes*, hailed as an accessible, comprehensive and interesting account of the patterns of drug use in Britain. A chapter was devoted to amphetamine that emphasized the epidemic nature of its use and ended on a rather optimistic note that the situation was better than it had been twenty years ago in the '60s outbreak and, although there were dangers in complacency, one could be consoled that epidemics do not continue to climb forever. No mention was made of an ongoing or growing problem.

There had been other signs. Pearson *et al.* (1985) in his study of heroin use among young people in the north of England saw the prevailing pattern there: "In many areas we were informed that heroin use was virtually unknown or that the pattern and scale of heroin use had not changed appreciably over recent years. The most significant drug problems in many of these areas were concerned with alcohol, solvents or amphetamines" (page 2). A few years later a conference organized in 1989 by the Standing Conference on Drug Abuse (SCODA), the national co-ordinating body for services to drug users in the UK, focused on treatment for amphetamine users. Noticeable increases in the use of amphetamine were reported. It was hypothesized that this might be preventing cocaine from achieving a significant foothold in the illicit market. In the opening to the summary of this conference (SCODA, 1990) the concern was made clear. "Stimulants, particularly amphetamine, are among the most commonly used drugs, yet get scant attention in the medical literature and in the lay press, which seems preoccupied with opiate use."

It is interesting to speculate on the reasons for the different degrees of concern. Could it be that amphetamine use was regarded as less problematic by some health professionals, that there was little that could be done about it, and that it would eventually decline? The concern of the Inspectorate was a reflection of the misgivings among drug workers in certain parts of the UK outside of London, particularly the South West of England and Wales, where the problems seemed particularly acute. Vindication of their suspicions came from an unexpected quarter when measures to combat the AIDS epidemic got underway.

Needle Exchanges and Harm Reduction

There is no doubt that the AIDS pandemic introduced another critically important dimension to the drug scene. In the mid 80s it became apparent that injecting drug users were at high risk of acquiring the viruses and could be instrumental in large-scale transmission of HIV to other populations. Almost by default, attention was fixed on injecting opiate or polydrug users and how to persuade them to stop sharing their equipment. An Advisory Council on the Misuse of Drugs report was highly influential in guiding such developments, emphasizing the urgency of dealing with the HIV problem as a matter of priority (ACMD, 1988). Resources to develop a national network of needle-exchanges schemes were made available and a monitoring exercise was quickly initiated to evaluate their impact on drug-injecting cultures (Stimson, *et al.*, 1988). It revealed unexpectedly high numbers of amphetamine injectors using them. Drug workers in several areas of the UK had their suspicions confirmed and amphetamine misuse edged a little more into the limelight. A study of the social and sexual lifestyles of amphetamine users in the Northwest of England subsequently revealed levels of injecting risk behaviour that far exceeded those of respondents who were opiate dependent, and also high levels of sexual risk (Klee, 1990; 1992; Klee *et al.*, 1990). The serious implications of amphetamine injecting became clear.

Outreach and Detached Drugs Work

To extend the harm reduction efforts to injectors not already in contact with drug agencies, several regional health authorities started to employ drug workers to work on the streets. Although this varied in its effectiveness, according to Stimson and his colleagues (1994), some were highly successful at reaching amphetamine users. How to attract the amphetamine users to treatment services surfaced on the agenda of many drug agencies in the early '90s and persists there without resolution. Information that was accumulating about users was informal, anecdotal and not disseminated to a wide audience. It was a poor basis on which to mount interventions. Despite seminars and conferences on the topic of amphetamine misuse there was still no guidance from government. "Since then (the 1960s) the abuse of amphetamines has continued to be a significant but largely unpublicized, and therefore not generally recognized, feature of the United Kingdom drug scene" (Spear, 1990).

A Problem Recognized or Ignored?

It seems that information about the problem use of amphetamine in England and Wales at varying levels of formality and from different sources has been available for many years. The inertia in tackling it can be attributed to a combination of many factors. The dominance of medical research that used readily available clinic patient samples and the corresponding lack of social research that sampled more widely, must be allocated a major role in contributing to neglect of amphetamine through ignorance (see Klee, 1992, for an expansion of this point).

Another reason could be the regional patterns of amphetamine misuse. An area seemingly least affected is London. Drug policy making is London based, with most serving members of committees of any seniority working in London and the Southeast of England. More provincial voices may have had fewer opportunities to be heard. In addition, older members of decision making groups may have been less than enthusiastic in their responses because of the implications for the provision of treatment for amphetamine users, remembering earlier failed attempts.

The problem may have seemed less urgent for a variety of reasons: the physical health hazards and social damage associated with amphetamine misuse are regarded as less severe than those associated with opiate use; the common mental health consequences for example, paranoid delusions and psychoses, are mostly short-lived; amphetamine users also seem able to exert a greater level of control over their drug use than opiate users; they also tend not to overdose because the purity level of street amphetamine is so low. Only with the injecting of amphetamine in the age of AIDS does the use of this drug assume importance at a level corresponding to that of heroin users. Large numbers of amphetamine users, particularly injecting users, are reported now in many parts of England and Wales. A critical feature is that few are in contact with agencies, and therefore represent a population out of reach of targeted HIV messages and harm reduction interventions. This is particularly important if sharing rates are inversely related to treatment. It should be no surprise that this implication seems to have raised the profile of amphetamine users.

Inadequate resources dedicated to drug treatment is one reason for ignoring the growing awareness of the problem. At the interface between carers and clients, agency personnel, already overstretched with caring for heroin addicts, are faced with the dilemma of whether to regard amphetamine users as potential clients. Understandably, they are ambivalent about increasing their case loads and waiting lists. There is also the uncertainty about what sort of treatment is appropriate. Substitute prescribing has considerable health and economic implications and remains a largely unresearched area. Alternatives are tried without much success and many clients disappear. Resource allocation may also be influenced at a higher level by the view that amphetamine use is epidemic in nature and hence may burn itself out naturally.

However, it seems that the issue of amphetamine misuse has finally emerged into the arena of policy development. The British Government is scrutinizing the effectiveness of the services available to drug users, and amphetamine users are now on the research agenda (Klee *et al.*, 1995). The

United Nations Drugs Control Programme is about to initiate an information-gathering exercise on amphetamines in 1996, a sign that perhaps those researchers and health professionals frustrated by the continuing neglect of this drug are at last about to see the issue of amphetamine misuse addressed.

Perhaps there is a lesson to be learned from the spasmodic progress towards recognition of amphetamine misuse. In their introduction to their monograph on Hidden Populations, (NIDA, 1990), Lambert and Wiebel equate the status of "hidden" with "the disadvantaged and disenfranchised: the homeless and transient, chronically mentally ill, high school dropouts, criminal offenders, prostitutes, juvenile delinquents, gang members, runaways and other street people". Despite the range of examples they give, this is too restrictive. The defining characteristic of a hidden population is not necessarily being part of an 'out-group'. Another definition is given in the first chapter of this monograph by Wiebel: "a subset of the general population whose membership is not readily distinguished or enumerated based on existing knowledge and/or sampling capabilities". More simply, the hidden are difficult to detect because we do not know enough about them, and the ways of finding them are deficient. As a general rule, a biased research methodology using restrictive sampling techniques will always lead to a distorted and incomplete picture of the phenomenon under observation. This has applied to drug use in the UK in the past and probably in most other nations too. However, the story of contemporary amphetamine misuse and its eventual surfacing in government circles is far more complex. Sampling bias is unlikely to be the whole answer. It has raised other questions: about the convenience of ignorance; the deficiencies in structural communication channels; resource implications, and estimates of success in dealing with the problem.

Fortunately, the incompleteness of our understanding about drug users is now exposed, and other 'hidden populations' — for example, the elusive ethnic minorities and drug-using mothers, are becoming popular topics for discussion. There will, no doubt, be others. The acknowledgement that there are major gaps in our understanding of the drug scene may ensure that few drug-using sub-cultures will be overlooked in future, that prevention interventions will be appropriately targeted and fully informed, and that the treatment needs of all misusers are met.

REFERENCES

ACMD (1988) AIDS and drug misuse: part 1. London: HMSO.

Annual Report: Drugs Branch Inspectorate (1987). London: Home Office.

Berridge, V. (1989) Historical Issues. In: S. MacGregor (ed.) *Drugs and British Society*. London: Routledge.

Davies, J.B. and Ditton, J. (1990) The 1990's: decade of the stimulants? *British Journal of Addiction*, **85**, pp. 811–813.

Donmall, M. (1990) The Drug Misuse Database: Local Monitoring of Presenting Problem Drug use. London: Department of Health H.M.S.O.

Greaves, G.B. (1980) Psychosocial aspects of amphetamines and related substance abuse. In: J. Caldwell (ed.) *Amphetamines and related stimulants: Chemical, biological, clinical and sociological aspects.* Florida: CRC Press Inc.

Hartnoll, R.L. and Mitcheson, M. (1973) Attitude of young people towards drug use. *Buletin of Narcotics,* **25**, pp. 9.

Hartnoll, R.L., Lewis, R.J. and Bryer, S. (1984) Recent trends in drug use in Britain. *Druglink,* pp. 22–24.

Hartnoll, R. (1989) The International Context. In: S. MacGregor (ed.) *Drugs and British Society.* London: Routledge.

Home Office, 1992; 1993. Regional Trends. London: HMSO.

ISDD (1992) National Audit of Drug Misuse in Britain 1992 Part 1: An overview. London: Institute for the Study of Drug Dependence.

ISDD (1994) Drug Misuse in Britain. London: Institute for the Study of Drug Dependence.

Klee, H. (1990) Some observations on the sexual activities of injecting drug users: implications for the spread of AIDS. In: P. Aggleton, P. Davies and G. Hart (eds.) *AIDS: Individual, Cultural and Policy Dimensions.* UK: Falmer Press.

Klee, H. (1992) A new target in behavioural research: Amphetamine misuse. *British Journal of Addiction,* **87**, pp. 439–446.

Klee, H., Faugier, J., Hayes, C., Boulton, T. and Morris, J. (1990) Factors associated with risk behaviour among injecting drug users. *AIDS Care,* **2(2)**, pp. 133–154.

Klee, H., Morris, J., Carnwath, T. and Merrill, J. (1995) Amphetamine misuse and treatment: An exploration of individual and policy impediments to effective service delivery. Interim Report to Department of Health UK.

Leitner, M., Shepland, J. and Wiles, P. (1993) Drug Usage and Drugs Prevention: the views and habits of the general public. London: HMSO (The Four Cities Survey).

MacGregor, S. (1989) Chapters I and II In: S. MacGregor (ed.) *Drugs in British Society.* London: Routledge.

McKim, N.A. (1986) *Drugs and Behaviour: An introduction to behavioural pharmology.* London: Prentice-Hall.

Marsh, C. (1986) Medicine and the media: government campaign on misuse of drugs report. *British Medical Journal,* **292**, p. 895.

Mitcheson, M., Edwards, G., Hawks, D. and Ogborne, A. (1976) Treatment of Methamphetamine users during the 1968 epidemic. In: G. Edwards, M. Russell, D. Hawks and M. McCaferty (eds.), *Drugs and Drugs Dependence.* London: Saxon House.

NIDA, (1990) The Collection and Interpretation of Data from Hidden Populations. *NIDA Research Monograph,* 98 Rockville MD: US Depart. Health and Human Services.

Pearson, G. (1987) The New Heroin Users. Oxford: Basil Blackwell.

Pearson, G., Gilman, M. and McIver, S. (1985) Young People and Heroin. Research Report No. 8. London: Health Education Council.

Power, R. (1989) Drugs and the media: prevention campaign and television. In: MacGregor (ed.) *Drugs and British Society.* London: Routledge.

Royal College of Psychiatrists (1987) *Drug Scenes.*

SCODA, (1990) Standing Conference on Drug Abuse. Report of Conference 'Working with Stimulant Users'. London: SCODA.

Spear, B. (1990) Introduction. SCODA, Report of Conference 'Working with Stimulant Users'. London: SCODA.

Stimson, G.V., Alldritt, L., Dolan, K. and Donoghoe, M. (1988) Injecting Equipment Exchange Schemes: Final Report. London: Goldsmith College.

Stimson, G.V., Eaton, G., Rhodes, T. and Power, R. (1994) Potential development of community oriented HIV outreach among drug injection in the UK. *Addiction,* **89**(12), pp. 1601–12.

Strang, J. (1989) A model service: turning the generalist on to drugs. In: MacGregor (ed.) *Drugs and British Society.* London: Routledge.

Teff, H. (1975) Drugs, Society and the Law. UK: Saxon House.

Wells, F. (1980) The effects of a voluntary ban on amphetamine prescribing by doctors on abuse patterns — experience in the United Kingdom. In: J. Caldwell (ed.) *Amphetamines and related stimulants: Chemical, biological, clinical and sociological aspects.* Florida: CRC Press Inc.

John Witton — personal communication (1995) ISDD Library.

3

A Typology of Amphetamine Users in the United Kingdom

HILARY KLEE

The title of this chapter may offend the highly tuned sensibilities of those who take it upon themselves to expose the dangers of labelling people and to challenge the assumptions on which this is based. Descriptors that gloss over human individuality and render a group of people homogeneous invites stereotyping. When some characteristics are stigmatized the door is open to active discrimination. Marginalized and disenfranchised groups are 'soft targets' for bigotry — they have little power and often no voice. Illicit drug users are by definition deviant. They are also responsible for a considerable proportion of property crime, a drain on the economy, lure children into drugs, neglect themselves, leave needles in the street, catch HIV, give it to others and so on ... and on. The vocabulary that perpetuates stereotyping tends to ensure that its targets retain the status of 'out-group'. The purpose of this chapter is not to obscure individuality, it is to promote understanding of the rich diversity to be found among those who use this particular stimulant. The variety, however, has to be documented in a structured way in order to be meaningful and communicable to others. A word such as taxonomy would have been preferable to typology, but this I feel should be reserved for an operation much more scientific than this.

The title may also catch the eye of those who are aware of the difficulties involved in producing a set of profiles that are both valid and recognizable to other observers. If they fail on either count, they will not provide information that is practically useful. Although I may not satisfy such potential critics, a description of the procedures involved in constructing these profiles will show their limitations and the results may then be judged in the context of such constraints.

THE DATA BASE

The typology is not the product of a piece of research dedicated to evaluating and measuring similarities and differences in a particular sample of amphetamine users. The data base is an amalgam of research studies that included amphetamine users in their samples. Five studies of drug-users' lifestyles that were carried out between 1990 and 1995 in the North-west of England contributed in this way. The majority of respondents were participants in studies specifically about primary amphetamine misusers — people for whom amphetamine was their preferred and most used drug — apart from cannabis and nicotine. There were also 30 polydrug injectors who used amphetamine daily as part of their repertoires. All involved face-to-face interviews and all interviews were recorded and transcribed. Both quantitative and qualitative data were collected. Formal, quantitative data were used in statistical analyses of data from 290 respondents and extended by purely qualitative analyses of a further 50. Field-notes and consultations with the research workers who did the field-work also contributed to the final profiles.

PROCEDURES

Over several years of contact with amphetamine users there were a number of fairly obvious groupings, for example: 'ravers' — young people using the drug at weekends for dancing and partying; 'drinkers' — young males using it in conjunction with alcohol; 'grafters' — young male burglars who described crime as a 'buzz'; 'young mums' — women with domestic responsibilities but who wanted some fun too; 'experimenters' — adolescent males who would try anything with their 'mates'. These were not systematized observations and were based on only a few, but prominent, features. There were five fairly clear 'types' and a few others that were discernible but less well defined.

A more reliable method of identifying such groups, though not without its problems, is cluster analysis. This is a statistical procedure that is used in social research and marketing and identifies people who are similar in some way. The aim in using it is to produce homogeneous groups. There are many forms of cluster analysis. The one chosen was the SPSS Quick Cluster for Windows. This can be used if the number of clusters can be specified in advance. It also handles large data sets. It is a method that selects k (the chosen number of clusters) that have well separated values as initial cluster centres. The program then passes through all cases (respondents) assigning them to the nearest cluster. The cluster centres are constantly updated as cases are added. In a final pass through the data the program assigns the cases to the cluster that has the closest centre. Another advantage of this method is that the number of clusters specified can be varied.

A decision about the variables that are to be used as the basis for cluster formation is the first, and possibly the most critical step. The choice needs to be fully justified, particularly when the number of variables are limited by the statistical analysis. The selection is done with care since the defining features of the final clusters can be based only on those variables. This sets inevitable limitations on interpretations.

There were several steps in the procedure adopted. The first step was to examine the groups already identified by informal inductive methods and identify the variables that were the defining features of those groups. The second step added other variables that were significant determiners of lifestyle variations. Variables, or groups of variables, were chosen that were statistically associated with many other important aspects of respondents lives. Many of them corresponded with those apparent in pre-defined groups. The final set were: age, gender, mode of administration (injecting or not), motives (why the drug is used), frequency of use, other drugs used, attitudes to amphetamine and other drugs, the social environment, employment status, psychological and physical health. Twenty variables were used in the cluster analysis. Seven clusters were specified for the first analysis but some proved to be unrelated to a clearly identifiable type. A second analysis was conducted with ten clusters specified. This illustrates the limitations of this method. The clusters produced may not be meaningful or useful, the program can generate clusters where no natural groups exist, and further validation procedures are required. Punj and Stewart (1983) suggest that the products of the analysis should be examined to determine whether the cluster solutions are interpretable in terms of differences on the variables used to arrive at them, whether they are related to variables other than those used in the analysis and whether they are useful.

The ten clusters were subjected to Chi-squared analyses as a validation procedure, and also to reveal patterns of associations between cluster type and a wide variety of other variables. There were many significant associations and the analyses were useful guides to important differences between clusters in the early development of fuller profiles.

The clusters were significantly different to each other on:

— demographic variables such as age, gender and parenthood

— the reasons for using amphetamine, for example, the 'buzz', socializing, going to clubs, relief from anxiety

— patterns of amphetamine use, for example, frequency, mode of administration, dose levels, binges

— the use of other drugs, for example, alcohol and heroin

— perceptions of dependence and control, the experience of withdrawal

— mental states, for example, depression, suicidal ideation, paranoid delusions

— the social context of drug use, whether alone, in company, or with a group

— activities with friends, for example, going to 'raves'/clubs and pubs, crime

Finally the transcripts of all respondents within each cluster were examined to evaluate the validity of the picture that was emerging. This most critical final stage resulted in one cluster (ravers) becoming subdivided when it became apparent that there were important differences in variables not used in the analysis. The end-product was ten main types which are presented below. The original six were there, now in much greater detail, the rest were new. The transcripts also revealed other groups, known to have some association with amphetamine use but with very few cases. Sampling strategies precluded greater numbers being recruited during field-work largely because of difficulty of access, for example 'new age travellers' and 'bikers'. These are mentioned briefly at the end of the chapter.

This analysis is not claimed to be comprehensive — there are likely to be other types of amphetamine users that would be revealed by research in different communities. The level of generality is also arbitrary, so that some 'types' are perhaps too broadly defined and so obscure interesting variations within them. Where this is known, the variations are also included. Some respondents were more central to the type, others were people who seemed in a state of transition — they had been more central but some modification of their behaviour, perhaps a major decrease in amphetamine use or forming an important relationship, indicated a potential change away from drug-related risk behaviour. This raises again the issue of labelling. Each respondent was located in a multi-dimensional space defined by the variables that were used. There are no boundaries in such space. Each individual occupies a unique location at a particular time in their lives and will be part of different clusters. A change in one of those variables — a move from non-injecting to injecting say, means a different location. If the cluster analysis is repeated they could be allocated to another type if there has been a slight change in lifestyle.

'RECREATIONAL' USERS

A dictionary definition of recreation is that it is an activity that refreshes spirits by relaxation and enjoyment (Collins, 1987). The use of a drug for recreational purposes could apply to many illicit drug users but perhaps is best typified by those who go out with friends and/or into social environments periodically to 'have a good time' — which can be defined in many ways.

Ravers

The 'rave' scene in the United Kingdom that was so much a part of the 1980s and early '90s was radically altered when prevention of the use of warehouses and other empty buildings for illegal dances became a major occupation for police. The collection of many hundreds, sometimes thousands, of young people in dilapidated buildings, without basic facilities involved health and safety risks that were unacceptable to adults although they seemed quite irrelevant to the participants. Their reputation for the use of drugs, particularly Ecstasy, was exploited ad nauseam by the tabloid press which no doubt contributed to their demise. However, while the spirit of adventure, associated with illegality, that was an intrinsic part of this era may be gone, there are similar outlets that offer various types of music and all-night dancing, and young people now go out to rave or dance parties, night-clubs or 'gigs' to hear bands and dance. (See Beck and Rosenbaum, 1994, for the equivalent phenomenon in the US.)

The term raver is a useful shorthand for a person who goes out, usually with friends on a Friday or Saturday night to dance more or less continuously until dawn. At one time the music was 'House' music and related styles — geared to dancing which is energetic and highly stylised. This has now diversified with increasing commercialization, for example 'Techno' is dominant in some areas. This means that there is greater heterogeneity now among ravers and this is often associated, not only with the type of music, but with age, social class and preferred drugs. There are rave magazines and commercial radio programmes devoted to them. One positive aspect of the rave scene — that of an uplifting and friendly atmosphere seems to be remaining relatively intact.

Ravers were defined in this typology by their age — mostly under 25 years, strictly weekend use of amphetamine and low dose levels — often sharing a gram of amphetamine between two or three friends. The purity of amphetamine sulphate sold on the streets has been about 5% since the research began in 1990 although occasionally this increases. The strength of dose typically used is, therefore, quite weak. There is little desire to increase it:

Interviewer   Do you think it improves your mood if you use more?

Respondent   No, I never go higher than what I normally have.
(Steve, 19 years)

This makes it a very cheap night out and attractive to unemployed or low paid youth and students. They tend to dislike alcohol, particularly in large quantities.

Respondent   I think drinking beer is pretty violent. Every time I've gone for a beer there's been trouble. It pisses you off ... when you can go out and have a gram of speed, get into the music an' have a brilliant night.
(Tanya, 19 years)

A highly valued characteristic of dance parties and similar gatherings is friendliness, and alcohol would spoil this.

Respondent   You socialise a lot better ... when you are at one of these parties, there's people from all over the country but you never see them fightin' or nothing.
(Mark, 23 years)

The dominant reason for using amphetamine is for the energy, the long term effects allowing continuous dancing for several hours.

Respondent   When there are parties I don't want to miss out ... an' I'm a bit tired so obviously if I didn't take it I wouldn't be able to last. I'd be sat in a corner while everyone else is dancing ... I don't like missing out on things.
(Mandy, 20 years)

Most of these young people take amphetamine orally — either 'dabbing' on their tongue or wrapping it up in a cigarette paper, or in an empty capsule shell and swallowing it, relatively few snort it. Some will administer it only once, just before they go into the party venue, others may take further doses later on in the night but this rather depends on the degree of security at the clubs. Most clubs try to disassociate themselves from the illicit drug scene.

Amphetamine seems to be an ideal antidote to adolescent anxiety about peer rejection and coping with social relationships. The next most commonly expressed reason for using amphetamine after energy is for the confidence to get up and dance uninhibitedly in front of others and be able to talk easily to others.

Respondent   I've noticed I can talk to anybody, even if I don't know them ... you make a lot of friends. I have to keep me mouth going unless I've got chewing gum.
(Andrew, 17 years)

Respondent   You have a brilliant time on speed ... you can get up an' dance. Some people go to a club an' can't get up an' dance because they're paranoid ... but I can, I don't care what people think. (Melanie, 17 years)

Most amphetamine using ravers like Ecstasy but can't afford it. It is more expensive than amphetamine and LSD and they tend to think it is a waste of money. Since it is also of uncertain quality, it is better to use amphetamine and LSD together. The more experienced believe this is an improvement in terms of the psychoactive state, others because the speed induces confidence that the hallucinogenic trip can be controlled. Some always 'trip and speed'.

Respondent   Speed and trip mainly because the Ecstasy's been crap. (Pete, 22 years)

Respondent   If I'm having trips I always have speed ... I think it helps me have confidence over the trip. (Robert, 19 years)

Generally there are few health problems among them, the dose and frequency levels are too low to cause health problems and even the comedown (withdrawal) well known to be very severe in terms of depression, is coped with fairly easily. Some simply sleep through it, those who can't sleep use cannabis. Cannabis is smoked regularly but heavier drugs like heroin and crack are rejected, as is injecting.

Respondent   I've seen people injecting at the raves but it makes me sick so I just walk away ... I wouldn't want to know about that. (Pete, 22 years)

The majority of respondents in this group live with their parents and they are concerned to conceal the effects from them. While many are employed or still in education, a surprising number are involved in minor crime of an opportunistic nature — shoplifting or theft from cars — to give them more spending money.

These users find very little that is bad about amphetamine and hence very little reason to stop — the few complaints are about depression when coming down and the after-effects of physical activity:

Interviewer   Are there any bad things about it?

Respondent   Coming down really — you're just worn out and your bones are aching because you've been on your feet all weekend but it's not seemed to hit you.

>Or you've not eaten all weekend so you feel pretty rough.
>(Tracey, 24 years)

Amphetamine is widely used at dance parties and clubs in the United Kingdom, sometimes under the guise of Ecstasy, for many ravers it is regarded as an essential and harmless part of their main leisure pursuit.

Older Hippie Ravers

These observations are more impressionistic and based on a qualitative examination of fairly small samples:

In the United Kingdom the contemporary rave scene is not a wholly new phenomenon. Many people of the 'sixties generation' have memories of getting together for all-night dancing and of using a stimulant for energy to keep going. This first generation of ravers was born out of the enthusiasm for Motown music imported from the United States. Black Rhythm n' Blues music was played all over the country, discs were released and live bands came on tour. In the 1970s it declined in London and the south but was taken up by devotees in the Midlands and North of England. Popular venues were in Stoke on Trent and Manchester, but the hub of it all was the Wigan Casino. The music was re-named 'Northern Soul' and developed a culture all of its own which was characterized by all-nighters at established night clubs or in hired halls, sometimes continuous through the day. These mostly occurred at weekends and a ritual developed that persists today of travelling to a venue for a weekend's dancing. The clientele are almost wholly white.

The scene then was similar to the current rave scene in being sustained by a stimulant — amphetamine. Then, as now, there was little use of alcohol, the atmosphere was friendly and trouble was rare. However, whereas injecting is not a part of the current rave scene, at one time it was in vogue on the Northern Soul scene with dancers queueing up in the toilets (bathrooms) to use injecting equipment that someone had brought in. There are other differences: the music of course, and also the style of dancing, the Northern Soul clientele are now older and more exclusive, the gatherings are smaller, except perhaps for major reunions, and most current ravers prefer Ecstasy.

With the resurgence of nostalgia for the 1960s recently some younger recruits are appearing although mostly among Mods in London. The majority of venues are still in the north and they are attended by devotees of very long standing who still use amphetamine only at weekends to go to these events. It was part of that scene and remains so for them.

Speeding Drinkers

A phenomenon well known to the amphetamine-using sub-culture is the drug's effect on the uptake of alcohol. Inebriation is difficult when a drinker has taken amphetamine. It is interesting that the women in our samples tended to feel that it was a waste of money to buy expensive alcohol if amphetamine was being used and it was more appropriate to drink soft drinks. Many young men however, who were part of drinking groups, used it regularly to go 'pubbing' with their friends at weekends. These were males between 16 and 30 years who found the drug a useful way of avoiding the social embarrassment of drunkenness and, for those who could not 'take their beer', the drug allowed them to keep up with friends:

Interviewer   Why do you use it?

Respondent   Because I like it. It's generally because I just want to be able to go out an' not end up with me head in a glass. Because by Friday I'm so tired (from working) and I know if I go out some-where there's going to be a lot going on ... so I don't want to end up like that.
(Malcolm, 25 years)

The drug also helps to make social interactions and sensible conversations possible:

Interviewer   What do you like about it?

Respondent   Well, it'll keep you drinking all night and talking away. If you go to a concert and that you can drink and dance all night ... you can talk and have a good time.
(Chris, 20 years)

Most speeding ravers also spontaneously mentioned confidence and this seemed a considerable bonus in the competitive male environment in which they found themselves.

Respondent   Well, I don't think I'm shy but it's just ... if you go into a pub and it's crowded you can't be bothered pushing through ... but when you're on speed you don't care.
(Chas, 22 years)

Confidence extended to going outside of the supporting environment of your own gang of friends and having the motivation and energy to do so.

Respondent   I know that if I have a bit of whizz I can piss off down town on me own 'cos I don't mind walking around on me own then ... and it gives me the energy to walk about an have a few drinks.
(John, 27 years)

There are consequences to the combining of amphetamine and alcohol however. The speeding drinker may be unaware of how much alcohol he is consuming.

Respondent   As soon as I come down off it, I've drunk that much that I'm sick. When I take speed … say I've got a pint in front of me … I'll drink some and, I don't know I've drunk it because, you know, me mouth's still dry.
(Dave, 18 years)

Many young male drinkers binge at the weekend, that is, non-stop drinking. They include a substantial minority of football supporters who like the confidence and composure induced by amphetamine when going to matches on other supporters' territory. Sometimes they anticipate trouble with rival gangs and look forward to it. A strong norm is apparent of not letting friends down through incapacity caused by drink.

Young Mums

The label here refers to women who had children while still in their teens, some of this group are now in their mid-twenties and the age range goes from 17 to about 25 years (see Klee and Reid, 1995). They have lived in their present area for many years, often since birth and have built up friendship groups, often with other mothers. There is usually contact with female friends every day — they share child-minding with their friends, have home selling parties of kitchenware or lingerie and so on. If their children are at school they often take part-time jobs. When they have a partner, that partner may be unemployed or work sporadically in casual labour. The partners also use drugs, sometimes heroin. The main aim of using amphetamine is to have enough energy to look after the children, do the housework and still have some leisure time. It seems that the responsibility of having babies at a young age, with the associated problem of confinement in the home until the children can be safely left with others, results later in a desire to have a good time while they are still young enough to enjoy it.

Respondent   I think the reason we use … we've all got kids … we don't go out until nine or ten at night … I mean, if we didn't take it (amphetamine), all right, we'd go out but we wouldn't enjoy ourselves as much, we'd be knackered (tired). Plus the fact that some of us have got work next morning and we take it for that as well.
(Pat, 24 years)

They will go out to clubs or pubs as a group without their partners, who tend, in any case, to go out with their 'mates'. There are gender-based norms governing male and female activities in these communities — the women going visiting their female friends or meeting at the shops, their partners going to the pubs, to score drugs or to play football. Going out is a fairly regular activity and amphetamine is used to lift their mood and replace the energy depleted by children and work, whether paid or housework. Pride is taken in the standards they achieve — clean children and houses.

A word often used is 'mission' and if a young mum wants to decorate the house or have a good clean out she may also take a little more in the week. It is never injected but put in drinks, dabbed, swallowed or snorted. Those who work tend to work part-time, during the day while the children are at school and/or in the evening if the children are looked after. Those who work tend to use more frequently so that they have the energy for the job too. They also use higher doses. Thus there is a wide range of use from very low dose, perhaps half a gram once a week to go out, up to several times a week using a gram or more a day. There is an obvious danger with these working women that they will suffer health problems. There was frequent mention in this sample of muscular strains that were related to lifting or continuous heavy work, and also accidents through tiredness. The jobs in which they are employed are low-paid and low status — house, office or school cleaning, and geriatric care.

The drug is functional in many other ways for these women, for example the desire to keep slim is important but seems secondary to the other benefits. However, an increase in weight seems to be the first disadvantage to be mentioned if a woman has cut down or stopped using amphetamine for a while.

Respondent   It keeps me nice and slim, but now (after a period of abstinence) I've put on a stone (6 kg) and it's cracking me up.
(Alison, 20 years)

Multiple benefits are attributed to amphetamine including general good health:

Respondent   I've got three kids and it makes me cope better. When I'm ill … say when I've got the 'flu and things like that, I take a bit of whizz and it sweats it out and gets rid of it. If I can't cope with the kids and I'm ill — if I take some of that I'm all right by the next day.
(Christine, 24 years)

Whether an occasional user or more frequent, they do not feel that the drug is easy to control and an increase in use often invokes warnings or counselling from friends. Trying to prevent uncalled for irritability with children when coming down is felt to be important and efforts are made to avoid unwanted effects. The allure of the drug is strongly felt although efforts at maintaining a 'normal' lifestyle are common.

Respondent   I've taught myself when I've had some to get the things done I want to do. That's why I have it to get the cleaning done and I'm not saying I can't control my little girl or nothing but I'm always nicer with her. But then I'll force myself to eat my tea or force myself to go to bed. I just use it to get things done in the day or if I'm going out.
(Marie, 20 years)

Respondent   I can get pretty bad tempered when I'm coming down, that's why I try an' have a smoke (cannabis) or get someone to take the kids out.
(Linda, 24 years)

Amphetamine is not regarded as a 'hard' drug like heroin or crack-cocaine and although some of their partners may use these drugs, they are considered unacceptable and dysfunctional by the women themselves:

Respondent   Out of all drug addicts heroin addicts are the worst. I can't stand them. I couldn't sit with a heroin addict … just the way they are. Frank (ex-partner) was older than me and we used to be on a different high, we'd be on completely different wavelengths. He'd be sat there with his head on his knees and I was there with the couch upside down cleaning it.
(Andrea, 21 years)

Alcohol is only rarely used, partly because it does not produce the right atmosphere, but mostly because it is expensive and regarded as a waste of money.

Respondent   I can have a drink with speed an' I never get drunk … but it's a waste of money really.

Interviewer   The speed or the drink?

Respondent   The drink … because you don't get drunk an' you're just drinking more … you might as well drink water.
(Pat, 24 years)

The attraction of amphetamine for these women is that they believe it meets so many of their needs and helps them enjoy what would otherwise be a restricted and tedious lifestyle. They are still young, interested in dancing, socialising and wanting to forget their domestic chores or work responsibilities. Since it is so very highly valued it is potentially dangerous and the dangers to health may fail to deter from more frequent use.

The Experimenters

These are mostly male adolescents who use amphetamine and a wide variety of other drugs to experience their effects. This is partly a game and diversion and often an intrinsic part of group activities. Their age range is 14 to 20 years and the drugs are used mostly at the weekends 'for a laugh' and always in the company of their 'mates'. The use of drugs or ways of combining drugs is discussed in advance and there is a 'macho' quality about decisions about trying the drug — usually ending with 'let's do it'. The group of friends is often not large but it is cohesive and the members tend to adhere strongly to the group norms. Drugs are shared and everyone is expected to contribute in some way.

Respondent   Everyone shares … we used to kick people out who weren't sharing — they were hangin' around trying to get what they could, then they'd be gone, next day they'd be back … we got sick of it so we just used to hide them and drop hints that they should go.
(James, 18 years)

The range of drugs is wide, they switch easily from one to another depending on the drug's availability and their mood. They will use an unknown drug, prescribed pharmaceuticals that they have been told about or read about, and they will mix drugs that they have used singly and believe they understand the effects.

Respondent   I'd probably try anything once.

Interviewer   Have you ever done crack?

Respondent   No, I haven't been offered it so I haven't had the chance … but I probably would do it.

Interviewer   And coke?

Respondent   I've never done that … it's a bit expensive really.
(Stuart, 18 years)

Interviewer   What about any other stuff?

Respondent   If there's anything going … if you're with your mates you'll have some.

Interviewer   What have you used in the last month?

Respondent   Speed, pot (cannabis), a bit of heroin ... I've had a go of that
             crack for the first time this month.

Interviewer   What did you think of that?

Respondent   It's no good ... it's a waste of money that ... £25 a go ... it
             wasn't worth it.
             (Steve, 17 years)

The younger experimenters are often naive about how to evaluate the quality of what they are buying and do not take the precaution of going to a
reliable dealer. They may not like to reveal that they do not know the drug
and if this is exposed some will turn it into a virtue — they will 'try anything'.
Despite the fact that they do not want to get 'ripped off' they are easy targets
for exploitation, especially since they tend to buy from different places and
in an opportunistic way. They therefore make mistakes:

Respondent   (About amphetamine of uncertain origin) You usually find out
             after you've taken it and you're just sat there after a couple of
             hours and not up and about.
             (Lewis, 20 years)

The drugs that were rejected were those that tended to interfere with social
interactions so that opiates, although tried, are regarded with extreme caution. Some will also try injecting and one suspects that they are most in
danger of progressing on to injecting polydrug use. However a decision to
inject will be a communal decision and the outcome of this is unpredictable.
Injecting may continue, be rejected democratically by all or individually by
some and not others, in which case it becomes divisive, introduces conflict,
and the group starts to break up.
    Another anti-social development is overuse of amphetamine, which in-
duces paranoid delusions that disrupt social interactions. There are normative mechanisms that seem to put brakes on this process and any obvious
lack of control:

Respondent   Last month we just went on a mad binge and everybody's head
             went ... well we all sat there doing silly things ... so we all
             decided to calm down ... I feel a lot better for it.
             (Malcolm, 18 years)

Many young experimenters are unemployed and living with their parents.
They are therefore keen to be out of the house and away from parental
supervision. They spend most of their time with their friends and have too
little money to afford alcohol, although those who are employed tend to slip

easily into 'pubbing' as an activity they do not need to conceal. The drugs they choose are those that are inexpensive — cannabis, amphetamine, LSD, psilobycin (magic mushrooms), prescribed pharmaceuticals such as analgesics and anti-emetics, volatile substances such as butane gas and glue. Experimenters do not take drugs seriously, they alleviate boredom, offer experiences that can be shared and that are affordable.

CONTROLLED AND UNCONTROLLED USERS

Amphetamine users range along a continuum of control. The majority are occasional users who will never experience the health and social problems of the daily injector. The extent of control is governed by both individual and environmental factors.

The Prudent User

For prudent users control is very important. It is not a characteristic necessarily acquired through personal experience but rather through an awareness of the consequences of excess, sometimes witnessed in friends or relatives. Addiction is to be avoided at all costs. Often highly informed, they will know the effects of drugs and should they fall victim to adverse symptoms, they will have strategies to counteract them. They are aware of the disadvantages of various modes of administration:

Respondent   I'm not saying I'm sensible, because no-one is sensible if they're taking drugs, but I do try to cut the risks. I'll say I'll do this because if I don't, this'll happen. If you're snorting it it's burning a hole in your nose for a kick-off and if you're injecting it isn't … but if you're injecting rubbish it's going to do you damage as well.
(Dave, 25 years)

The use of amphetamine is occasional and is used for a particular purpose, for example, playing football, decorating, house-cleaning, driving a long distance, going to an all-night party, or even staying up to watch television. Some employed people would fall into this category and use amphetamine when working.

There has to be some value associated with using the drug — it is not driven by pure hedonism. The age range of this group is wide, it seems more that personality characteristics define this type than age, gender or group membership, though there were fewer women than men in this cluster.

Prudent users dislike the unpredictability of purity levels and are suspicious of additives in amphetamine. They are unwilling to try new drugs, particularly if they are expensive and contributing to the high earnings of dealers.

Interviewer   Have you ever done Ecstasy?

Respondent   No … at £20 a go I wouldn't bother.

Interviewer   What about coke? Would you try it if it was offered you?

Respondent   No, I don't think so … it's only supposed to last 20 minutes.
(Mark, 23 years)

They will use amphetamine if they can afford it. Since most are not involved in criminal activities they cannot often afford more, but even with more money it is unlikely that they would increase their use:

Respondent   I've never been badly into anything for the simple reason that I've never wanted to spend me money on it … a great deal of money on it.
(Alan, 30 years)

Drinking with friends is not a part of their social life, partly because of the cost but also because of the potential lack of control in public:

Respondent   I don't like alcohol at all. I used to find that I could easily get drunk an' that. I liked the feeling but I overdid it. I don't like drinking, I think it's anti-social.

Interviewer   In terms of sociability speed is better than alcohol?

Respondent   Definitely. I think most drugs are if they're taken when you're in the right mood … if I'm feeling down or anything I wouldn't touch them.
(Mike, 20 years)

Prudent users take amphetamine occasionally and at low doses. They are concerned about their health — 'I hate to abuse my body' — and often about their reputation too.

Interviewer   So you can't afford it?

Respondent   There are people I know an' I could go down there an' get it but then I'll get a reputation for owing money an' things so that tends to stop me.
(Steve, 34 years)

There were injectors included in this cluster. They tend to dislike the taste of amphetamine when snorted and turned straight to injecting on the advice of friends.

Respondent   When I try taking it in a drink, or just throwing it in my mouth it nearly makes me throw up ... just the smell of it.
(Tanya, 22 years)

The cautious approach to life is apparent in prudent users, they dislike excess because it means lack of control. Experimentation is dangerous and value for money is very important. It is unlikely that they will become problem users.

The Isolate

The isolated user of amphetamine is comparatively rare. There are sub-types but all have certain characteristics in common — they will use the drug when alone, which is incomprehensible to many amphetamine users, have little confidence, very low self-esteem and tend to have few friends. The majority are male and injecting. He may be a long term user who has been through the early stages of functional use of the drug for giving confidence in social environments or for the 'buzz' and has now become more introspective (see Morgan and Beck Chapter 7, this volume, on paradoxical effects). There are some who are attempting to stay away from other users to avoid being lured back into activities that they fear will be harmful to their health or to their relationship with their partner and family. There are others who need to conceal their use from parents, partners and friends. There are also those who have endemic mental problems and tend to have problems with aggression.

Respondent   I feel like killing people sometimes.

Interviewer   What would make you feel like that?

Respondent   It just happens.
(Justin, 20 years)

It tends to be isolated users who go for treatment. Almost all respondents who were attending a drug agency were in this cluster. Sometimes they may be prescribed dexamphetamine, but more often they find the agency has nothing for them — which many drug workers freely admit. 'She said there's no help for it'. They have often sought help because of paranoia and violent reactions to imaginary criticisms.
    The isolate will rarely drink in company:

Interviewer   Do you drink?

Respondent   Yeh ... but I never go out to the pub. If I drink I get a few cans in.
(Stuart, 27 years)

Sometimes this is because the isolate has lost friends 'A lot of people don't want to know you if you're sticking needles in yourself'.

There are more employed people who are isolates.

Respondent   (Describing his regular binges) I wouldn't sleep at all. Some times I start Friday night and I'm wrecked by Monday morning. I'd go to work in a real state. I thought everybody knew I'd been on speed an' I wouldn't look anyone in the eye … I wouldn't talk to anybody. I'd keep myself busy so I didn't have any contact with anyone.

The same man spent long hours trying to sort out problems:

Respondent   Most nights I'm on me own … an' you tend to sit an' think. It's like, really intense thinking an' I might work out the same problem fifty different times in me head. But when I go to bed, the following night I've forgotten what I've tried to work out in me bloody head anyway.

He had reasons for avoiding people:

> I try not to mix with anybody who's on the gear really because then you get yourself noticed if they get pulled (arrested by police).
> (Daniel, 28 years)

Many long term users comment on the change in the effects of amphetamine which they themselves find rather strange:

Respondent   It's different effects now. When I used to have a hit … it'd be up, get changed and go out. But sometimes it's just like it gets rid of the aches and pains, and sometimes I can just sit and be relaxed and not get excited. It's all different now I've been using a long time.
(Barry, 26 years)

For some it seems that extended heavy use has failed them in no longer giving them the confidence to socialize:

Interviewer   Are you quite happy being on your own now?

Respondent   I miss the relationship part, like when I was with me girl-friend … I miss that a lot. And like I say, I still don't feel I've got the confidence to go out with a group of people and I'd have to be desperate before I'd turn to friends for help.
(Robert, 22 years)

It seems that many amphetamine users become isolates when they find that the drug no longer deals with a particular condition that is associated with social interaction, for example, confidence and aggression. If the condition has become acute they may then turn to drug agencies or their doctor for help. They do not feel particularly dependent on amphetamine, they know of no other way of tackling their problem. Many started the use of amphetamine very early in adolescence and it has provided a solution for many years — a good mood replaces depression or aggression, confidence replaces awkwardness. But heavy use brings other effects and the earlier symptoms return with a vengeance. They do not know how to cope. Their friends are either rejected, avoided or alienated.

Polydrug/Phasic Users

This typology used data from studies of primary amphetamine users, but some samples included polydrug users for whom amphetamine was a part of their repertoires. This could be concurrent use, for example using amphetamine to lift the effects of heroin or in conjunction with a diet of prescribed pharmaceuticals, or consecutively as drugs became available or of good quality. As one respondent put it when asked what was his preferred drug 'Whatever I happen to be using at the time'. Most of them inject a least one drug.

Some polydrug users are early experimenters but a few years on. Often they are driven by drug availability and finances and seem not to have strong preferences:

Respondent   It all depends … like this week all I've had is smack. Another week all I'll have is speed, an' just hammer the speed. Or sometimes I'll have both. If I get pot there's no point in getting speed 'cos speed's an upper an' pot is a downer.
(Mark, 20 years)

This respondent injected amphetamine but smoked heroin, a fairly common practice. He also liked to use a small dose of amphetamine in the morning before work to give him energy. Even when bingeing, usually with friends, several drugs were used.

Other polydrug users inject more than one drug and this respondent was typical of others in using a drug that matched his mood at the time.

Interviewer   Do you inject the heroin?

Respondent   Yeah, as I say like, I've injected quite a lot of drugs … I don't see the point anymore in swallowing it or something 'cos you don't get the full benefit of the drug.

Interviewer   Have you done tranquilisers and things like that recently?

Respondent   I'd say that if it's there an' I was in the right mood for that
             particular drug, then I'll have it.
             (Dave, 19 years)

Amphetamine using polydrug users in this sample tended to have started to
use drugs very young, perhaps cannabis at eleven or twelve, progressing on to
other cheap drugs such as amphetamine and LSD two or three years later. If
they were also early experimenters they had acquired a considerable amount
of knowledge and sophistication about drugs and how to control their effects.

This type of polydrug user is not primarily oriented to sedative effects.
Their drug career does not follow the path of opiate and tranquillizer use
with the decline into physical addiction. However they sometimes have
problems in balancing the 'uppers and downers'. They may learn from the
experience and subsequently control them:

Respondent   I got myself in a mess … I was addicted to all the drugs in one
             go. Like I was on speed … I was coming down off speed an' I
             had to have some downers … I was taking a lot of downers on
             top of a lot of speed … an' I was taking a lot of gear at the
             same time as well. So I messed up on everything at the same
             time really. It just made me a physical wreck. So I went into
             hospital an' got the drugs out me system … but it never really
             got me off the drugs you know.
             (Danny, 20 years)

Some polydrug users, after cannabis, atypically progress onto heroin and
that is an important drug in their repertoire. The cost and its addictive qualities make it unattractive however and amphetamine replaces it for a variety
of reasons, a principal one being to counteract the heroin addiction and
perhaps also, get out of debt. They may then feel strongly attached to amphetamine but occasionally use heroin or a tranquilliser to come down. Balancing drugs becomes a way of life for some:

Interviewer   And when you're actually using speed are you using other
              things at the same time, actually at the same time?

Respondent   Yeah, sometimes I use heroin at the same time, an' all the time
              I use valium because I really need that, but if I'm on speed I
              try to cut down on the valium because it seems pointless be-
              cause valium gives me the same sort of feeling to speed … it
              gives me a lift. I mean, I've had 50 mg of valium an' I've not
              been able to sleep all night. But it's the heroin I need really.
              You really miss the one you've not got. It's like anything, even
              when you're taking speed you miss your other drugs.
              (Christine, 28 years)

Amphetamine is part of most polydrug repertoires — it may be appreciated for particular properties: the 'rush' when injecting, the lifting of mood, the energy and so on, it may be valued for performing certain functions, for example as an antidote to heroin addiction, it is a more socially acceptable drug than heroin, is believed to be easier to control than heroin, and is less expensive. Concurrent use of many drugs is a risky business and while some polydrug users seem to have control, there are many others who are in danger of serious damage to health.

The Modified User

Since amphetamine is second to cannabis in terms of popularity in the United Kingdom, it is inevitable that there are many modified users around. These are people who are at a later stage of their drug 'career', have experienced the first excitement of amphetamine and what it can do for them, increased the frequency and dose levels, may have moved to injecting, developed various health and psychological symptoms, perhaps lost their job or were caught by the police for property crime, were deserted by a friend or threatened with the departure of a partner, and have decided to take themselves in hand. The pattern is very common and follows a similar course, although there is often one factor that seems particularly critical in initiating such a change.

Going to prison seems to be a major motive to modify drug-taking behaviour. However it is not the unpleasantness of the experience that is its only or even main impact, but its associated effects. A desire to settle down with a partner, a fear of losing the partner while in prison, being available for the children, are some common positive pressures towards change.

Children are an important motivator, partly because of the difficulty of concealing drug use from them as they get older and partly because of the effects on them when a parent is away in prison:

Respondent   I've learnt me lesson. With having three kids, married … I've been inside just recently an' I've found out how much it does to your family.

The same man was concerned to protect his children from the consequences of his mood when coming down from amphetamine:

Respondent   I can get bad-tempered, and if me kids are messing about I snap at them, so when that starts I piss off so I don't batter me kids or anything … I don't want to do that. I just get me head down upstairs and get it sorted, then I come down an' I'm great with them then.
(Barry, 23 years)

If the partner uses the drug it often means that some agreement has to be made that they both cut down or stop. It is recognized that unilateral action is difficult to sustain. Such pacts are more likely if a child's welfare is at risk:

Respondent   (With a pregnant partner) Years ago we used to be into it more than we are now ... we used to be up for weeks on end. Now we realise we have to eat and sleep.
(Bob, 38 years)

For some the experience of prison and the enforced abstinence (stimulants are not as popular in prisons as cannabis and heroin) allow time for reflection and result in an awareness of the slide into an unacceptable lifestyle:

Respondent   Well I've been out since September an' I've had it ten times at the most.

Interviewer   So it's only an occasional thing for you now?

Respondent   Yeah, an' that's how I'm going to keep it as well. I was using it for three months every day ... diggin it every day ... three digs a day an' like when I look back at it I know what it did to me ... it just took me over.
(Jack, 20 years)

Interviewer   So how come you haven't got back into it since you've been inside?

Respondent   Before I got sent down I wasn't realising what it was doing to me. I was losing weight all the time, thin as a rake and all me face was all drawn. I didn't realise like until I got out ... till I'd put a load of weight on and stuff like that ... so I thought 'I won't use that again'.
(Stuart, 21 years)

The criminal life itself becomes too wearing for some:

Respondent   I just got pissed off with it, going out robbing to get the money ... and I ended up owing money.

Interviewer   So it got a bit out of hand?

Respondent   It just gets too much of a hassle.
(Will, 21 years)

The reason why many women cut down or abstain temporarily is because they get pregnant. There is often pressure from partners, family and friends. Although the main reason for modifying amphetamine use is to avoid damage to the foetus and have a normal birth, there is concern that ante-natal care will reveal their use of drugs. Some will go to considerable lengths to produce the right environment to help them change their behaviour:

Interviewer   So what made you stop?

Respondent   I was pregnant. I'd already had about four miscarriages 'cos I was using, an' I wanted this one. I moved away from all me friends … cos' that's the only way you can do it.
(Helen, 26 years)

Other women cut down at times when their children have been removed into care and they are attempting to get them back. Some leave their children in the care of their mother when they feel they cannot cope and then try to restore their control so that they can have them back:

Respondent   She's with my mum now … just for the time being. As soon as I get off I'm going to get it all sorted and get me daughter back. Me mum doesn't know I'm on drugs … she's no idea. But if I don't come off then I don't want her back 'cos I know if I still took speed and I didn't have none I'd take it out on me daughter.
(Jenny, 21 years)

The example they set their children concerns many women and while they want to go on using for as long as possible, as the children get older it is increasingly difficult to conceal it from them:

Respondent   What makes me stop a lot of things is me kids … I just think 'I don't want them to grow up like that'. It would kill me if my kids ever went near drugs.
(Tracy, 22 years)

Some older users notice and fear the effects on their health:

Interviewer   So you're a bit wary now of using too much?

Respondent   Yeah, because of the effect it has on me body … I can't take it as much now … the way it messes me body up. I don't like what it's doing to me. It's probably shortened me life … probably brain damage, quite a lot of the brain cells gone missing … you don't eat, you lose weight. You see, I never wanted to get past thirty. The motto of my generation was don't trust anyone over thirty an' when I got to thirty I realised why. Now I've got to the grand old age of forty … life begins again … I believe it begins for me again and I want to live as long as possible.
(Gerry, 42 years)

Younger people dislike other aspects of slipping into regular use — appearance plays a major role. Spots are commonly mentioned but more alarming is the increased 'scruffiness' when they come to resemble their own stereotype of a 'smack-head' (heroin user). This is a major contrast to the earlier days of obsessive attention to cleanliness. The changes they see in themselves seem to come as a surprise:

Respondent   The next time I have it I won't dig it … I'll never dig it again.

Interviewer   Why?

Respondent   Because I've gone scruffy, I've got scruffy with everything, not having clean clothes all the time like I used to. I've gone like a tramp. And I've lost about two stone (12 kg) in the past three months. I never thought I'd get to the stage when I'd have to try an' get off it.
(Kevin, 19 years)

Others fear that psychological effects will become permanent:

Respondent   I've got to get out of this otherwise I'm going to be cabbaged for the rest of me life'.
(Dennis, 19 years)

A sudden resolution to change does not necessarily indicate a serious intent to give up amphetamine completely. Many modified users yearn for the earlier stages when they used less frequently, their lives were more under control and they were less likely to attract the attention of the police. They are ambivalent about the prospect of total and permanent abstinence:

Interviewer   Do you think you'll ever stop completely?

Respondent   I'd like to, but I don't know … I don't think I would … I don't know though … when I'm a bit older I might think 'forget it'. But it's good so you take it.
(Robert, 20 years)

There are many health and social factors that push a heavy user of amphetamine towards restraint, the modified user is at a crossroad in his or her drug career and one path leads out of illicit drug use. Unfortunately good intentions do not guarantee success and we found that older modified users had been down this path many times before.

CRIMINAL USERS

There are higher proportions of males taken into custody and imprisoned than females, and one would expect that there would be more males who are criminally oriented in our sample than females. However, in all of our studies we found no gender differences in self-reported criminal activity among amphetamine users although with the overall proportion of reported crime typically around 90% a 'ceiling effect' would preclude the opportunity of finding a difference. Any differences between men and women lie in the type of crime they commit, with women preferring shop-lifting and fraud, and men responsible for burglary and theft from cars. Indeed, among some amphetamine using males, shoplifting is a low grade activity to be disdained.

The majority of amphetamine users in our samples reported that property crime preceded the use of drugs (Klee, 1994) and claim that their criminal activities have little or nothing to do with the use of amphetamine. The samples comprised mostly young people, average age 22 years and included many recreational users whose expenditure on drugs was very low. Amphetamine is cheap and obtained in many ways and crime is unlikely to be seen as essential for funding drug use. One gender difference was observed in the cluster that generated this type. This was associated with friendship patterns. Males tended to belong to groups and the activities of such groups were focused on communal speed use and crime. These groups were very prominent in our field work and were found on all the public-sector housing estates where youth unemployment is high and facilities for youth are poor. Women seemed to be the outliers in this cluster, although there were female members of criminal groups. The analysis generated only one clear, criminally oriented cluster, though criminal activity was a part of the profile of all the rest.

Grafters

In the UK the term 'grafter' refers to "the acquisition of money, power etc. by dishonest means" (Collins, 1986). Amphetamine is regarded as functional by many grafters, mainly because it keeps them awake and alert, particularly at night, they run faster if pursued and it gives them confidence.

Respondent   It just gives you guts … it's as though everything's yours. (Jenny, 18 years).

This may turn into over-confidence however:

Respondent   While you're robbin', like you think you're totally on the ball on the whizz but you've got that much confidence you don't really know whether you're taking a risk, whereas if you were straight you'd know.
(Chas, 21 years)

Most seem to experience feelings of paranoia when out intending to rob, but a part of a professional approach is to know that this is drug-induced and therefore to be controlled. It is often paranoia that is offered as a reason for not using amphetamine when out stealing. However, the crime tends to be described in a positive way as a 'buzz' by young grafters, while some time later in their drug careers older grafters find little excitement in it.

Respondent   Up until getting in a place and actually doing a job, then you're on edge all the time. But after you've got in there you're buzzin. It's a really unusual feeling when you know you've got away with it … the adrenalin flowing through you is unbeliev-able. I used to do it for fun … it was more fun than anything. (Billy, 21 years)

Some women are useful members of groups and find the activity as exciting as the men.

Respondent   It's dead exciting.

Interviewer   What happened?

Respondent   Me, Danny and Paul, we took the windowpanes out an' there was a great big stack (Hi Fi) there. An' they said 'if you get it we'll give you speed for it plus £80. But I couldn't get it out of the window an' the busies (police) were coming round so I just had to do a runner out through the garden. (Dawn, 19 years)

Most young grafters work with a friend or two, and a larger group may burgle a factory or warehouse, but most will rob houses and garden sheds by themselves if they look safe. Some prefer to work alone however:

Respondent   I'd sooner work on my own, then you can't get grassed on … if you're caught it's your own fault. (Mandy, 21 years)

The use of amphetamine by grafters covered the range from orally adminis-tered low doses to frequent injecting. Groups tended to be fairly homogene-ous in terms of the mode of administration. The injecting grafter seeks stimulation through the 'rush' and through crime associated risks and 'mis-sions' most of the time — planning and setting goals, working out strategies and says that this is as much a buzz as the crime itself. Some are sexually highly active. The vocabulary reflects the lifestyle — words like mission, power-charge, whizzing:

Respondent   (Charismatic leader of one inner-city gang) When you're whiz-zing and you've had some good whizz and you feel powerful, you capture people, you make everybody round you do exactly what you want ... you make them go places, you make them do things ... like a puppet master. People who aren't on whizz just can't say no to you, they don't even know how to say no ... you're in control, you're nearly telepathic sometimes. (Chris, 23 years)

SELF-MEDICATORS

While self-medication of health symptoms is a common practice for both men and women there are significant gender differences, with women buying more over the counter medicines (although this may partly be accounted for by their role as the guardian of the family's health) and receiving a much higher proportion of prescriptions for tranquillizers (Lader, 1991; Vogt, 1995). A type emerged from the analysis that comprised mostly women who had started to take amphetamine for specific physical or mental health symptoms. The men were less likely to identify these symptoms as factors that led to their use of the drug, though there is no reason to suppose that they do not self-medicate.

Self-Medicating Women

Amphetamine in moderation is capable of treating effectively a variety of disorders, which is why it is so alluring to many people. Since the early days of prescribing (see Chapter 4 this volume) its appetite suppressant and anti-depressant capacities have been particularly valuable to women who suffer from depression and obesity (real or imagined). Women confined to the home by children, who have several small children and other responsibilities and are tired, find that not only is their depression lifted, but they have more motivation and energy. It is not surprising that amphetamine is particularly attractive to them, and perhaps gives rise to the reputation of this drug as 'a woman's drug'.

Some women start their drug career early with a prescription from their doctor for dexamphetamine or get the tablets from relatives or friends and then move on to street amphetamine:

Respondent   The very first drug I ever took was D_____ (an appetite suppressant) when I moved over here. After me third child I'd gone really fat. I've been the same on all me pregnancies and I've lost it but it was hard to this time so I went to me doctor an' he gave me diet sheets an' some tablets an' they used to give me some side effects so he said 'Well, we'll try this one but it's addictive so you can only go on it for so many weeks'. So I tried it an' it were brilliant ... I like it, it's brilliant, I've

been on it twelve months, but he's told me he's taking me off it so I'll be doing me speed full-time then ... 'cos I took it in between with me D_____.
(Pat, 22 years)

The same woman was lured into using street amphetamine in order to get an added boost of energy.

Respondent   I was going through court to get me child back and I eventually got him back that Christmas but I was so low in morale an' I needed something to liven me up for when he came home, because then I would have the three of them you see. So a friend of mine offered me some, she said 'Just try it, it might give you a bit of energy'. Because the D_____ only works if you're in a confident mood, but if you're feelin' down it'll put you to sleep. She said 'This probably won't last long it'll just keep you goin' for the time you need'. But you get to like it ... you get to need that energy.

Tiredness and depression are the critical features of a self-medicating female amphetamine user. The tiredness is often associated with children:

Respondent   It makes you feel more awake ... like with having the children I'm knackered all the time so it makes me feel not tired so much.
(Jenny, 21 years)

However, weight control can be important too.

Respondent   I do it really to get me weight down, 'cos I'm very conscious of me weight ... but a lot of it is because I'm tired.
(Linda, 22 years)

The younger women with partners may be criticised by them for putting on weight, which threatens their fragile self-esteem further. It is difficult to determine how body image interacts with depression — the women get depressed when they put on weight but frequently they have eating habits strongly influenced by depression that cause obesity and the pattern becomes cyclic. Most self-medicating women have a history of depression from traumatic life events in childhood or adolescence. However, not all women are introduced to amphetamine by a medical prescription — doctors are extremely reluctant to prescribe dexamphetamine. The majority start their use, like most amphetamine users, by being offered street drugs.

Once introduced to the drug, it is so valuable to such women as a source of energy and an antidote for their problems that there is considerable danger of them increasing the frequency and dose. This pressure is particularly acute if a child is taken into care. If, in addition, oral administration combined with poor eating habits gives rise to gastric problems or there is a need for a 'quick fix' they may turn to injecting. It is easy for them to get out of control:

Respondent   It keeps you awake you know. Like in the morning if you get up an' you feel tired you just have another hit. That's how it works for me anyway. I know the baby will be up at seven an' if I've been up speeding an got tired about four say, I'll have another hit to keep awake until he's up. Then another at about one … he won't go to bed until seven an' it'll keep me awake until then. If I want to sleep, I'll sleep then.
(Linda, 21 years)

When confined to the house by children, and the use of amphetamine has increased over many months or even years, there are none of the social effects of the drug:

Respondent   (Single parent) Before, I wouldn't take it unless somebody was here. I thought 'What's the fun on your own?'… but now I buy it, take it and sit here on my own talking to the wallpaper.
(Jane, 27 years)

The self-medicating woman may be treating depression that is consequent on such childhood traumata as parental drug or alcohol abuse and/or child abuse, sometimes sexual abuse. The problems are frequently multiple since a cycle develops of depression, drug use, problems with child care, relationship problems with a partner, more depression and more drugs. Some eventually proceed to the use of benzodiazepines and heroin in order to sleep and to deal with the hyperactivity when speeding, and aggression or acute depression when coming down. This type had the highest rate of attempted suicide in the analyses.

Self-medicating women regard themselves as dependent on the drug and believe they would not cope without it. They also know that it is not the answer to their problems, although not all are as articulate as this woman:

Respondent   I think it affected me psychologically when I was younger because I wasn't confronting the issues that were going on … my whole mind was telling me to be depressed because of the circumstances I was in and because I was taking speed I was blocking that out. So it made it worse I think, really.
(Aileen, 29 years)

If the process starts at an early age, it has consequences for ideas about self-identity:

Interviewer   Would you say you were a depressed sort of person?

Respondent   I don't know 'cos I'm on drugs that often I don't know what me personality is any more. That sounds terrible … me saying that, but it's true.
(Jane, 27 years)

The increasing doses are usually to attenuate the depression associated with coming down, which are severe for most people, but are particularly acute for women with few alternative coping strategies. It is made worse if, in addition to the unwelcome return to reality, there is a tendency to become irritable or aggressive and thus impact on the lives of those around them:

Respondent   I get really violent when I come down and he (boyfriend) hates me like that … he can't handle me like that.
(Carol, 25 years)

Most women, (and men too), make efforts not to allow this to affect the children but their solution to the problem is recognized as far from ideal:

Respondent   I shouted at me son … I shouted at him, yeah, but I don't smack him or nothin' because I've wanted a kid for so long … you know what I mean. I shouted at him when I was comin' down an' I felt dead guilty … I went into the other room an' started cryin' an' I thought it's not his fault I haven't got any whizz. So now when I haven't got any I let him do what he wants … wreck me house or whatever. I give in to him too much because it's not his fault I haven't got me whizz, why should I take it out on me son?
(Diane, 28 years)

Guilt over children is common though most attempt to be good mothers. Women whose children suffer harm through lack of care in watching over them can be very self-critical if they usually take a pride in the way they maintain standards.

Respondent   He (toddler, about 2 years) fell and hurt his head today an' split his head open so he's getting spoiled today … he's had presents an' that. All his face was a mess an' I was really frightened … I felt really guilty.
(Tracy, 21 years)

If the woman's partner is using amphetamine her control is usually affected. He may restrain her from excessive consumption, but may be using heavily himself. Unless an agreement is made between them, it can be difficult for her to moderate her use and the feeling of failure lowers self-esteem further and adds to the depression.

Fortunately not all self-medicating women get to such damaging stages. Remedial measures are possible and are put into effect. The use of cannabis attenuates withdrawal in a relatively harmless way and softens the resurgence of chronic problems. Eating regularly, using vitamin supplements and not going too long without sleep are also common. They have friends or family to take the children out when they themselves are low and so on.

Those women with a long history of severe psychological and social problems are most at risk of becoming chaotic, but there are many others who start by regarding amphetamine as a harmless panacea for all ills. They are unaware that increasing the frequency or dose will not increase its effectiveness, and eventually they may become enmeshed in a downward spiral that is only temporarily arrested by another dose of amphetamine. Other drugs are tried to restore the balance but this may fail. This pattern is, of course, not confined to amphetamine users.

CONCLUSIONS AND IMPLICATIONS FOR INTERVENTIONS

There are types that may be associated with amphetamine use that are not included here. The construction of a hypothetical list of types based on hearsay may be easy, but if the basic data are lacking, to implicate them in illicit drug use through statements unsupported by evidence would be ethically unacceptable. The types that have been identified have the advantage of a basis in a formal system of classification. The variability observable within types provides information about the range of behaviours, attitudes and values that can be expected about a person who seems to conform to a type. This may be helpful to drug workers when approaching new clients, but there is a danger of making unwarranted assumptions. Typological characteristics would need to be used only as heuristic devices, that is, to suggest lines of enquiry when seeking information.

The value to drug prevention initiatives, health promotion workers, and enforcers of social order lies in the extent to which identifiable patterns can suggest effective interventions. The data suggest that certain groups, most notably young mums, self-medicating women, young experimenters, some isolates and uncontrolled polydrug users are in particular danger of becoming victim to the health damaging effects of amphetamine but in different ways and for different reasons.

Crime control measures need to take into account why amphetamine users commit crimes and what effects amphetamine has on the criminal user.

For many of them, particularly those carrying out burglaries, crime is a 'buzz'. This is less often described in these terms by shoplifters who, presumably because they are in public, are more prey to paranoia. In both cases it is rare that obtaining money for drugs is the primary motive.

Health interventions also need comprehensive information about the target group in order to be effective. Each of the types identified here display areas of vulnerability that could suggest ways of attempting to change their behaviour. Many young amphetamine using ravers already know about the variable quality of Ecstasy and some believe they can avoid mishap, and spend less if they use amphetamine, which is rather strange since the quality of amphetamine has been consistently poor for several years now. This may the group of people who will be most resistant to prevention messages, since it is both highly functional and a part of the culture, but they are likely to be very responsive to harm reduction messages about safe dancing, particularly if facilities are provided as a matter of course at clubs and other venues.

For speeding drinkers the main problem is alcohol, but the combination can pose problems for police who have to cope with 'macho' confidence and the potential for violence by these young men. However, it seems that lack of confidence in living up to the demands of the group is a strong motivator and this may be useful in developing appropriate health messages for them.

Young mums are vulnerable through the allure of the drug in offering ways of being better mums and having a more interesting lifestyle. Being able to look after the children and the house and even a part-time job is very gratifying and boosts self-esteem. Yet many will initially be unaware of the irritability and other effects of the comedown on their children as well as themselves, which most would seek to avoid. This could be a very useful Achilles Heel for those who want to increase their awareness of such dangers.

The experimenters are the most likely to be influenced by group norms. The leader of the group is pivotal and will be the most knowledgeable, the most enterprising, attractive and so on. He or she may have acquired their status among their peers by being prepared to take more risks. Any intervention will need to focus on the leader and is more likely to be successful if harm reduction is the aim rather than prevention (Klee and Reid, 1995). A particular issue that would need to be addressed is the likely transition to regular polydrug use by some members of experimenting groups. Starting to inject any of the drugs would be a signal that more serious problems can be expected.

Isolates seem to have become isolated for one of three main reasons: first, the need for concealment from employers, family or friends; second, through circumstances forced upon them, such as single parents without the support of partner or family, and third, as a consequence of a long history of misuse which has brought about a change in the effects of the drug, both on themselves and their social relationships. In the last of these there may have been rejection by friends because of persistent paranoia and aggressiveness and there will be those with underlying mental health problems. The heterogeneous nature of those identified as an isolate means that each sub-type needs a different approach by helping agencies.

Polydrug users and phasic users, who have no particular allegiances for specific drugs are also sub-types. The polydrug user with a wide repertoire of drugs is subject to risks through combining drugs and/or using them concurrently and the risks are considerably increased if the drugs are injected, (Klee, Morris and Ruben, 1993). Chaotic patterns of use can emerge during attempts to balance the drugs and this type is then one that is in most serious danger of harm. Information about the hazards in making up drugs cocktails and using certain drugs concurrently should be emphasized since the majority of illicit drug users now tend to be polydrug users. The phasic user who switches drugs over time is less at risk.

The self-medicating woman is potentially a problem user if the symptoms she is treating are of a long-lasting or recurrent nature. A variety of personal and environmental variables may limit her options, for example, a drug using and/or dominant partner, or a fear of seeking help because this risks exposure to the authorities and may lead to her children being taken into care. The causes of her depression or her negative self-image are the obvious targets in any intervention, but depend upon her becoming visible to those who could help. Access therefore is a primary issue.

From a health perspective, the construction of a typology of drug users has value only insofar as it indicates those most in need of help, can suggest ways of helping those in need, and can be used to prevent others from reaching a stage where they need help. They are, however, only rough guides to targetted educational and health interventions among the drug users who have the characteristics identified. Each type comprises individuals with their own complex patterns of motivational, social and environmental factors that give rise to their behaviour at a particular stage in their lives. The real problems come in attempting to assess current and potential damage and developing an appropriate strategy.

ACKNOWLEDGEMENTS

I am indebted to Anthony Thorley, Senior Medical Officer, Health Promotion Division at the Department of Health for the idea of constructing this typology. It was commissioned by the Task Force to Review Services for Drug Misusers and I am grateful for their support and that of The Economic and Social Research Council, the Department of Health, the Home Office and The Higher Education Funding Council.

The data are drawn from the following projects:

Klee, H. and Faugier, J. Intravenous Drug Users: their role in the sexual mediation of HIV. 1989–1990. The Economic and Social Research Council (ESRC).

Klee, H. and Ruben, S. Amphetamine Misuse: a study of social and sexual lifestyles. 1990–1992. (ESRC).

Klee, H., Morris, J. and Ruben, S. A Study of Polydrug Misuse: health risk and implications for HIV transmission. 1991–1993. The Department of Health.

Klee, H. and Reid, P. Amphetamine Misusing Groups: a feasibility study of the use of peer group leaders for drug prevention work among their associates. 1993. Home Office, Central Drugs Prevention Unit.

Klee, H. and Lewis, S. Drugs in the Work-Place. Higher Education Funding Council for England (HEFCE).

REFERENCES

Beck, J. and Rosenbaum, M. (1994) Pursuit of Ecstasy. NY: State University of New York Press.

Collins (1986) Collins Dictionary of the English Language. London: Collins.

Klee, H. (1994) Crime and drug misuse: economic and psychological aspects of the criminal activities of heroin and amphetamine injectors. *Addiction Research,* **1**(4), pp. 377–386.

Klee, H., Morris, J. and Ruben, S. (1993) Polydrug Misuse: Health Risks and Implications for HIV transmission. Final Report to Department of Health, U.K.

Klee, H. and Reid, P. (1995) Amphetamine Misusing Groups: A feasibility study of the use of peer group leaders for drug prevention work among their associates. Paper 3. London: Home Office Drugs Prevention Initiative.

Lader, M. (1991) History of benzodiazepine dependence. In: Miller, N.S. (ed.) *Comprehensive Handbook of Drug and Alcohol Addiction.* New York.

Punj, G. and Stewart, D.W. (1983) Cluster analysis in marketing research: Review and suggestions for applications. *Journal of Marketing Research,* **20**(2), May.

Vogt, I. (1995) Women and Addiction: A frame of reference for theory and practice. In: *Proceedings: Women and Drugs, Council of Europe Seminar.* Council of Europe Publishing.

4

Treatment for Amphetamine Misuse in the United Kingdom

JUDITH MYLES

HISTORY OF AMPHETAMINE USE IN THE UNITED KINGDOM

Amphetamines have been prescribed to treat medical conditions in the UK since the 1920s (see Chapter 2). However, their use became increasingly popular among groups seeking the stimulant effect rather than needing treatment for a psychological or physical disorder, particularly in combination with barbiturates, such combination becoming known colloquially as 'purple hearts'. Such social groups perceived amphetamines as attractive as a recreational mood enhancer and an instrument in which periods of recreation could be extended without the need for sleep. Amphetamine preparations had also become attractive to those in occupations that required long periods of wakefulness, for example long distance lorry drivers, doctors, nurses, and students.

The first reference to the adverse effects of amphetamine appeared in the *Pharmaceutical Journal* of 20th June, 1936, quoting a report that the drug produced hypertension (high blood pressure). In the same journal on 22nd May, 1937, there appeared a comment on references in the daily newspapers to the misuse of Benzedrine (amphetamine) by the general public. By that time one major company of multiple chemists had already decided to supply the drug to the general public only on prescription, this was even though the law at the time allowed for its free sale. In June 1939, the British Government placed Benzedrine on Part I of the Poisons List with the proviso that the drug should be labelled "Caution/it is dangerous to take this preparation except under medical supervision".

By 1954 the demand for amphetamine had increased and pharmacists were responding to demands for its provision. It was at this time that reports appeared of the misuse in the UK of nasal amphetamine-based inhalers. Amphetamine and its compounds were placed in Schedule IV of the Poisons Rules and could only be obtained on prescription except for preparations in an inhaler. This only served to encourage the misuse of inhalers and the manufacturers responded either by withdrawing their products from the market or by altering the formulation.

The misuse of amphetamine was not the only cause for concern. In 1958 a monograph on amphetamine psychosis (Connell, 1958) was published which described an amphetamine psychosis that mimicked schizophrenia. The author reported that this could occur with low doses of amphetamine in some patients. In the following years mounting concern over the increasing misuse, by young persons, of drugs containing amphetamine, either alone or in combination with barbiturates, became a matter for debate in the Houses of Parliament and in the press. At the same time the Police became aware of widespread use of these drugs and evidence was appearing that importation of amphetamines had commenced.

In March 1964 the Drugs (Prevention of Misuse) Act was introduced. It then became illegal to be in unauthorized possession of drugs of the amphetamine type or to import them without a licence. Amphetamines, being Schedule II controlled drugs are now only legally obtainable on prescription in the UK.

EPIDEMIC AMPHETAMINE USE AND ITS CONTROL

In the summer of 1968, London experienced a methyl amphetamine epidemic. A small number of doctors were prescribing large quantities of injectable amphetamines (methyl amphetamine), which were being diverted onto the black market. Although problem amphetamine users were referred to a number of drugs agencies, it proved difficult to sustain continuing contact. In the course of epidemiological research (Hawks *et al.*, 1969) a number of amphetamine users were interviewed and it was deemed necessary to offer a treatment intervention.

A treatment service offering prescribed methyl amphetamine treatment was initiated and subsequently reported (Mitcheson *et al.*, 1976). It is noteworthy that within the group treated (all injecting, high dose amphetamine users), amphetamine psychosis as described by Connell in 1958 was so frequent as to be accepted as the norm.

The results of the treatment group indeed of only 12 patients, were viewed pessimistically at the time, but, when viewed in retrospect, were perhaps better than had been appreciated. Two of the patients achieved abstinence whilst another showed improvements in social stability. The conclusion included a comment that remains relevant today; "we should be resistant to the notion that the addict is a sick person with the implication that the Doctor has total responsibility for dealing with the sickness and providing a prescription, whilst society itself does little to prevent the endless production of new patients. The need for controlled clinical experiments and, in the absence of such work, over-confident championing of a particular method of treatment, must be avoided."

It is evident, that, over two decades later, little has changed.

ISSUES FOR THE TREATMENT OF AMPHETAMINE MISUSERS

Dependency and Withdrawal

The prescription of stimulant drugs to amphetamine users remains more contentious than the prescribing of long acting methadone or indeed shorter acting opiates, for example Diamorphine. This is because the opiates/opioids are basically sedative and do not present the same risk of increasing behavioural disturbance as do the amphetamines. Neither do they bear the same risk of psychosis as amphetamine. Furthermore, while there is a clearly defined physical withdrawal syndrome on withdrawal from opiates, a clear withdrawal syndrome is not evident on cessation of amphetamines. This continues to be an issue, even though the former view of addictive behaviour, placing greater emphasis on withdrawal has now progressed to the view where the compulsive use of a particular substance is deemed to be of greater importance. Indeed at one time it was widely believed that the presence of a physical withdrawal syndrome was the defining feature of drug addiction (WHO, 1964) and amphetamines were classified as drugs of habituation.

Whilst withdrawal from all drugs of dependence results in mood disturbance, the characterization of stimulant withdrawal is still uncertain. Sleep disturbance is widely reported, although direct links with the pharmacological actions of the withdrawn drug have not been established. Some researchers believe that depression in the withdrawal stage of stimulants occurs as a result of a physiological rebound, and although less well studied than opiate withdrawal, amphetamine withdrawal appears to have symptoms similar to cocaine withdrawal.

Amphetamine withdrawal is described in DSM/III/R (the Diagnostic Statistical Manual, which defines internationally agreed diagnostic categories in psychiatry) as the cessation of the consumption of amphetamine, after at least several days of heavy use, followed by depression, irritability and anxiety, and at least one of the following which persist for more than 24 hours after the last use of amphetamines: fatigue, insomnia or hypersomnia, and psychomotor agitation. DSM/IV proposes two changes to this withdrawal description. Firstly the depression, irritability and anxiety phase, or dysphoric phase, be typified by sadness as opposed to depression. Secondly it adds drug craving, increased appetite, psychomotor retardation and vivid unpleasant dreams to the previously identified symptoms of fatigue, sleeplessness, and agitation. These symptoms are referred to as physiological changes and have probably resulted from the increasing awareness by clinicians and researchers of the symptoms observed after cessation of prolonged cocaine use. However, they have also been assumed to characterize withdrawal from other stimulants such as amphetamine.

In areas of the UK where daily consumption of amphetamines by injection is common, clinicians are gaining further experience in the pattern of symptoms experienced on cessation of consumption of amphetamine. Subjectively patients complain of fatigue and inertia, an initial period of hypersomnia followed by protracted insomnia and an onset of agitation, usually within 36 hours of cessation, that exists for between 3–5 days. The degree of mood disturbance, while influenced by the previous level of consumption, ranges from dysphoria to severe clinical depression. Subjectively such patients report symptoms that, although differing from those of opiate withdrawal, require support, and in some cases, urgent psychiatric intervention.

EVIDENCE OF A NEED FOR TREATMENT SERVICES FOR AMPHETAMINE MISUSERS

Is Such a Need Demonstrable?

While the numbers of amphetamine misusers presenting to drug treatment services is low when compared to opiate users, it is noteworthy that drug seizures of amphetamines continue to be very high. Indeed amphetamine is the second most common illicit drug recovered in the UK after cannabis. Therefore it is evident that there is a market for amphetamines despite the legal restrictions referred to above.

Amphetamine use in the UK is largely restricted to amphetamine sulphate or 'speed'. Such amphetamine sulphate is of very low purity, consistently reported, on analysis of supplies seized, at between 2% and 5% purity. It is apparent, particularly in rural areas, where a regular supply of opiates is unreliable, that local production of amphetamine sulphate has existed over the past two decades.

The prevalence of local production is revealed again by drug seizures data. Much of the amphetamine sulphate that is seized, is not imported, but is locally produced. In practice an amphetamine user, at the present time in the UK who is using four grams of 'street' amphetamine sulphate by injection daily, is probably using an equivalent of 10 to 15 mgs. of dexamphetamine orally daily. This bears no comparison to the levels of amphetamine being consumed, either in combination with barbiturates (purple hearts), or by intravenous methamphetamine users, in London, in the 1960s.

Large numbers of people using amphetamines are administering the drug by injection, as evidenced by the high rate of contact of this group with Needle Exchanges in the UK. However, few amphetamine misusers seek drug clinic or medical treatment for their amphetamine problem. Therefore the issues of personal and public risk of such injecting behaviour remain largely unaddressed by treatment agencies. Klee (1992) reported a readier distribution of used injecting equipment amongst a group of amphetamine users when compared to opiate users.

Amphetamines, being stimulants, may be used as an adjunct to sexual activity whilst opiates, being sedative, do not lead to such increased sexual activity. Klee (1993) reported levels of sociability and higher levels of sexual activity amongst the same cohort of amphetamine users when compared to opiate users as referred to above. The age distribution of injecting amphetamine users, reported to the Regional Databases in the UK, is comparable to a similar cohort using opiates and therefore falls within a sexually active age-band. It is obvious that intravenous amphetamine use in a sexually active population carries concomitant risks of HIV infection and hepatitis B or C infection. This is a group that is, in the main, not in touch with specialist drug services.

DEVELOPMENT OF SERVICES FOR AMPHETAMINE MISUSERS

Changes in Service Delivery

Significant change has taken place in the provision of specialist drug services during the 1980s in the UK. These changes are directly related to the concerns of transmission of the HIV virus. In 1988, the Advisory Council on the Misuse of Drugs published a report entitled *Aids and Drug Misuse* (ACMD, 1988). Its first conclusion was that "HIV is a greater threat to public and individual health than drug misuse", and continues, "abstinence remains the ultimate goal but efforts to bring it about in individual cases must not jeopardise any reduction in HIV risk behaviour which has already been achieved". The same report recommended expansion of community based drug services to ensure that accessible and attractive services were available to drug users throughout the country. The report further recommended that a range of responses be provided to maximise the reduction in risk behaviour.

Monies were subsequently made available to increase drug services provision. This enabled the development of services in the regions and, for the first time, allowed for a more local delivery of services, particularly in the more rural areas. It placed an emphasis on the training of drugs workers and psychiatrists specialising in drug dependence and promoted an assessment of the individual drug user, in terms of risk taking behaviour as well as evidence of physical dependence, and the delivery of treatment. Drug services accepted that engagement in treatment, and retention within treatment of the drug taking population was of greater importance than treatment aimed solely at abstinence. Drug services began to place emphasis on harm reduction principles including the provision of information, education and on-going treatment to drug users. In the case of opiate users, methadone maintenance again became acceptable alongside detoxification where indicated. However, the absence of a clearly defined withdrawal syndrome from amphetamines and clinically accepted replacement medication, left most services unable to offer a treatment intervention that amphetamine users perceived as attractive.

While there has been a clear emphasis on attracting those drug users engaging in most high risk activity into services, the rate of demand for services for opiate users has continued to increase in a linear fashion over the past 10 years in the UK. Therefore services that were developed to provide replacement opiate treatments, i.e., methadone, have had little opportunity to develop services for other cohorts of drugs misusers. The Drugs Services that have developed since the mid 1980s, particularly those outwith the main urban areas in the UK, have had a greater opportunity to develop according to local patterns of need and have therefore attracted a relatively larger proportion of stimulant users.

Involvement in Criminal Activity

Since possession of amphetamines, other than on prescription, is illegal in the UK, those involved in amphetamine use are, by definition, engaging in an illegal activity. This may perpetuate contact with others involved in illegal activity. The psycho-active effects of stimulants may increase the risk of criminal activity since the consequent disinhibition may remove normal social controls. It is of note that heroin is much more expensive than amphetamine sulphate. However, the rate of criminal activity observed in amphetamine users is similar to the rate of criminal activity observed in heroin users (Klee, 1993). This suggests that the stimulant effect, rather than the cost of the amphetamine, is having a direct effect on behaviour.

The Maturation Effect

It is often stated that amphetamines are used by a younger population than opiates. They are used for a limited period of time and then the user either moves away from the drug culture with maturation, or moves on to consistent use of a more sedative drug like heroin. However in areas of the South West of England, mid-Wales, Wessex, East Anglia and the West Midlands, drugs services, in particular Needle Exchanges and non-statutory drugs services, are in contact with large cohorts of amphetamine users who have used amphetamine as their preferred drug for many years. Indeed, amongst such groups there are individuals who have experimented with opiates and disliked its effects.

The drugs misusers in London in the 1960s, who used injectable methyl amphetamine, bear little resemblance to contemporary amphetamine injectors in terms of their behaviour or their incidence of psychosis. Contemporary amphetamine users who are in contact with services mostly report amphetamine use on a daily basis, many of them by injection, many having used the drug for many years and not solely for occasional recreational purposes.

The Future of Drug Services

Those agencies in the UK, particularly outside London, who have been confronted by large numbers of injecting amphetamine users, have shown a variable response. In some districts the response has been that the service is for opiate users and therefore there is no treatment available for amphetamine users.

In some districts, drugs counselling and support towards abstinence has been offered to amphetamine users without substitute prescribing. The retention rates in such treatment interventions have been very low. In a minority of cases in the UK, treatment for injecting amphetamine users that includes substitute prescribing with oral dexamphetamine has been instituted.

In the guidelines on the Clinical Management of Drug Dependence (HMSO, 1991), it is advised that the most appropriate treatment for amphetamine users is abrupt cessation of amphetamines without substitute prescribing. It has also been the consistent view, held by many statutory drugs agencies in the UK, that developing interventions that involve substitute prescribing for amphetamine users, is only prolonging and expanding the extent of amphetamine use generally. It has further been the view, that to prescribe a stimulant drug is dangerous in terms of the anticipated behavioural consequences and may induce more cases of amphetamine psychosis.

The services that have attracted amphetamine users have tended to be in areas where there is active working collaboration between the voluntary and statutory agencies. Common to all of these services is a view that this type of intervention should only be offered to those patients whose pattern of amphetamine use is prolonged, intravenous, and significant in amount. Their common objective is to encourage injecting amphetamine users into the service, in order to reduce their injecting behaviour, and ultimately to reduce the spread of HIV and other infections. The subsidiary objectives are to stabilise users' lifestyles, educate them in health awareness, and encourage harm reduction.

Furthermore, it is recognised that the specialist service should be offered to those described above but not to those who report occasional recreational use of amphetamines.

Evaluation of Treatment Interventions

Some services in the UK have received short term funding to evaluate the outcomes for patients with problematic amphetamine use. In the case of some services the prescribing intervention was a local agreement, in response to a need to improve the social, psychological and physical well-being, of the stimulant users in their area. In either case it is quite apparent that there was a genuine commitment to evaluate the effectiveness of the intervention and adapt the service delivery accordingly. A common anxiety was that the prescription of amphetamine would increase the risk of precipitating psychotic illness and, to that end, the patients were closely monitored in terms of their mental health.

In common with all other medical treatment interventions in the UK, it is accepted by medical practitioners working in the field of drug dependency, that the key to good treatment lies in a thorough assessment which then leads to the establishment of an individual treatment plan. The assessment of amphetamine users therefore usually includes a full drug history, establishment of current injecting practice and evaluation of the risk of such practice, the social, forensic and physical health of the individual, and a full assessment of the underlying personality and the current mental state. Particular attention is paid to previous episodes of psychiatric illness and the relationship of such episodes to drug use. Such mental state assessment is possible in the UK as specialist doctors in drug dependency are members of the Royal College of Psychiatrists and therefore have completed their psychiatric training.

Within statutory drugs agencies several disciplines will be involved in discussion and establishment of a treatment plan, with clear identification of treatment goals. The multi-disciplinary team within a specialist drugs service usually comprises a Consultant Psychiatrist, Community Psychiatric Nurses, a Clinical Psychologist and sometimes a Social Worker and/or a Probation Officer. It is accepted that discussion of treatment plans that involve the prescription of controlled drugs should follow discussion of each case across disciplines. The existence of an ethical prescribing protocol and a regular review system, following such multi-disciplinary discussion and mental health assessment, provides a setting within which substitute prescription of amphetamines can be provided, with as high a degree of safety as an opiate prescription. Daily dispensing arrangements, and (ideally) supervised consumption of such daily dispensing, reduce the possibility of the diversion of supplies of amphetamines to the black market.

A prescribing protocol that designates criteria for the initiation of a prescription, the maintenance of a prescription, and the termination of a prescription, would be negotiated in the following way. A treatment plan or contract would be agreed as being acceptable to the service, the prescriber, and the patient. Such agreement would include an acceptance of appropriate levels of prescribed drug, appropriate behaviour, both personally and generally during treatment, the provision of urine samples for urinalysis on request, and a commitment to areas of therapy to enable the patient to move beyond a drug-taking lifestyle.

The maintenance of the prescription is determined primarily by the ability of the service to offer treatment. In the case of some of the services offering substitute prescribing of amphetamines over the past few years, this has been time limited by research protocol and research funding. Continuance of the prescription is determined by its continuing capacity to improve health and the patient's compliance with treatment goals.

The termination of the prescription may be at the point of an achieved state of abstinence, or determined by a deterioration in health or social functioning, or by the practitioner if it is evident that the treatment goals are unobtainable.

Experience of Prescribing Services in the United Kingdom

There is little to be found in the published literature during the 1990s in the UK on the topic of substitute prescribing of amphetamines. However there have been both national and local professional conferences addressing the issue. These meetings have included contributions from specialists in Drug Dependency in Wales, South West England, Wessex, and Manchester. Prescribing services have reported careful assessment, particularly of injecting practice, physical health, and mental health in amphetamine users presenting for treatment. They included urine drug screens, both in the assessment process and during treatment.

Presentations clearly demonstrated certain outcomes of treatment, most notably that drug users engaged in services when they became aware that a substitute prescribing intervention might be available and that those patients taken on for treatment, showed a high rate of retention in treatment. Additionally they demonstrated a marked decrease in injecting practice, increased social stability and a marked reduction in criminal activity.

In one area in the South West of England, there were reports on the rates of illicit benzodiazepine use in an amphetamine treated group compared to an opiate treated group (Myles, 1993), in which the rates of benzodiazapine use were similar in both groups. Services reported no evidence of the precipitation of psychotic illness and indeed demonstrated that patients who had used large quantities of illegal amphetamine sulphate by injection prior to being engaged in treatment, and who had suffered periods of psychosis in the past, were managed with no further recurrence of psychotic illness (Fleming, 1994). It was considered essential to avoid the diversion of prescribed amphetamines onto the black market as had occurred previously in London in the 1960s. Interval dispensing, through retail pharmacists, or the supervised consumption of amphetamines where facilities allowed was arranged. Dosage levels in some reports (Fleming, 1994) were fixed between

20 and 30 mg. of dexamphetamine daily. In other services doses were not fixed but rarely exceeded 50 mg. of Dexamphetamine daily.

Perhaps one of the most interesting features of those receiving prescriptions of dexamphetamine lies in the individual amphetamine user's reasons for using a stimulant (Myles, 1993). None of this group were using amphetamines recreationally. Many had been using amphetamines for many years and many had underlying phobic disorders or anxiety states. Additionally a proportion of these patients had a marked wish to remain very thin and a minority had a diagnosable eating disorder.

In the assessment of patients seeking treatment with substitute amphetamines, it was apparent that several suffered from a major mental illness, in particular schizophrenia. Those patients were not prescribed amphetamines, but were actively treated for their underlying mental illness.

Concerns continue that patients, who would have spontaneously ended their amphetamine sulphate consumption, have continued to use amphetamines on prescription by drugs agencies. However, reports from various oral presentations at conferences in the early years of the 1990s in the UK, show an abstinence rate during treatment, of about 25%. Additionally, there are concerns that amphetamines, being stimulants, will perpetuate disinhibited and reactive behaviour, leaving the patients or the public at risk. However, Fleming (1994) found a reduction in offending behaviour, whether violent or non-violent in character, in those treated with substitute dexamphetamine. The balance of risks associated with prescribing dexamphetamine when compared with the alternatives — irresponsible injecting behaviour, lack of retention of stimulant users in drug services, unplanned sexual activity, and recurrent episodes of psychosis — suggests that a well controlled prescribing intervention could quite reasonably be recommended.

THE IMPLICATIONS OF TREATING AMPHETAMINE USERS

If many more drug users, not previously in contact with drug services, are to be treated in future by existing agencies, the financial implications are considerable. In 1988, the report by the Advisory Council on the Misuse of Drugs, to the Department of Health and Social Security, concluded "that a change in professional and public attitudes to drug misuse is necessary, as attitudes and policies which lead to drug misusers remaining hidden, will impair the effectiveness of measures to combat the spread of HIV".

As was noted in 1976 by Mitcheson *et al.* (a) "the client has to be reached" and (b) "there may be a place for very carefully considered prescribing of amphetamines".

It is evident that further research into the extent and nature of stimulant misuse in the UK is urgently required. It is also evident that research into the effectiveness and outcomes in prescribing interventions for amphetamine users is a matter of priority. During 1995 a Department of Health Task Force commissioned research specifically to look at services for cocaine and amphetamine users.

It is, however, with regret that the author, in 1995, acknowledges that interventions for stimulant users are little better researched and developed now than in 1968.

REFERENCES

Advisory Council on Misuse of Drugs (1988) *Aids and Drug Misuse: Part 1.* London: HMSO.

Connell, P.H. (1958) Amphetamine Psychosis, *Maudsley Monograph No. 5.* London: Chapman and Hall Ltd., for the Institute of Psychiatry.

Department of Health (1991) *Guidelines on Clinical Management.* London: HMSO.

Fleming, P. and Roberts, D. (1994) Is the prescription of Amphetamine justified as a harm reduction measure? *Journal of the Royal Society of Health,* pp. 127–131.

Hawks, D., Mitcheson, M., Ogborne, A. and Edwards, G. (1969) Abuse of Methylamphetamine, *British Medical Journal,* **2**, pp. 715–721.

Klee, H. (1993) Sexual risk among amphetamine misusers, prospects for change. In: Aggleton, P., Davies, P. and Hart, G. (eds.) *Aids, Rights, Risk and Reason.* London: The Falmer Press.

Klee, H. (1992) A new target for behavioural research — amphetamine misuse, *British Journal of Addiction,* **87**, pp. 439–446.

Mitcheson, M., Edwards, G., Hawks, D. and Ogbourne, A., (1976) Treatment of Methylamphetamine users during the 1968 epidemic. In: Edwards, G., Russell, M.A.H., Hawks, A. and Maccafferty, M. (eds.) *Drugs and Drug Dependence,* London: Saxon House Publishers.

5

Patterns of Amphetamine Use in Australia

JULIE HANDO and WAYNE HALL

National household surveys from 1985 to 1993 show that amphetamine[1] is the most widely used illicit drug after cannabis (Table 1). A variety of other indicators suggest that amphetamine use has increased in prevalence since the mid 1980s, including police seizures of amphetamine, users presenting to treatment services and findings from studies of illicit drug users (e.g. Spooner, Flaherty and Homel, 1993; Tebbutt, Muir and Heather, 1990; National Drug Abuse Information Centre, 1991). Such increasing use has occurred in context of widespread availability and low cost of amphetamine in Australia, due to the relative ease of local manufacture in the absence until recently of controls on the supply of the precursor chemicals used to produce the drug. During this period there has been an increase in sociological, epidemiological and clinical research which has provided valuable information about the patterns of amphetamine use and related harms.

The research reviewed in this chapter has been restricted in three main ways. First, the focus is on the 'recreational' use of amphetamine, that is, its use for purposes connected with recreation such as party-going and

---

[1] The term 'amphetamine' and 'speed' are commonly used street names in Australia for illicit substances which may chemically contain methylamphetamine, amphetamine sulphate, dexamphetamine hydrochloride, ephedrine, pseudoephedrine and other non-identified compounds and adulterants. The most popular forms of amphetamine are as a powder or crystal, though liquid amphetamine had also been identified along with some 'new' amphetamine analogues. The use of mdma (methylene dioxymethylamphetamine; ecstasy), an amphetamine analogue, has not been included as amphetamine in this report, though patterns of Ecstasy use are noted separately in the text.

Table 1 Prevalence of ever having used various illicit drugs in Australia in 1985, 1988, 1991, 1993 among persons aged 14+ years (%)

Year	1985	1988	1991	1993
Sample size	2796	1830	2483	3500
Cannabis	28	28	32	34
Amphetamine	9	6	8	8
Hallucinogens	8	7	7	7
Cocaine	4	3	3	2
Heroin	1	2	2	2
Ecstasy	*	1	2	3

* not available
Source: Commonwealth Department of Health, Housing, Local Government and Community Services 1985 Social Issues Survey and 1988–1993 NCADA and NDS National Household Surveys.

weekend social activity among young adults, rather than its use in an occupational context. Briefly, the occupational use of amphetamine (e.g. by heavy transport drivers and shiftworkers) became an issue of public concern in the early 1990s in the state of New South Wales because of horrific motor vehicle accidents involving heavy transport vehicles in which some of the drivers had taken excessive amounts of the stimulant ephedrine (Staysafe Committee, 1992). The reader is referred to Haworth (1989), Haworth *et al.* (1991) and Hensher *et al.* (1991) for further information.

Second, research has largely been confined to the major capital cities in Australia because that is where substantial numbers of illicit drug users congregate, making the phenomena of illicit drug use relatively easy to study. Third, the review has been limited to the period from 1985 to 1994 since there was little systematic research on illicit drug use in Australia before funding became available for such research with the establishment of the National Campaign Against Drug Abuse in 1985.

HISTORICAL BACKGROUND

There are indications of a small epidemic[2] of amphetamine use in Australia in the late 1960s and early 1970s which resembled similar epidemics that

---

[2] An epidemic here is defined as an episodic occurrence with rapid and substantial increases in the prevalence of use, often but not invariably accompanied by an increase in drug-related problems. Both use and problems often equally quickly subside. Our use of the term 'epidemic' is not meant to imply that illicit amphetamine use is a 'disease', it is only used to capture the contagious character of the spread of amphetamine use.

occurred in Japan, Sweden, the United States and the United Kingdom around this time. The Australian epidemic was facilitated by a large increase in the prescription of amphetamine by general practitioners (Baume, 1977), and manifested in an increased use of amphetamine among young offenders and young adults attending psychiatric hospitals (Briscoe and Hinterberger, 1968; Healy, 1978), and an increase in the prevalence of persons diagnosed with amphetamine psychoses (Bell, 1973). As with the epidemics in other countries, it was fuelled by a combination of ready availability, and the perceived safety of amphetamine by the medical profession and users (Ellinwood, 1974).

This epidemic lasted for several years before largely disappearing. The reasons for its disappearance are uncertain but at least two processes appear to have played a part. First, once the epidemic became apparent, some years after the increased prevalence of use, the governments introduced restrictions on the conditions for which they could be prescribed, decreasing their availability, making them scarce and driving up their price, thereby deterring the less committed users, as has been documented in Britain by De Alarcon (1972). Second, the decline of the epidemic appears to have been accelerated by the rediscovery and dissemination of information within the drug culture about the adverse health and psychological effects of chronic heavy amphetamine use (Chesher, 1991).

In the middle of the 1980s there seems to have been a recurrence of epidemic amphetamine use, again occurring at around the same time as a recurrence in Britain (Klee, 1992) and the United States (Morgan, personal communication). It seems as though each new generation of illicit drug users rediscovers the euphoric effects of amphetamine in the absence of any subcultural memory of the hazards of their use. Amphetamines then enjoy a vogue among injecting drug users because they are cheaper and easy to produce locally.

AMPHETAMINE AND OTHER ILLICIT DRUG USE IN AUSTRALIA SINCE THE 1980s

Concern about a looming cocaine epidemic similar to that which was occurring in the United States (e.g. Pierce and Levy, 1986) distracted attention from an emerging home grown amphetamine epidemic. As a consequence, most of what is known about amphetamine use in Australia during this period has been gathered *en passant* in the course of research on the use of cocaine (Homel *et al.*, 1990; Hall *et al.*, 1991), or on the risks of HIV transmission among injecting heroin users (Hall *et al.*, 1992). The following review begins with information gleaned on amphetamine use from surveys of drug use in the general population, among students, and high risk populations such as recreational drug users, injecting drug users, street youth, young offenders and sex workers. Then follows a more detailed review of research studies that have specifically investigated patterns of amphetamine use.

The General Population

Apart from the use of cannabis which has increased, illicit drug use overall in Australia remains at fairly low levels. The prevalence of illicit drug use is generally higher among males than females across all age groups and for most drug types. Marijuana is the most common illicit drug used in Australia (Table 1), with almost one in three persons aged 14 and over having ever tried it (Donnelly and Hall, 1994). Amphetamine remains the second most popular illicit drug in Australia: 8% of the general population have used it at some time, and this is several times greater than the proportion which has used cocaine (2–3%) or heroin (1–2%). The proportions who had used amphetamines in the year prior to interview ranged between 2 and 3%.

Amphetamine was most often tried by males and those aged in their 20s and 30s (Table 2). An increase in amphetamine use was noted among males aged 25–39 years (from 12 to 19%) and females aged 14–24 years (from 4 to 11%) between 1988 and 1991. In 1993, 24% of males aged 20–24 years and 16% of 25–34 year old males had tried amphetamine. For females, 16% of those aged 20–24 had tried the drug and 10% of 25–34 years olds. The average age of first amphetamine use in the most recent household survey was 19.2 years (CDHHCSLG, 1993). Around 12–13% of the population reported being offered amphetamines in all surveys except 1988 when only 9% had been offered amphetamine. In addition, five percent of people in later surveys (CDHHCSLG, 1991, 1993) thought that the regular use of amphetamines was acceptable. Highest rates of use which were above the national figure of 8% of people ever trying amphetamine were noted in Sydney (10%), Adelaide (12%), Canberra (9%) and Darwin (13%) in the 1991 survey. In the later surveys, respondents were asked whether they had ever injected illicit drugs: this figure increased from 1% in 1988 to 2% in the 1991 and 1993 surveys.

Table 2   Lifetime prevalence of amphetamine use amongst the general population by gender within age, Australia, 1993

Age	14–19		20–24		25–34		35–54	
Sex	M	F	M	F	M	F	M	F
%	5	8	24	16	16	10	7	4

Source: Commonwealth Department of Health, Housing, Local Government and Community Services, NDS National Household Survey 1993.

Students

Surveys of secondary school students show low levels of amphetamine and other stimulant use. In 1992, a survey of 3,828 New South Wales secondary school students (Cooney, Dobbinson and Flaherty, 1993) found that 7% had used stimulants. While this figure potentially includes the use of cocaine and amphetamine, it probably reflects the use of amphetamine more than cocaine due to its greater availability and cheaper price. A comparable survey of 9,513 students in Victoria in 1992 (Roy Morgan Research Centre, 1993) found that 10% had used stimulants. No information has been obtained on the frequency or recency of these forms of drug use. Prevalence is higher among older students in post-secondary training courses. In 1992, for example, the proportion of 3,489 post-secondary school Technical and Further Education students (aged 16 to 25) who had ever tried stimulants ranged from 14–19% for males and 10–20% for females (Keys Young, 1993).

Recreational Drug Users

Amphetamine has been consistently identified as the most commonly used illicit drug after cannabis in a number of surveys of recreational drug users (e.g., Reilly and Homel, 1988; Homel *et al.*, 1990; Hall *et al.*, 1991; Mugford and Cohen, 1989; Spooner, Flaherty and Homel, 1993). Reilly and Homel (1988), for example, interviewed 1071 recreational drug users (aged 15–18 years) in 1986 who were contacted in public places around Sydney such as beaches and shopping centres. Their sample included only respondents who had used illicit drugs other than cannabis. The prevalence of illicit drug use was accordingly high: 92% of the sample had used cannabis, 72% had tried amphetamine and 45% had tried cocaine. Respondents who preferred stimulants (amphetamines, cocaine, ecstasy, hallucinogens) reported using them in pursuit of a 'high'.

Spooner, Flaherty and Homel (1992) repeated this street intercept survey in 1990, interviewing 581 young adults between the ages of 16 and 21 years. The subjects again had to have used at least one illicit drug other than cannabis. Amphetamines remained the most popular illicit drug after cannabis, with 75% having used amphetamines at least once. Over a third (36%) had used amphetamines within the last month and 14% had used it within the last week. A third of amphetamine users had injected the drug at some time.

A secondary analysis of data from a telephone survey of 499 young Sydney adults among whom recreational drug users were over-represented (Homel *et al.*, 1990; Hall *et al.*, 1991) indicated that amphetamine users were more likely to be male, were less well educated and had a lower median income than those who had not used amphetamines. They were also more likely to have tried a variety of other illicit drugs, particularly those perceived to be 'harder' and riskier, such as cocaine, heroin and ecstasy.

More recently, Ovenden and Loxely (1994) conducted a qualitative face-to-face survey of 105 young illicit drug users in Perth about their patterns of drug consumption. The median age of the sample was 18 years, over half were male (52%), half (51%) were unemployed and 26% were students. A quarter of the sample had previously sought counselling for a drug problem, and 8% had been to a detoxification program. Three-quarters of the sample (74%) were classified as 'bingers' either by the subject or by the researchers' definition (namely, repeated use of drugs for 36 to 48 hours before 'crashing' followed by a period of four or more days of abstinence). Injectors were more likely to binge (81%) than non-injectors (54%). Amphetamines were the predominant drug used in binges, having been used by two-thirds (65%) of bingers in the month prior to interview. Amphetamine was often used in binges to avoid the 'coming down' effects. Tolerance to the effects of amphetamine also led to frequent administration.

Injecting Drug Users

Several studies have found that a substantial minority of injecting drug users use amphetamine. Regular amphetamine injection was reported by a third of 1245 injecting drug users recruited through advertisements in a 1989 Australian National AIDS and Injecting Drug Use Study (ANAIDUS) conducted in Sydney (Hall *et al.*, 1992). The sample comprised 73% males and had a mean age of 27.5 years. Although opioid drugs were still the drug of preference for the majority of the sample, there was a smaller group who were primarily using amphetamines and 6% of the total sample injected amphetamines on a daily basis. The daily opioid injectors who comprised 38% of the sample were on average older (28.7 years vs 25.5 years), better educated and more likely to have been in treatment (78% vs 41%) than the daily amphetamine users.

The broad pattern of injecting amphetamine use in the ANAIDUS Sydney cohort was confirmed in a smaller Sydney study of 352 injecting drug users using needle and syringe exchanges and pharmacies (MSJ Keys Young, 1989). A secondary analysis of these data indicated that although heroin was the preferred drug (79%), a substantial minority (18%) injected amphetamine, and the latter were more likely to be younger and male, and less likely to be daily users.

Similar findings have been reported from the Melbourne ANAIDUS cohort of 356 injecting drug users (Lewis, Monheit and Mijch, 1991). While more females (46%) were recruited in this study than in the Sydney cohort, the average age composition (mean age 27.1 years) and age of initiation of injecting drug use (18.6 years in Melbourne and 18.4 years in Sydney) were similar in both studies. The prevalence of ever having injected amphetamine was higher in Melbourne than Sydney (93% and 73% respectively), as was the proportion of daily amphetamine injectors in the sample (20% in Melbourne and 6% in Sydney). Nevertheless, the characteristics that distinguished primary amphetamine from heroin users were the same in both cities: amphetamine users were younger and less likely to have had any treatment contact.

Loxely and Marsh (1990) examined the risk behaviour of a sample of 195 injecting drug users in the Perth ANAIDUS cohort. Respondents were drawn from both treatment and non-treatment sources. Analysis by age showed that more younger users had used amphetamines and amphetamine analogues such as ecstasy, and younger users were more likely to inject amphetamines. Younger users were also less likely to have been in treatment, to have started injecting at a younger age, and were more likely to inject other illicit drugs.

Other Populations

Amphetamine use is prevalent among populations such as prisoners, street youth and sex workers. For example, amphetamine use was surveyed among 279 young detainees in nine New South Wales Juvenile Justice Centres (Zibert, Hando and Howard, 1994). The mean age of this sample was 17 years, and ranged from 12 to 21 years. The sample was mostly male (96%) and over one-third were Aboriginal. Three-quarters were serving a sentence (75%), 24% were on remand and the remaining 1% were on a warrant. One-third had tried amphetamine, more than half (55%) of whom had used it more than 10 times. Eighteen percent of the sample had used amphetamine in the month prior to incarceration, and 13% had used it in the week prior to incarceration. A higher prevalence of use was reported in a 1990 survey of 181 new adult prisoners (mean age 28 years) in eight New South Wales correctional centres (Stathis, Eyland and Bertram, 1991): 43% had tried amphetamine, and 25% had used in the year prior to incarceration, mostly on a weekly or monthly basis. The average age they commenced amphetamine use was 19 years.

The main reasons given for the use of amphetamine by juvenile offenders were similar to those given by recreational users, namely, to party and have fun (24%), to feel good (23%), to satisfy curiosity about the drug (19%) and to increase energy and stay awake (18%). Over half (54%) usually administered amphetamine by injection, the remainder using it intranasally or by mouth. The average age of first using amphetamine was 14.4 years. Most of the sample (63%) consumed amphetamine in their own home or a friend's home and 24% always used it in a public setting such as a nightclub. More than two-thirds (71%) usually consumed amphetamine with other people. Most of the amphetamine users (82%) knew other similar users, with over half (59%) reporting that they knew at least 50 other users.

Less is known about amphetamine use among other populations who are seen as 'at-risk' of engaging in illicit drug use, such as street youth and sex workers. In 1991, a subsample of 82 street youth aged 14–19 were interviewed in the National Household Survey (Commonwealth Department of

Health, Housing and Community Services, 1992). It found that 82% had ever used amphetamines (as against only 7% of their peers), and almost two thirds (62%) had injected drugs. A subsequent study of 192 Sydney street youth by Howard (1993) obtained similar findings. This sample, which was recruited between 1989 and 1991 from treatment agencies, other services for homeless youth and snowball methods, had a mean age of 17 years (range 13–20 years) and comprised 71% males. High levels of stimulant use were again found, with between 64% and 76% having ever tried stimulants,[3] half of whom (51%) had injected them.

Surveys of sex workers show that a substantial minority use amphetamine. A 1986 survey of 128 female sex workers in Sydney found that one-third (33%) had used amphetamine, which was again the most commonly tried illicit drug among this population after cannabis (Perkins, 1991). A later survey of 78 private prostitutes and 124 brothel workers found that 21% and 45% respectively had used amphetamine (Perkins, 1994). Illicit drug use is, however, more likely to occur among the more marginalised street sex workers, with some sources suggesting that around 80% of these women regularly use illicit and licit drugs (Parliament of New South Wales, 1986). A recent key informant study of drug use among these women in Sydney has found that they are more likely to prefer heroin and cocaine to amphetamine, even though the latter is more readily available and cheaper (Hando, 1994).

Amphetamine-Specific Research

National surveys

National surveys of amphetamine use and attitudes towards such use among young adults have been conducted in the course of developing a mass media strategy to reduce the harms associated with the use of this drug ('Speed Catches Up With You' Campaign) (see also Table 4). The first of these surveys in 1991 involved a national probability sample of 1004 people aged 14 to 35 years (Commonwealth Department of Health, Housing, Community Services and Local Government, 1993). Ten percent were aged 14 to 16 years, 17% were 17–20 years, 23% were 21–25 years, a further 23% were 26–30 years and the remaining 27% were aged 31–35. Fifty-three percent of interviews were conducted in city locations, the remaining conducted in rural sites. Interviews were conducted in all Australian States and Territories. Respondents were either students (14%), unemployed (12%), employed part-time (16%) full-time (43%) or had some other employment status (15%) such as working at home or not actively seeking employment.

Almost all respondents had heard of amphetamines (92%). One in three people (33%) were able to report at least one positive aspect of using am-

---

[3] Includes amphetamine and/or cocaine.

phetamine, among which the most common were: a feeling of alertness (3%), increased energy (7%) and that 'everything happens quickly' (4%). In comparison, three-quarters (75%) were able to name at least one negative aspect of using amphetamine, most commonly that it could damage health both physically and mentally (38%) and lead to addiction (31%).

Twelve percent of the sample had used amphetamines, with slightly more city (14%) than country residents (10%) having used it. Those aged 21–30 years were also more likely to try the drug (15%), compared to 14–16 year olds (5%) and 17–20 year olds (11%). Very few (2.5%) had ever injected amphetamine (4% for males and 0.6% for females) and this was also slightly higher among city residents. Fourteen percent stated they would be likely to use amphetamines if it was offered to them by a friend or acquaintance.

A second survey was conducted in February 1993 to establish baseline measures of attitudes, intentions and behaviours among amphetamine users prior to the launch of the media campaign (Commonwealth Department of Health, Housing, Community Services and Local Government, 1993). In this survey, 1206 people were interviewed using similar methodology as the first. This survey differed from the first in that it sampled a smaller range of age groups (15–30 years olds): 15% of the sample were 15–16 years old, 29% were 17–20, 32% were 21–25 years and 25% were 26–30. Slightly more city (65%) than country (35%) residents were recruited than in the 1991 survey. Respondents were also more likely to be students (28%) or unemployed (22%) than in the earlier study. The remaining were employed part-time (14%) or full-time (33%).

Again, most of those surveyed had heard of amphetamine (95%), and the proportion of positive and negative perceptions of amphetamine had remained stable over time. Somewhat more people reported ever trying amphetamine (15%), with half of these (51%) saying that they had used amphetamines on only a few occasions and did not intend to continue with use. One-fifth (20%) of those who had tried amphetamines reported doing so on an occasional or regular basis. Use among city residents remained stable between the two surveys although use by country residents had increased to 18% in the 1993 study. Males in the 21–25 year age group were the most likely group to use amphetamine (25%) and this had increased since 1991. In 1993, almost twice the number of respondents had injected amphetamine (4.2%, 5.5% males and 2.9% females), the highest prevalence of which was observed among 26–30 year old males (10%), those unemployed (7%) and city residents. A similar proportion of people (15%) said they would accept offers of amphetamine as in the 1991 survey.

Special populations

In response to indications of increased amphetamine use Hando and Hall (1993) surveyed 231 amphetamine users in Sydney to determine their characteristics, their patterns of use, the contexts within which amphetamine were used, and the potentially adverse consequences of amphetamine use. In-depth, structured interviews were conducted with users who were recruited from a broad range of sources including drug treatment centres, other health services, advertisements, peer referral and other non-treatment sources.

The survey sample consisted of two-thirds (66%) males and one-third females, with a median age of 24 years. Subjects resided mostly in the inner city of Sydney (39%) and in the outer western and south-western suburbs (51%). Three-quarters of the sample were Australian born from an English-speaking background, a further 11% were born in another English-speaking country, 9% were of non-English-speaking background, and 5% were Australian Aboriginals. The median years of education in the sample was 10 years. A third were in full-time (17%) or part-time employment (11%), or were full-time students (8%), and 57% were unemployed. The median income was $12,700 (typical of low income earners), reflecting the high level of unemployment. Only one in ten participants had dependent children. Two-thirds (66%) of the sample had never received any drug treatment.

All participants had used amphetamine prior to the interview. The median age at which amphetamine was first used was 17 years and most respondents (75%) initiated their amphetamine use between the years 1981 and 1989. The frequency of current use varied from two or more times per week (30%), to once a week (13%), and once or twice a month or less (57%). The typical quantity used was a quarter to half a 'street gram' over a period of 24 hours. Snorting (61%) or swallowing (22%) were the most common methods of first use but two-thirds (69%) had injected amphetamine at some time, and just over half of the sample (55%) usually injected the drug.

Amphetamine injectors were older, less well educated, more likely to be unemployed, and more likely to reside in the outer south-western and western Sydney suburbs than non-injectors. They were also more likely: to have injected amphetamine on their first occasion of use; to have used amphetamine on a daily basis for at least three months; to have used amphetamine two or three times a week or more; to have used a gram or more of amphetamine within a day; to have first used an illicit drug at an earlier age, and be polydrug users.

Amphetamine was most often used with other people and in a social setting such as a pub or nightclub. The main reasons for starting to use amphetamines were: curiosity about the drug's effects; to party and have fun; to feel like one of the group; to feel good; and to have more energy. The main reasons for continuing to use amphetamine were much the same although substantial minorities reported using amphetamine to help with their work or studies, or because they could drink more alcohol without feeling intoxicated.

Subjects had a substantial history of other illicit drug use. All had used cannabis, 93% had used hallucinogens, 73% had used minor tranquillisers,

62% had used cocaine, 58% had used ecstasy, and 55% had used heroin. Amphetamine was the preferred drug of 29%, followed by cannabis (28%), heroin (17%) and hallucinogens (9%). Experimentation with illicit drugs on average began at 13.5 years, and an average of 9 different drug types had been tried. Over half of the sample (60%) had injected two other drug types, most often heroin (52%), cocaine (36%), and other opiates (31%).

The major drugs that were used in combination with amphetamine were: cannabis (71%), alcohol (66%), and tobacco (42%). More than half usually consumed five or more standard drinks while using amphetamine. The most common drugs used to manage the 'come-down' were: cannabis (48%), tobacco (31%), sedatives (30%), and alcohol (15%). Over half of the sample also used methods besides drugs to help manage the negative effects of coming down from amphetamine.

Regional differences were noted among the Sydney amphetamine users. Users residing in the outer western and south western suburbs were younger, less likely to be of English speaking background, had fewer years of education, were more likely to be unemployed and had lower median incomes than their inner city counterparts. Clear differences in drug use patterns were also found. Those from the west typically used more amphetamine per hit or snort, used fewer types of other drugs, and experienced significantly more health-related consequences from their use of amphetamine compared to those in the inner city.

The amphetamine users differed from other samples of illicit drug users in Sydney, such as recreational illicit drug users (Spooner, Flaherty and Homel, 1993), injecting drug users (Hall *et al.*, 1992) and detained youth (Zibert, Hando and Howard, 1994) (Table 3). They were on average eight years older than the sample of detained youth, six years older than the recreational drug users and two years younger than the injecting drug user cohort. They had a higher rate of unemployment than both the injecting cohort (over half of which were on government pensions) and the recreational drug users. They also had much less drug treatment contact than the injecting cohort but more than the recreational drug users and detained youth. All four samples had consumed a number of different substances in the previous month, the most common being alcohol and cannabis. Substantial minorities of each had also consumed tranquillisers and heroin during this time. Finally, the amphetamine cohort not surprisingly contained fewer injectors than the injecting cohort but more than the samples of detained youth and recreational drug users.

Transitions to injecting

A second study of amphetamine use was conducted in Sydney in 1993 to examine user characteristics and situational factors that predicted transitions to injecting amphetamine use (Darke *et al.*, 1994). A sample of 301 amphetamine

Table 3   Comparison of recent drug use surveys conducted in Sydney

Variable	Injecting drug users (a)	Recreational drug users (b)	Detained youth (c)	Amphetamine users (d)
Sample size (no.)	1245	581	279	231
Mean age (yrs)	27	19	17	25
% Males	73	59	96	66
Employment: (%)				
F/T employed	9	34	na	24
P/T employed	9	29	na	11
Student	3	14	na	8
Unemployed	18	20	na	57
Pension	59	4	na	–
Drug use in: (%)	Typical month	Last month	Last month*	Last month
Alcohol	66	94	76	77
Cannabis	64	85	75	86
Amphetamine	34	36	18	100
Hallucinogens	4	22	18	30
Ecstasy	3	23	7	15
Tranquillisers	38	22	19	32
Inhalants	–	12	7	16
Cocaine	9	11	7	13
Heroin	67	12	10	22
% Injectors	100	28	24	34
% Drug treatment contact	62	11	25	34

* Drugs consumed in the month prior to detention
na = not available
Sources: (a) Hall *et al.*, 1992; (b) Spooner, Flaherty and Homel, 1993; (c) Zibert, Hando and Howard, 1994; (d) Hando and Hall, 1993.

users who had used amphetamines at least monthly for the preceding six months were recruited using similar methods to the first study. The sample was also demographically similar to that recruited by Hando and Hall (1993) except for a greater proportion of female respondents (47%). The mean age was 24.7 years and the mean number of years of schooling was 10.6. Twelve percent of subjects were in full-time paid employment, with a further 19% in part-time or casual employment. The majority were not currently enrolled in any drug treatment, and two-thirds (68%) had never been in drug treatment.

The mean age of first amphetamine use was 17.4 years and 19.2 years for the commencement of regular amphetamine use. The mean length of time since first amphetamine use was 7.3 years. The median number of days on which amphetamines were used in the 6 months preceding interview was 24, approximating weekly use. Less than one in ten had used amphetamines six times during the preceding 6 months, with a quarter of subjects (23%) reporting use on 60 or more days, and 13% on 90 or more days. Only 2% of subjects reported daily use over the preceding 6 months.

Polydrug use was common. The average number of drug classes ever used was 8, with 6 drug classes having been used in the 6 months preceding interview. The most commonly used drugs in the previous six months were: cannabis (93%), hallucinogens (64%), opiates (61%), benzodiazepines (56%), and cocaine (35%). Among those who had injected amphetamine, two thirds had injected three other drug classes.

Two-thirds of the sample had injected amphetamine during the six months preceding interview, with 42% only injecting amphetamines in that period, 24% using both injecting and non-injecting methods, and the remaining third (34%) only snorting or swallowing the drug. Overall, two thirds reported that they had injected amphetamine at some time. The mean age of first amphetamine injection was 18.8 years. For those that did not inject on the first occasion of use, the average time to first injection was 2.5 years.

As in the earlier study, less than a quarter (23%) reported that they injected amphetamines the first time that they used them. Snorting was the most common first route of administration (58%), with the remainder either swallowing (19%) or smoking (1%) the drug. Forty percent, however, made a transition to regular amphetamine injecting, in that they injected on four or more occasions of use. Males were more likely than females to report such a transition (47% vs 32%). The median number of transitions to injecting was one and the mean age at first transition was 19.7 years. The majority of subjects (69%) reported that they used more amphetamines after beginning to inject, and almost half (44%) reported that they used larger quantities of other drugs, and injected other drugs that they had not previously injected (46%).

The most common reasons given for changing to amphetamine injecting was liking the 'rush' associated with injecting (88%). The next two most popular responses were that injecting was more economical (23%), and a 'healthier', 'cleaner' way of using amphetamines than snorting (22%) which caused nasal ulcers. The latter reasons are contradicted by the finding that users typically used larger quantities of amphetamines after moving to injection, and so spent more money on the drug, and by the health risks of injecting amphetamine (e.g. HIV, vascular problems, psychological problems) which are far greater than for snorting or swallowing amphetamine.

One in eight of the regular injectors (12%) said they were likely to change to routes other than injecting, the main reason being concern about their veins (26%). A small proportion of injectors (9%) had already done so because of concerns about vascular damage (39%), fears of contracting HIV (23%) or feeling addicted to amphetamines (19%). A third (32%) of the sample reported only ever swallowing or snorting amphetamines, with females more likely to have never injected than males. The main reasons for not having injected were a hatred or fear of needles (72%) and a fear of addiction (23%).

It is difficult to determine how representative these findings of amphetamine users are, given that the parameters of the population are unknown. While both Sydney studies were essentially self-selected, multiple recruitment methods were used to obtain a broad spectrum of amphetamine users. In addition, many of the findings from earlier study of amphetamine use (Hando and Hall, 1993) were consistent with those of the second study focusing on transitions in routes of administration. The similarities include: the fact that both samples represent a younger population than that of the widely researched opiate users; the low levels of education and high rates of unemployment; the high proportions of subjects injecting amphetamines; the social context of amphetamine use; and correlates between frequency of amphetamine use, route of administration and negative consequences of use, which will be expanded upon in the next section.

Other studies

Studies in other States suggest similar patterns of amphetamine use among young people (Ross and Miller, 1994; Moore, 1993). Moore (1993) conducted ethnographic studies of a small network of psychostimulant users in Perth, Western Australia during 1990 and 1991 which have borne out the findings of quantitative surveys. In addition, a quantitative survey of 197 amphetamine users was conducted in Melbourne in the early 1990s (Ross and Miller, 1994) using similar methods as the Sydney surveys and with similar findings. The samples differed in the proportion who had ever injected amphetamine: 78% of the Melbourne sample compared to 69% in Sydney (Hando and Hall, 1993).

INDICATORS OF AMPHETAMINE-RELATED PROBLEMS

Morbidity and Mortality

In 1990, 21% of the 120,062 deaths in Australia were estimated to be associated with drug use. Of these, 1% were attributable to amphetamines, cocaine, cannabis, hallucinogens and pharmaceuticals. Tobacco and alcohol resulted in the greatest number of deaths of Australians, at 71% and 26% respectively (Commonwealth Department of Health, Housing and Community Services, 1992). In NSW, amphetamines were detected in 2% (9 deaths) of deaths referred to the coroner for investigation in the second half of 1987, and in 3% (37 deaths) of cases in 1988. These amphetamine-related deaths tended to be in the younger age group (below 29 years) and typically resulted from motor vehicle accidents or other accidents, including homicides, drownings and falls (Tebbutt, Muir and Heather, 1990).

The New South Wales Health Department has collected information on drug-related hospital admissions from public hospitals, private hospitals and psychiatric hospitals in NSW. In 1986, 81 hospital admissions caused by amphetamines were recorded, and this figure has remained stable until 1991 except for 1989/90 when only 57 were recorded. Accidental poisonings from stimulants (including amphetamine and cocaine) ranged from 36 in 1986 to 39 in 1991.

Treatment Service Utilisation

There are no specialist drug and alcohol services in Australia that deal exclusively with individuals who experience problems with their amphetamine use. There are instead a wide range of alcohol and other drug treatment agencies, and most of these agencies treat amphetamine users when they present. Public and private services include general hospital accident and emergency treatment for overdose or crisis presentations, general hospital admissions for patients withdrawing from alcohol/drugs, particularly within the country areas, admission in psychiatric hosptials for those with dual psychiatric and alcohol/drug dependence problems, short term (three to twelve week) residential post-detoxification educational and therapeutic programmes with both group and individual counselling, and therapeutic communities and rehabilitation centres for chronic alcohol/drug using individuals who require a longer term (greater than three months) social and environmental structure to promote lifestyle and behavioural changes.

Public community based alcohol and other drug units providing inpatient and outpatient services are available in most major cities, and alcohol and other drug counsellors are based in many community health centres in both city and country areas. Private practice general practitioners, psychiatrists and alternative medical practitioners may also provide health services to individuals including drug users. Self-help organisations such as Narcotics Anonymous are also available.

Wickes (1993) outlines the range of treatment approaches available to users experiencing problems from pychostimulants. These include pharmacological interventions which may be used as an aid in obtaining and sustaining abstinence and lessening the discomfort of withdrawal. These medications include tricyclic antidepressants, bromocriptine and amantadine. Their use is currently minimal and at the discretion of individual medical practitioners.

Early and brief interventions, motivational interviewing, cognitive-behavioural therapies and relapse prevention techniques are gaining more currency as appropriate interventions within the alcohol and other drug treatment field (Ali *et al.*, 1992). As such they may be on offer at different centres to amphetamine users. Supportive outpatient counselling is the most widely available intervention offered, with few therapists engaging in psycho-dynamic counselling. Abstinence is still the most common long-term aim of many treatment centres and, whilst some centres offer controlled drinking programmes, and methadone substitution is widely available for opioid users, there has only been one practitioner offering dexamphetamine substitution for amphetamine use. Psycho-surgery is not practised in this country as a treatment for drug dependency.

The indications are that the number of amphetamine users presenting to such treatment services is still low compared to those with alcohol and opiate problems, although there is suggestive evidence of an increase in numbers during the 1980s.

Two national one day surveys of the characteristics of clients in drug treatment agencies were conducted in 1990 and 1992 (Webster, Mattick and Baillie, 1992; Chen, Mattick and Baillie, 1993). These surveys included any agency that "specialised in the care, treatment or rehabilitation of persons requiring assistance because of problems caused or exacerbated by the use of substances, including alcohol" (Webster *et al.*, 1992, p. 112). The 1990 survey found that 4% of the 5,583 clients seen on the census day presented for problems primarily caused by amphetamine use, ten times more than the number of clients presenting with cocaine problems. More people, however, sought treatment from the use of alcohol (55%), opiates (27%), opiates/polydrug (7%) and tobacco (8%). Similar findings were reported in the 1992 survey of 5,730 clients, with 4.3% of people seeking treatment for amphetamine problems.

Clearer evidence of an increase in presentations of amphetamine users comes from profiles of admissions to two New South Wales therapeutic communities. The first was compiled on the inner city Sydney therapeutic community 'We Help Ourselves' between 1985 and 1991 (Swift, Darke, Hall and Popple, 1993). During this seven year period there were 4,792 admissions, including 1,676 readmissions. A small increase was noted in the number of clients nominating amphetamine as a problem drug, from 35% in 1985 to 43% in 1987. However, during 1985 to 1987 clients were able to nominate more than one problem drug, and high rates were noted for several drugs including alcohol, tobacco, opiates, cannabis and benzodiazepines. From 1988 to 1991 clients were only able to nominate one problem drug, with 11% reporting amphetamine as against 72% for opiates.

The second study reported on the characteristics of persons admitted to 'the Buttery' situated on the Far North Coast of NSW between 1980 and 1992 (Hall, Chen and Evans, 1993). There were 1219 admissions during this period, including 89 readmissions. Twenty percent nominated stimulants as their drug of choice, with others nominating opiates (85%), alcohol (37%) and benzodiazepines (11%). The proportion of people reporting stimulant problems increased from less than 5% in 1980 to 30% in 1991. These findings were consistent with the results of a survey of key informants in the treatment and law enforcement fields conducted by the National Drug Abuse Information Centre (1991) which indicated that most States reported a small increase in both use of amphetamines and problems in 1990.

Self-Reported Problems

The 1992 survey of Sydney amphetamine users (Hando and Hall, 1993) inquired about the occurrence of various amphetamine-related problems. Several physical and psychological health symptoms related to amphetamine use were reported by subjects. The most common physical symptoms of amphetamine use were: tiredness (89%), loss of appetite (85%), dehydration (73%), jaw clenching (73%), headaches (62%), muscle pain (58%), shortness of breath (55%), and tremors (55%). The most common psychological symptoms were: mood swings (80%), sleep problems (78%), anxiety (72%), difficulty concentrating (71%), depression (71%), and paranoia (71%). Hallucinations, and episodes of aggression and violence were reported by 46% and 43% respectively.

The number of symptoms reported was correlated with: being male, unemployed, daily amphetamine use, using a gram or more on an occasion of use, and using more drug types. Separate analyses of three psychological symptoms which have been previously reported to occur with high prevalence among regular injecting amphetamine users, namely, hallucinations, aggression, and paranoia showed that all three were related to injecting as a route of administration, symptoms of dependence upon amphetamine, and to a history of daily amphetamine use.

Using a stringent cut-off of 8 or more on the 28 item General Health Questionnaire (Goldberg and Williams, 1988), 35% of the sample would be regarded as suffering from a psychiatric disorder if seen by a psychiatrist. These scores were correlated with: being female, unemployed, and a polydrug user, and the number of health problems experienced from amphetamine use.

The use of a cut-off score of 4 or more on the Severity of Dependence Scale (Gossop *et al.*, 1992) classified 36% of the sample as dependent on amphetamine. Dependence was correlated with the use of amphetamine two or more times per week, injection as a usual route of administration, and a history of daily amphetamine use. It was most strongly predicted by: having fewer years of education, being unemployed, living in south-western and western Sydney, and having a family history of alcohol or drug dependence.

Given the high prevalence of psychological symptoms and dependence, it was unsurprising that a third of the sample (34%) had received treatment for a drug or alcohol problem, and one in four (24%) were currently receiving some form of drug treatment, most often methadone maintenance. Moreover, 41% of the sample had felt a need for treatment for an amphetamine-related problem, and about two-thirds of these had sought help from a drug and alcohol treatment service (12%), a general practitioner (10%), or a psychiatrist (2%). It was not clear, however, how often these problems were presented, or recognised by health workers, as being related to the use of amphetamine. Seeking treatment for amphetamine-related problems was related to: being older, less well educated, unemployed, having a family history of alcohol and drug dependence, being an injecting drug user, using amphetamines frequently in the previous six months, especially daily use, being dependent on amphetamine and injecting and using more other drug types.

Criminal Behaviour

There was a considerable amount of criminal activity within the sample, though this tended to be lower than for comparative samples of primary heroin users (eg. Darke *et al.*, 1992). A quarter of the sample (26%) had been imprisoned previously, 21% had been in a juvenile institution, and 39% had been arrested for a drug-related offence. More than half of the sample had engaged in criminal activity such as: dealing in drugs (61%); property offences (e.g. shoplifting, break and enter) (54% of males and 42% of females); fraud offences (33% of males and 40% of females); and offences involving violence against persons (e.g. armed robbery, assault) (31% of males and 22% of females).

The range of offences were predicted by a variety of factors. In all cases the strongest predictor of having committed an offence after using amphetamine was a history of having committed the same type of offence before using amphetamine. In addition, property and fraud offences were best predicted by the experience of four or more health complications of injecting drug use. Drug dealing was best predicted by: injection as the usual route of administration of amphetamine, the use of amphetamine two or more times per week, and being dependent on amphetamines. Crimes of violence were best predicted by: fewer years of education, a history of daily amphetamine use, and a history of having injected drugs other than amphetamine.

HIV Risk

The level of HIV risk-taking by the sample was also assessed because of concerns about the potential for the transmission of HIV and hepatitis C. A third of those who had injected amphetamine (35%) in the last 6 months had shared a needle, most often with a friend (53%) if male, and with a sexual partner (61%) if female. Those who shared were more likely to: have a sexual partner who was an injecting drug user, to have health complications related to injecting drug use, to report symptoms of dependence upon amphetamine, and to have sought treatment for an amphetamine-related problem. Only a small proportion of those cleaning needles before or after sharing did so using the recommended procedure with bleach. Needles and syringes were often obtained from needle and syringe exchange programs (65%), chemists (58%) and friends (11%).

In terms of sexual behaviour, the majority of the sample were heterosexual (82%), with the remainder identifying as gay, lesbian or bisexual. Two thirds (63%) reported that amphetamine increased their sexual desire, but up to half of those in sexual relationships reported that it impaired sexual performance. Sexually risky behaviour was evident in the sample. A third (32%) reported using condoms with regular partners during penetrative sex, two-thirds (68%) with casual partners, and most (88%) with clients for the few participants who worked in the sex industry. A significant proportion of those with regular sexual partners were non-monogamous, and 44% reported having at least one casual sexual partner in the month prior to interview. The average length of regular relationships was 20 months.

Two thirds of the sample reported that they had been tested for HIV infection (76% of women and 65% of men) of whom 7% reported that they were HIV positive. Subjects were well informed about the risks of HIV infection from needle-sharing and sex without condoms, but a substantial minority (22%) did not believe that bleach killed HIV.

Studies of HIV risk-taking behaviour among other amphetamine users and opioid users have reported similar findings (Darke *et al.*, 1994; Hall *et al.*, 1992; Lewis *et al.*, 1991). For example, a comparison of risky behaviour among daily injectors of opioids and amphetamines indicated very few differences in high risk injecting behaviour such as needle sharing, and unprotected sex with multiple partners (Hall *et al.*, 1992).

HARM MINIMISATION EFFORTS

The National Campaign Against Drug Abuse which was introduced in 1985 made the minimisation of drug-related harm its key goal (Blewett, 1990). While maintaining restrictions on the supply of illegal drugs it placed an increased emphasis on demand reduction strategies by increasing spending on education, treatment and rehabilitation programs for illicit drug users. Almost a decade later, supply reduction and demand reduction efforts continue but with little integration between these two approaches (Wardlaw, 1993). In the case of the amphetamines, the major demand reduction responses have been media and educational campaigns while law enforcement efforts to reduce their supply have primarily focused on controlling precursor chemicals. There have been, in addition, some efforts to improve the responses of generalist health services and specialist drug and alcohol treatment services to persons seeking help with amphetamine-related problems.

Supply Reduction Measures

Until relatively recently, the manufacture of amphetamine in Australia has been an easy task, the requirements of which included a basic knowledge of chemistry, possession of a "recipe" and access to precursor chemicals. Australia had a well organised system of illicit manufacture and distribution which has developed because amphetamines have been easy to manufacture in the absence of controls on the supply of precursor chemicals. Most chemical precursors for amphetamine manufacture were legally imported from the United States and Europe for use in chemical and industrial applications. There were a large number of outlets in Australia from which such chemicals could be obtained, 550 in NSW alone. Amphetamine manufacturers were also able to import precursor chemicals directly from countries other than the US where legislation exists which makes this difficult.

A National Working Party on Amphetamine Control established by the Police Ministers Council recommended in 1990 that a number of amphetamine precursors should be scheduled for control and monitoring. This recommendation was implemented in March 1992 in NSW with new regulations being added to the Poisons Act (1966). A code of conduct was devised by the NSW and Victorian Police Forces in conjunction with the Australian Chemical Industry Council and the Scientific Suppliers Association of Australia to monitor the disbursement of precursors, chemicals and equipment used in amphetamine manufacture. All transactions of the precursor chemicals above a specified quantity require notification to the Commissioner of Police. The supplier is required to obtain evidence of the purchaser's identity and address and to forward this information each month, together with the full details of the transactions involved. An offence is also created of supplying a precursor knowing or suspecting it will or may be used to manufacture an illicit substance (Wardlaw, 1993). Other States and Territories are in the process of or have already enacted this legislation and code of conduct. The Australian Customs Service has also listed some of the more amphetamine-specific chemicals in the Customs (Prohibited) Imports Regulations, including ephedrine and pseudoephedrine. Legitimate importers of such products must be licensed by the Department of Health, Housing and Community Services and permits issued for each importation.

Police report that precursor legislation has reduced the availability of chemicals and precursors required for the illicit manufacture of amphetamines at the possible cost of a rise in diversion of supplies, thefts or illegal imports (Australian Bureau of Criminal Intelligence (ABCI), 1993). All jurisdictions with precursor legislation have seen a decrease in the purity of street level amphetamine which may reflect greater adulteration as the precursor chemicals become harder to obtain. In South Australia, reports from police sources note that amphetamine containing contaminants and diluents have recently caused medical problems for users (ABCI, 1993). In addition, South Australian authorities have also identified two new varieties of amphetamine on the market; these are chemical analogues of amphetamine that are thought to be an attempt to circumvent the precursor legislation (ABCI, 1993). Seizures of clandestine laboratories have occurred in most States in recent years, and this has become one of the major police tactics to reduce the availability of the drug at street level.

Other supply reduction strategies are less often used. Targeting high level distributors, for example, is less effective in Australian because of the larger number of manufacturers of amphetamines which exist at various levels of sophistication and size. It is doubtful that the removal of manufacturers would make a significant impact on the amphetamine market (Wardlaw, 1993). Opportunities for targeting 'street' level distributors and users of amphetamine are also limited since there are no public amphetamine markets in Australia (like those among heroin users in the United States). Most amphetamine transactions occur in private places, usually between people who have had prior contact such as friends and acquaintances, and the lower rate of daily amphetamine use reduces users' needs to purchase the drug frequently (Wardlaw, 1993).

Amphetamine markets

Law enforcement indicators suggest that the availability and use of amphetamine has increased in most Australian States and Territories since 1990. The Australian Bureau of Criminal Intelligence received reports of 3,705 amphetamine-related arrests in 1993 which accounted for about 9% of the total drug arrests in Australia. As in 1992, Victoria led NSW in the number of arrests relating to amphetamine. Males comprised the highest number of those arrested, accounting for about 79%. Those charged with providing the drug accounted for 28% of those charged, users comprising the other 72% and this is only a slight variation on the 1992 figure (Australian Bureau of Criminal Intelligence, 1993).

During 1993, the ABCI also received reports of 3,141 seizures totalling 280,770 grams.[4] 68% of the weight seized was in Victoria. In comparison, the total weight of amphetamine seized at the Customs barrier for 1993 was 854 grams, representing 26 seizures. The methods of trafficking included on the person, in cargo and by the postal system. The top three countries in 1993 from which these drugs originated were Thailand, the Netherlands and Papua New Guinea. While law enforcement data is limited prior to 1990, a general trend of increasing seizures of amphetamine has been noted in Australia from the mid 1980s (Tebbutt, Muir and Heather, 1990). Seizures of liquid amphetamine have occurred during the 1990s in some States, though usually at a lower level than the traditional powder or crystal forms of the drug. There is little information which suggests that the smokeable form of amphetamine 'ice'[5] is available in Australia (ABCI, 1993).

In 1993, a gram of amphetamine at street level ranged between $40 to $120 in Australia. The prices remain comparable to those in 1992 despite an overall apparent decrease in the purity of the product (ABCI, 1993). The price and purity of illicit amphetamines varies by geographical location but purity levels on the street are typically low (in the range 1–10%, and most often consisting of 2–5% of methamphetamine).

The law enforcement data are consistent with the reports of amphetamine users (Hando and Hall, 1993). Nearly all respondents in the 1992 amphetamine study conducted in Sydney reported that amphetamines were easy to

---

[4] Includes seizures of clandestine laboratories and Ecstasy.
[5] Crystalline methylamphetamine hydrochloride.

obtain (94%). Most purchased their amphetamine from dealers (66%) and/or friends (40%) for a price usually in the range of $80–$100 a gram. Amphetamine was most often used as a powder (98%), with a quarter (26%) having tried liquid amphetamine. The majority (60%) of the sample were unaware of the chemical composition of the "amphetamine" that they used, although all agreed that it had probably been adulterated.

Demand Reduction Efforts

"Speed catches up with you" campaign

In 1991–1992 a National Action Plan on Amphetamines was implemented which included the development and evaluation of a national media campaign. Two national, representative surveys of young people in 1991 and 1993 were used to inform the design of the campaign, the components of which were extensively tested by qualitative research methods prior to their introduction (Commonwealth Department of Health, Housing, Community Services and Local Government, 1993). The campaign comprised television and cinema advertisements, billboards and other signs, a radio advertisement, sponsorship of Drug Offensive Video Smash Hits Dance Parties, distribution of almost 100,000 "Dance Offensive" Magazines and 136,000 campaign information brochures, the production of a popular record album, a school teaching kit and two monographs outlining the project. The themes highlighted health risks of amphetamine use, namely, overdose, dependence ("Speed catches up with you"), HIV risk ("AIDS hits speed users too"), and the effects of adulterants and contaminants ("The people who make speed don't test it on animals — they use people"). It was launched in June 1993 and has been conducted at regular intervals since then.

The impact of the campaign was evaluated by a survey of 1212 people aged 15–30 years conducted in August 1993 (Commonwealth Department of Health, Housing, Local Government and Community Services, 1994). This sample was demographically similar to the baseline survey sample conducted earlier in the year (Commonwealth Department of Health, Housing, Community Services and Local Government, 1993; Table 4). The research showed that awareness of the campaign was high, with between a quarter (24%) and 91% of the target group recalling at least one element of it. Three quarters of respondents said that the Campaign had made them more aware of the negative effects of amphetamine, and there was an increase in the proportion listing negative consequences of use (90% as against 75% in the previous survey). The level of amphetamine use remained steady with only a small decrease in the proportion who used amphetamines regularly, although the sample size was probably too small to detect all but major changes in the frequency of amphetamine use.

Table 4   A comparison of the three national amphetamine campaigns

Variable	October 1991 (a)	February 1993 (b)	August 1993 (c)
Sample size (no.)	1004	1206	1212
% Male	50	49	50
Ages: (yrs)			
15–16	10	15	15
17–20	17	29	31
21–25	23	32	29
26–30	23	25	26
31–35	27	–	–
Location:			
City	53	65	65
Country	47	35	35
Employment status:			
Employed F/T	13	33	33
Employed P/T	16	14	12
Student	14	28	28
Unemployed	12	22	28
Other*	15	6	–
Awareness of negative effects of amphetamine (%)#	75	78	90
Awareness of positive effects of amphetamine (%)#	33	33	33
% Ever tried amphetamine	12	15	15
% Ever injected amphetamine	2.5	4	5

* Includes working at home and not actively seeking employment. In the August 1993 survey this was included in the unemployment category
# Indicates awareness of at least one effect
(a) Survey to determine the target population, objectives and strategies of the mass media campaign
(b) Survey to establish baseline measures of attitudes, intentions and behaviours of target population
(c) Survey to evaluate the impact of the mass media campaign
Source: Commonwealth Department of Health, Housing, Local Government and Community Services, 1993 and 1994)

"Speedwise-speedsafe" campaign

In 1993 the NSW Drug and Alcohol Directorate developed a more limited educational campaign that provided harm reduction messages to amphetamine users. The material was based upon the Hando and Hall (1992) survey of Sydney amphetamine users, with contributions from injecting drug user groups and health educators. The campaign was 'narrowcast', using pamphlets that were distributed at night-clubs, dance-party venues and pubs in combination with advertisements on the radio stations favoured by the target group. The content of the material stressed the need for users to keep hydrated and well nourished, to avoid binge use, not to combine intoxicating doses of alcohol and amphetamine, and to observe standard precautions against HIV infection if injecting. The impact of the campaign was evaluated with mainly positive outcomes: most of the target sample recognised the campaign logo, and substantial numbers were familiar with the specific campaign messages. The campaign has since been adopted by other States and jurisdictions.

Treatment responses

The lack of experience of many health workers in dealing with the problems of stimulant users prompted the Federal Government to commission and publish a booklet on the management of these drugs (Wickes, 1993). This was widely distributed throughout the generalist and specialist health services. A monograph was also prepared to provide an overview of the current situation on psychostimulant issues from an Australian perspective (Burrows, Flaherty and MacAvoy, 1993). More recently, a national health education strategy on amphetamine for health workers has been developed.

TRENDS IN AMPHETAMINE USE: PAST AND FUTURE

There are consistent indications from research studies and official statistics that amphetamine use increased among young Australian adults during the middle 1980s, probably because of their widespread availability, their lower cost by comparison with heroin and cocaine, and their relatively benign reputation. Amphetamines appear to be primarily used for recreational purposes in social settings where young people gather to 'party' and have a good time; amphetamines providing pharmacological assistance in achieving the latter goals.

From a public health perspective, one of the most worrisome features of the current epidemic has been the relatively high rates of experimentation with injecting as a route of administration. This has obvious relevance to the risks of infectious disease transmission but there is also an increased risk of problems of dependence and psychological disorders arising from daily amphetamine injection. The indications are that these problems are being experienced by regular users, especially injectors, although they are not as yet reflected in a substantial increase in the number of users seeking help.

What about the future? Amphetamine fads exemplify the cyclical pattern that Kleiman (1992) has argued characterise most epidemics of illicit drug use. During the early period of an illicit drug use fad there is a bias in favour of positive effects which encourages more people to use the drug. Most users are new, their initial drug experiences are largely positive, and few have had a chance to develop tolerance or dependence, or to experience the adverse effects of hazardous patterns of use (such as injecting large quantities at frequent intervals). The rare adverse effects that do occur are either not recognised, or their connection with drug use is discounted as due to the peculiarities of affected users.

Only as the new drug use fashion saturates the market of potential users are adverse drug effects noticed. As the number of new recruits decreases, and existing users stop or moderate their use, the problem users become visible to other drug users, reducing new recruits and encouraging more users to moderate their use. Given the time it takes to develop problems, it is not until after the recruitment of users has peaked that damaged and dependent users come to the attention of treatment agencies and drug researchers. Subsequent media attention to such casualties of illicit drug use produce inflated estimates of the particular form of drug use and its associated problems. Because of these cycles drug policy responses usually lag some time behind drug use trends, as has been the case with amphetamines in Australia where harm minimisation efforts have followed four or five years after the peak period of uptake.

If Kleiman's analysis is correct, then one would predict that amphetamine use in Australia will decline over the next few years as news about users' experience of adverse health and psychological effects spreads. Its spread may be facilitated and perhaps reinforced by targeted media advertisements and other interventions designed specifically for the populations that use these substances. A variety of such interventions have already been conducted in most Australian States and Territories with varying levels of success, and other interventions are currently being planned. The decline in use may also be accelerated if precursor controls are effective in reducing availability, increasing price and decreasing quality, and to the extent that there are no other widely available drugs to take up the market niche currently occupied by amphetamines. Surveys of drug use over the next several years will see whether these predictions are correct. Other things are less certain. Will the disappearing amphetamine epidemic leave in its wake a cohort of amphetamine-dependent individuals who are difficult to treat? How many of these individuals will abandon amphetamine in favour of the more traditional opioid drugs? In the event that treatment agencies do see an increase in amphetamine users seeking assistance, a national health education strategy on recognising and managing such users is currently being prepared for health practitioners. However, the lack of effective amphetamine-specific treatment still remains.

REFERENCES

Ali, R., Miller, M. and Cormack, S. (eds.) (1992) *Future Directions for Alcohol and Other Drug Treatment in Australia.* National Campaign Against Drug Abuse Monograph Series No. 17. Canberra: Australian Government Publishing Service.

Australian Bureau of Criminal Intelligence (1993) *Australian Drug Intelligence Assessment, 1993.* Canberra: Australian Bureau of Criminal Intelligence.

Baume, P. (1977) *Drug problems in Australia: An intoxicated society?* Report from the Senate Standing Committee on Social Welfare. Canberra: Australian Government Publishing Service.

Bell, D. (1973) The experimental reproduction of amphetamine psychosis. *Archives of General Psychiatry,* **29**, pp. 35–40.

Blewett, N. (1990) *National Campaign Against Drug Abuse: Assumptions, arguments and aspirations.* NCADA Monograph Series No. 1. Canberra: Australian Government Publishing Service.

Briscoe, O.V. and Hinterberger, H. (1968) A survey of the usage of amphetamines in parts of the Sydney community. *Medical Journal of Australia,* **12**, pp. 480–485.

Burrows, D., Flaherty, B. and MacAvoy, M. (eds.) (1993) *Illicit Psychostimulant Use in Australia.* Canberra: Australian Government Publishing Service.

Chen, R., Mattick, R.P. and Baillie, A. (1993) *Clients of treatment service agencies: March 1992 Census findings.* Department of Health, Housing, Local Government and Community Services. Canberra: Australian Government Publishing Service.

Chesher, G.B. (1991) Hazardous amphetamine use: The need to consider dosage. *Drug and Alcohol Review,* **10**, pp. 299–303.

Commonwealth Department of Community Services and Health (1990) *Statistics on Drug Abuse in Australia, 1989.* Canberra: Australian Government Publishing Service.

Commonwealth Department of Health, Housing and Community Services (1992) *Statistics on Drug Abuse in Australia, 1992.* Canberra: Australian Government Publishing Service.

Commonwealth Department of Health, Housing, Local Government and Community Services (1993) *National Drug Household Survey.* Canberra: Australian Government Publishing Service.

Commonwealth Department of Health, Housing, Local Government and Community Services (1993) *Amphetamines Campaign Benchmark Report.* Canberra: The Drug Offensive.

Commonwealth Department of Health, Housing, Local Government and Community Services (1994) *Amphetamines Campaign Tracking Study Report.* Canberra: The Drug Offensive.

Cooney, A., Dobbinson, S. and Flaherty, B. (1993) *Drug use by NSW secondary school students: 1992 survey.* Drug and Alcohol Directorate, New South Wales Health Department Report Series. No. 93–98. Sydney.

Darke, S., Hall, W., Wodak, A., Heather, N. and Ward, J. (1992) Development and validation of a multi-dimensional instrument for assessing outcome of treatment among opiate users: The Opiate Treatment Index. *British Journal of Addiction,* **87**, pp. 733–742.

Darke, S., Cohen, J., Ross, J., Hando, J. and Hall, W. (1994) Transitions between routes of administration of regular amphetamine users. *Addiction,* **89**, pp. 1077–1083.

De Alarcon, R. (1972) An epidemiological evaluation of a public health measure aimed at reducing the availability of methylamphetamine. *Psychological Medicine,* **2**, pp. 293–300.

Donnelly, N. and Hall, W. (1994) *Patterns of cannabis use in Australia.* National Drug Strategy Monograph Series No. 27. Canberra: Australian Government Publishing Service.

Ellinwood, E.H. (1974) The epidemiology of stimulant abuse. In E. Josephson and E.E. Carroll, (eds.). *Drug use: Epidemiological and sociological perspectives.* New York: John Wiley and Sons.

Goldberg, D. and Williams, P. (1988) *A User's Guide to the General Health Questionnaire.* Berkshire: NFER-Nelson.

Gossop, M., Griffiths, P., Powis, B. and Strang, J. (1992) Severity of dependence and route of administration of cocaine, heroin and amphetamines. *British Journal of Addiction,* **87**, pp. 1527–1536.

Hall, W., Carless, J., Homel, P., Flaherty, B. and Reilly, C. (1991) The characteristics of cocaine users among young adults in Sydney. *Medical Journal of Australia,* **155**, pp. 11–14.

Hall, W., Chen, R. and Evans, B. (1993) *Clients admitted to "The Buttery", A therapeutic community, 1980–1992.* National Drug and Alcohol Research Centre Technical Report No. 18. Sydney: National Drug and Alcohol Research Centre, University of NSW.

Hall, W., Darke, S., Ross, M. and Wodak, A. (1992) Patterns of drug use and risk-taking behaviour among opioid and amphetamine injecting drug users in Sydney. *Addiction,* **88**, pp. 509–516.

Hando, J. (1994) *World Health Organisation Initiative on Cocaine: Sydney Key Informant Study.* Drug and Alcohol Directorate, New South Wales Health Department Research Grant Report Series. No. B94/6. Sydney.

Hando, J. and Hall, W. (1993) *Amphetamine use among young adults in Sydney, Australia.* Drug and Alcohol Directorate, New South Wales Health Department Research Grant Report Series. No. B93/2. Sydney.

Haworth, N.L. (1989) *Driver fatigue and stimulants.* Report No. MR5. Department of Transport and Communications. Canberra: Federal Office of Road Safety.

Haworth, N.L., Vulcan, P., Schulze, M.T. and Foddy, B. (1991). *Truck driver behaviour and perceptions study.* Report No. 18. Melbourne: Monash University Accident Research Centre.

Healy, P. (1978) *Patterns of drug use in Australia: 1970–1977.* Sydney: NSW Health Commission.

Hensher, D.A., Battellino, H.C., Gee, J.L. and Daniels, R.F. (1991) *Long-distance truck drivers: On road performance and economic reward.* Report No. CR99. Department of Transport and Communications. Canberra: Federal Office of Road Safety.

Homel, P., Flaherty, B., Reilly, C., Hall, W. and Carless, J. (1990) The drug market position of cocaine among young adults in Sydney. *British Journal of Addiction,* **85**, pp. 891–897.

Howard, J. (1993) Taking a chance on love: Risk behaviour of Sydney street youth. *Journal of Paediatric Child Health Care, 29* (Supplement 1), S60–S65.

Keys Young (1993) *Quantitative survey of NSW TAFE students' alcohol, tobacco and other drug use.* Sydney: A report prepared by Keys Young.

Klee, H. (1992) A new target for behavioural research — amphetamine misuse. *British Journal of Addiction,* **87**, pp. 439–446.

Kleiman, M. (1993) *Against excess: Drug policy for results.* Sydney: Basic books.

Lewis, L., Monheit, B. and Mijch, A. (1991) *Report of the Melbourne Centre of the Australian National AIDS and Injecting Drug Use Study.* Sydney: National Centre for Social and Behavioural Research into Human Immunodeficiency Virus.

Loxley, W. and Marsh, A. (1990) *Nodding and speeding: Age and injecting drug use in Perth.* National Centre for Research into the Prevention of Drug Abuse. Perth: Curtin University.

Moore, D. (1993) 'Speeding, ecking and tripping': Ethnographic notes from a small world of psychostimulant use. In: *Illicit Psychostimulant Use in Australia.* D. Burrows, B. Flaherty and M. MacAvoy (eds.). Canberra: Australian Government Publishing Service.

Morgan, P. (1994) Personal communication.

MSJ Keys Young (1989) *Evaluation of the New South Wales Needle and Syringe Exchange Program.* AIDS Bureau. Sydney: NSW Department of Health.

Mugford, S. and Cohen, P. (1989) *Drug use, social relations and commodity consumption: A study of recreational cocaine users in Sydney, Canberra and Melbourne.* A Report to the Research into Drug Abuse Advisory Committee. Canberra: National Campaign Against Drug Abuse.

National Drug Abuse Information Centre (1991) *Statistical update No. 13 May 1991.* Canberra: Department of Community Services and Health.

Ovenden, C. and Loxely, W. (1994) Binging on psychostimulants: What's it like for young users? Perth: National Centre for Research into the Prevention of Drug Abuse. Curtin University.

Parliament of NSW (1986) Report of the Select Committee of the Legislative Assembly upon Prostitution.

Perkins, R. (1991) *Working Girls: Prostitutes, Their Life and Social Control.* Canberra: Australian Institute of Criminology.

Perkins, R. (1994) Health Aspects of Female Private Prostitutes in New South Wales. Canberra: Report to the National Health and Medical Research Council.

Pierce, J.P. and Levy, S. (1986) The looming cocaine problem in Australia. *Medical Journal of Australia,* **144**, pp. 562–563.

Reilly, C. and Homel, P. (1988) Teenage drug use: A study of drug use patterns and attitudes of a subgroup of Sydney adolescents. *Australian Drug and Alcohol Review,* **7**, pp. 167–174.

Ross, J. and Miller, S. (1994) Hidden use of amphetamine in metropolitan Melbourne. In R. Godding and G. Whelan (eds.) *The Proceedings of the 1994 Autumn School of Studies on Alcohol and Drugs.* Melbourne: St Vincent's Hospital.

Roy Morgan Research Centre (1993) *1992 Survey of alcohol, tobacco and other drug use among Victorian secondary school students.* A report prepared for the Department of Health and Community Services, Victorian Drug Strategy Unit. Melbourne: The Roy Morgan Research Centre Party Ltd.

Spooner, C., Flaherty, B. and Homel, P. (1993) Illicit drug use by young people: Results of a street intercept survey. *Drug and Alcohol Review,* **12**, pp. 159–168.

Stathis, H., Bertram, S. and Eyland, S. (1991). *Patterns of drug use amongst New South Wales prison receptions.* NSW Department of Corrective Services, Research and Statistics Branch, Sydney: Strategic Services Division.

Staysafe Committee of New South Wales (1992) *Staysafe 19: Alcohol and other drugs on New South Wales roads 1. The problem and counter-measures.* NSW Parliament. Sydney.

Swift, W., Darke, S., Hall, W. and Popple, G. (1993) *Who's Who? A report on the characteristics of clients seen at We Help Ourselves (WHOS), 1985–1991.* National Drug and Alcohol Research Centre Technical Report No. 18. Sydney. National Drug and Alcohol Research Centre, University of NSW.

Tebbutt, J., Muir, C. and Heather, N. (1990) *Drug trends in New South Wales: A Report to the WHO Collaborative Study on World Trends in Drug Abuse.* Monograph No. 13. Sydney: National Drug and Alcohol Research Centre.

Wardlaw, G. (1993). Supply reduction (law enforcement) strategies pertaining to illicit use of psychostimulants. In: *Illicit Psychostimulant Use in Australia.* D. Burrows, B. Flaherty and M. MacAvoy (eds.). Australian Government Publishing Service. Canberra.

Webster, P., Mattick, R.P. and Baillie, A.J. (1992) Characteristics of clients receiving treatment in Australian drug and alcohol agencies: A national census. *Drug and Alcohol Review,* **11**, pp. 111–119.

Wickes, W.A. (1993) *Amphetamines and Other Psychostimulants: A Guide to the Management of Users.* Canberra: Australian Government Publishing Service.

Zibert, E., Hando, J. and Howard, J. (1994) *Patterns of drug use and indicators of harm among persons detained in New South Wales Juvenile Justice Centres.* A Report Prepared for the New South Wales Department of Juvenile Justice. Sydney: NSW Department of Juvenile Justice.

Introduction to Section 2: United States of America

To the rest of the world the contemporary drug scene in the United States is overwhelmingly dominated by cocaine. Methamphetamine abuse in the US has a long history however and is still the drug of choice in certain areas on the West Coast. It now seems to be on the increase and spreading. After Miller's concise overview of history and trends, Morgan and Beck examine in more detail the varying patterns of abuse in the three cities of San Francisco, San Diego and Honolulu — well known for their traditional interest in methamphetamine.

The special case of Hawaii is taken up by Joe-Laidler and Morgan. 'Ice' is a form of methamphetamine that at one time was predicted to replace inject-able methamphetamine in the US and elsewhere in the world. It seems to have remained confined to Hawaii and areas in South East Asia where much of the supply comes from and there seems to have been little spread to mainland states. If this is an example of containment or of market failure, an analysis of the reasons for this could be instructive. On the other hand, the islands of Hawaii, their geographical position, cultural and political history may make them a unique case. The rise in crystal methamphetamine use as a consequence of increased law enforcement against marijuana is a telling example of market fluidity and flexibility that is an increasingly common characteristic of drug markets.

In the final chapter of this section Anderson and Flynn address directly the potential transmission of HIV infection, a problem associated elsewhere in the world with heroin and cocaine. The findings of greater HIV-related injec-tion and sexual risk among methamphetamine users than heroin users are

111

comparable to those in the UK (Chapter 2) despite the cultural differences. Such commonalities suggest several avenues for more detailed research — on the impact of amphetamine on sexuality and sociability, and the reasons for lack of contact with treatment services. However, there are also implications for future trends in the AIDS epidemic among younger drug users world-wide if amphetamine use, particularly the injection of amphetamine, increases and no preventive interventions are initiated.

6

History and Epidemiology of Amphetamine Abuse in The United States

MARISSA A. MILLER

INTRODUCTION

Trends in drug abuse are influenced by many factors including properties of the drug, characteristics of the abusing population, the environment within which the abuse occurs, as well as broader issues related to drug manufacturing, marketing, and distribution. Many complex and interrelated elements have converged in promulgating past and present epidemics of amphetamine abuse. This chapter will: chronicle the unique history of the development of amphetamine and methamphetamine, the medical and nonmedical use of these drugs, and subsequent epidemics of abuse in the United States; describe current patterns and trends of abuse and factors influencing these trends; explain how legal control of the manufacture and distribution has influenced the availability and propelled the patterns of abuse; and consider the potential for future abuse of methamphetamine and related substances.

Background

Amphetamines are a class of synthetic stimulants that include several specific chemical agents the most common of which are: amphetamine (Benzedrine), methamphetamine (Desoxyn), dextroamphetamine (Dexadrine), and benzphetamine (Didrex), plus the combination amphetamine and dextroamphetamine (Biphetamine) (King and Coleman, 1987). Amphetamines were first manufactured in 1887 (Caldwell, 1980). Methamphetamine was first synthesized in 1919 and closely resembles amphetamine in chemical structure and pharmacologic action. Today the term amphetamine refers generally to popular pharmaceutical pills and capsules used licitly and illicitly. Methamphetamine is a related compound that generally is more sought after due to its long lasting high. Methamphetamine is the only compound in this class of stimulants that is manufactured to any significant extent in clandestine laboratories in the United States and currently is a more prevalent drug of abuse than amphetamine.

Speed is a term used to describe all the synthetic stimulants including amphetamine and methamphetamine. Illicit methamphetamine is known by names such as 'meth', 'crystal', and 'crank'. Amphetamine pills and capsules that have found their way onto the streets are commonly referred to as 'denies', 'dexies', 'bennies', and 'uppers'. Street drug terminology is very location specific and not standardized, so wherever possible any new term will be defined in the text.

History of Early Use

Historically, use of the synthetically manufactured amphetamines and methamphetamine can be traced back to the early 1930s when medicinally useful attributes of these compounds were discovered. Amphetamine and the closely related methamphetamine exhibited bronchodilator and hypertensive properties, they reversed barbiturate anesthesia, and treated lung congestion. Between 1932 and 1946, the pharmaceutical industry developed a list of 39 generally accepted clinical uses for these drugs, including the treatment of schizophrenia, morphine and codeine addiction, tobacco smoking, heart block, head injuries, radiation sickness, low blood pressure, and persistent hiccups (Lucas, 1985). They were promoted as being safe without risks (Grinspoon and Hedblom, 1975). From the time of early use the existence of psychoactive properties were also identified in association with these substances. Extensive use, combined with the inherent properties of the drugs set the stage for later widespread abuse.

Amphetamines rapidly became popular in the U.S. amphetamine tablets could be obtained without prescription until 1951, and amphetamine inhalers were available until 1959. Amphetamines and methamphetamine were widely marketed during the 1950s and 1960s for obesity, narcolepsy, hyperkinesis, and depression. Housewives were prescribed amphetamines for weight loss; others including students, businessmen, and truck drivers used them for their anti-fatigue effects (Ellinwood, 1974). Their popularity was bolstered by low cost and long duration of effect (Fischman, 1990). During World War II amphetamines were used extensively by the American, British, German, and Japanese military as stimulants and insomniacs. An estimated 200 million tablets and pills were supplied to American troops during World War II (Grinspoon and Hedblom, 1975). Some of the American soldiers returned home following the war and continued to use stimulants.

The popularity of amphetamines drove production, and production levels served ultimately to drive popularity. Legal production soared from approximately 3.5 billion tablets in 1958, to 10 billion tablets by 1970 (Grinspoon and Hedblom, 1975). During the 1960s 20 million prescriptions were written each year predominantly for weight reduction purposes (Ellinwood, 1979; Spotts and Spotts, 1980). Prescribing practices escalated until 1967 when 31 million scripts were written. The prevalence of use was much higher among younger adults and in certain areas of the country such as San Francisco (Mellinger *et al.*, 1971).

In the late 1950s some physicians began prescribing intravenously administered methamphetamine as a treatment for heroin addiction. Other doctors and pharmacists became involved in writing illegal prescriptions for liquid amphetamine ampoules (Lake and Quirk, 1984). These practices contributed to the origination of new abuse patterns involving intravenous injection of methamphetamine. The most popular of the injectable ampoules were made by Abbott (Desoxyn) and Burroughs Wellcome (Methedrine). During the first half of 1962 over 500,000 ampules were prescribed (Brecher, 1972; Smith, 1969).

During the 1960s speed use spread to a variety of groups throughout the San Francisco Bay area. Haight-Ashbury, a neighbourhood of the Bay area, epitomized the 1960s drug subculture. In Haight-Ashbury speed began to replace hallucinogenic drugs such as LSD in popularity (Pittel and Hofer, 1970). Speed use escalated and a shift from oral preparations to intravenous abuse occurred. By the early 1960s the San Francisco Bay area was home to a large and increasing number of intravenous methamphetamine users. Intravenous use combined with the development of tolerance, led to escalating use. Serial intravenous speed users became known as 'speed freaks'. A public campaign in response to this trend warned that 'speed kills' (Lucas, 1985). As a result of law enforcement targeting activities, the public health campaign, user demographic changes, and other factors, the prevalence of methamphetamine and amphetamine use dropped after 1972 (Newmeyer, 1988).

Manufacture, Distribution, and Diversion

During the 1960s pharmaceutical amphetamine production soared with the demand from widespread use. However, production levels grew at a rate that far exceeded medical use. One consequence of excessive production combined with widespread popularity was diversion of pharmaceutical grade drugs to illegal traffic and use. The black market in amphetamines involved diversions from pharmaceutical companies, wholesalers, pharmacists, and physicians. It is estimated that up until 1971 between one half to two thirds of the 100,000 pounds of pharmaceutical amphetamine produced each year were diverted to black market channels (Grinspoon and Hedblom, 1975). In 1971 the Justice Department began imposing quotas on legal amphetamine production.

The Department of Justice (DOJ) became aware of the magnitude of dispensation of intravenous methamphetamine through illegal prescription writing. The DOJ intervened and pharmaceutical manufacturers voluntarily removed methamphetamine ampoules from the outpatient prescription marketplace (Spotts and Spotts, 1980). Abbott withdrew Desoxyn in 1962 and Burroughs Wellcome withdrew Methedrine in 1963. This action left intravenous methamphetamine users without a product which could be readily injected. Demand was created for an inexpensive water-soluble powder product.

What resulted was the emergence of the first illicit 'bathtub' methamphetamine laboratories in late 1962 in San Francisco to satisfy the demand for a user friendly product (Morgan *et al.*, 1994). The early illicit methamphetamine was synthesized from phenyl-2-propanone (P-2-P) and methylamine by a process referred to as the amalgam method resulting in a racemic mixture of d (the more pharmacologically active form) and l-isomer methamphetamine. A few legitimate chemists are believed to have helped several groups develop this manufacturing process (Morgan *et al.*, 1994). The illicit product was less potent and less pure than the pharmaceutical product which is all d-isomer methamphetamine. The newly manufactured product became known by a number of street names such as: 'crank', 'bathtub crank', 'biker crank', 'peanut butter', 'prope-dope', and 'wire'.

Whereas prior to 1962 the quality and purity of methamphetamine was defined by pharmaceutical supplies, after 1962 the availability and quality of the illicit product was unpredictable. Up until 1974 only 30% of street samples purported to be methamphetamine truly were methamphetamine. 'Look-alike' speed, a combination of phenylpropanolamine, ephedrine, and caffeine, sometimes with other constituents, flooded the street market (Lake and Quirk, 1984). From 1975 to 1983 the meth content of street samples increased from 60 percent to over 90 percent. Overtime clandestinely manufactured methamphetamine came to dominate the street speed market (Puder *et al.*, 1988).

With the escalation of use during the 1960s came an increase in violence and a diffusion of clandestine manufacturing and distribution of speed outward from Haight-Ashbury to other areas along the West Coast (Smith, 1970). By 1965 outlaw motorcycle gangs, notorious for their depraved and unlawful activities, realizing there was profit to be made began manufacturing and distributing speed (NNICC, 1993). Crank became regarded as the best speed for the biker lifestyle, which emphasized fast high-risk motorcycling, fighting, heavy drinking, partying, and barbiturate use (Thompson, 1967). The combination of the affinity of bikers and their lifestyle for the drug, and the sizeable profits to be made from its manufacture and distribution, led to increasing involvement and dominance over distribution by mid 1960. Biker distribution of crank diffused north to Oregon and Washington State and into southern California. The laboratories were located primarily in rural areas.

The Department of Justice recognized the involvement of outlaw biker groups in particular the Hell's Angels, in methamphetamine manufacture and distribution and began targeting these groups. During the 1980s the law enforcement pressure combined with the dissemination of a new method of synthesis led to significant changes in methamphetamine distribution networks. The shift was to smaller producers and groups of friends or family who cooperated to produce small amounts of methamphetamine in low-tech labs (NNICC, 1993). Beginning around 1980 methamphetamine laboratories began to proliferate around San Diego and use in that area escalated.

The illicit manufacture of methamphetamine is relatively simple and can be carried out by individuals without special knowledge or expertise provided a detailed recipe is available (Irvine and Chin, 1991; BJS, 1992). Laboratory operators include high school dropouts and highly educated chemists. Clandestine laboratories are commonly operated on an irregular basis — frequently a batch of product is produced and the laboratory is disassembled, stored, or moved to a new location. Sites for laboratories vary from sophisticated underground hideaways to motel rooms, kitchens, or garages (NNICC, 1993). Laboratories tend to be located in more secluded rural sites, initially to avoid discovery due to fumes and odours vented during the production process (Irvine and Chin, 1991). The precursors and methods used in methamphetamine synthesis can vary from laboratory to laboratory. In many cases the producers possess insufficient knowledge and skill to carry out the synthesis appropriately and completely. In these cases the purity and quality of the end product suffer with the output containing large levels of contaminants and unreacted precursors.

The DEA reports that methamphetamine is the most prevalent clandestinely manufactured controlled substance in the US (DEA, 1993). The number of clandestine methamphetamine laboratories seized rose dramatically during the 1980s from 88 in 1981 to 652 in 1989. This dramatic increase reflects both increased law enforcement pursuit of clandestine laboratories and the expansion of clandestine production. Since 1989 there has been a decrease in laboratory seizures to 429 in 1990, 315 in 1991 and 288 in 1992. Consistent with previous years the clandestine manufacture of methamphetamine was located primarily in the West and Southwest of the US. During 1992, 78% of the laboratories seized were located in the Denver, Los Angeles, Phoenix, San Diego, San Francisco, and Seattle DEA field areas (NNICC 1993). Methamphetamine laboratories accounted for more than 87% of all clandestine laboratory seizures during 1992. The decrease in the number of methamphetamine laboratories seized in the United States during the 1990s as compared to the large number of laboratory seizures during 1989 is believed to be largely a result of the enactment and enforcement of the Chemical Diversion and Trafficking Act of 1988, which placed the distribution of 12 precursor and 8 essential chemicals used in the production of illicit drugs under federal control (DEA, 1993).

Currently the ephedrine reduction method is the principal means employed in the manufacture of methamphetamine. This relatively simple process originated in Southern California and now is widespread throughout the United States (NNICC, 1993). The resulting product is the d-isomer of methamphetamine. Reportedly, new and altered chemical processes for clandestine manufacturing of methamphetamine are emerging on the West Coast including the tetrahydrofuran (THF) synthesis (Wrede and Murphy, 1994), and a relatively simple synthesis procedure that is a variation of the ephedrine reduction method that is called 'cold cook' because no external heat source is required for the synthesis to proceed (Dode and Dye, 1994; DEA, 1993).

During 1992 the individuals and groups involved in manufacture and distribution of methamphetamine were diverse and numerous and included independent entrepreneurs, outlaw motorcycle gangs, and Hispanic polydrug trafficking organizations (NNICC, 1993). Independent entrepreneur involvement was broad and distributed nationally. Motorcycle gangs influenced production in select areas and Mexican traffickers dominated the large-scale production and distribution in San Diego, Riverside, San Bernardino, and Fresno areas of California (NNICC, 1993; DEA, 1993). The Mexican traffickers typically manufacture large quantities of methamphetamine in Mexico and smuggle the finished product into California through heroin and marijuana trafficking routes with the potential for distribution throughout the United States. Mexican smuggling of precursor chemicals such as ephedrine into California also provides evidence of their domination of methamphetamine production in the West (DEA, 1993). The emergence of this new trafficking and distribution scheme involving large quantities of methamphetamine may serve to drive a new widespread epidemic of use in endemic regions and new areas. Increases in methamphetamine use in Phoenix are attributed to a newly forged trafficking relationship between Mexican nationals and local Hispanics (Dode and Dye, 1994).

This brief but significant history of use and abuse of amphetamine and methamphetamine (decades rather than centuries) has laid the foundation for continued abuse of methamphetamine, the arrival of new dosage forms, and the emergence of new chemically-related analogues.

Current Trends of Methamphetamine Abuse

Due to its illicit and illegal nature, the direct, reliable, and consistent measurement of substance abuse is difficult, if not impossible. As a result, the description of patterns and trends of drug abuse are derived from a variety of data sources, some more scientifically rigorous than others. These sources of information are interpreted as available and patterns and trends inferred from them. Data sources include national probability surveys such as the Monitoring the Future study (MTF), nationally representative surveillance systems akin to the Drug Abuse Warning Network (DAWN) and the Drug Use Forecasting system (DUF), State-based treatment data, small-scale field studies, and ethnographic observational research.

DAWN data

The first measured surge in methamphetamine use following what has been described historically in Haight-Ashbury during the 1960s and early 1970s, occurred during the mid-1980s among metropolitan areas primarily along the West Coast. These increases were first picked up through ethnographic research and field studies (NIDA, 1986; NIDA, 1989), and later recognized through the Drug Abuse Warning Network (DAWN) system and reported through the Community Epidemiology Work Group, a network of researchers from major metropolitan areas of the U.S. who provide ongoing community level surveillance of drug abuse.

The DAWN is a national surveillance system that monitors hospital emergencies and deaths associated with drug abuse. The DAWN system was begun in the early 1970s as a random sample of hospital emergency departments, over time the number and type of participating hospitals changed and the representativeness of the sample was compromised. The current system was revitalized and a new sample drawn in 1986 to represent all hospital emergency departments in the coterminous United States. Non-Federal, short-stay, general hospitals with a 24 hour emergency department are eligible for inclusion in DAWN. Twenty-one Metropolitan Statistical Areas (MSAs) are designated for oversampling. Hospitals outside of these 21 areas are assigned to a National Panel and sampled. A total of 685 hospitals was selected for the sample and 508 hospitals (74%) participated in the survey in 1993 (OAS, 1994a). Participation in DAWN is voluntary and involves a designated reporter within each facility reviewing hospital emergency department (ED) admission records.

An episode report is submitted each time a patient visits a DAWN hospital with problems relating to their own drug use. The case definition involves four criteria, all of which must be met: the patient must be treated in the hospital's ED, the presenting complaint must have been induced by or related to drug use at anytime preceding the episode, the case must involve the nonmedical use of a legal drug or any use of an illegal drug, and the patient's reason for taking the drug/drugs include dependence, suicide attempt, or psychic effect. If all the above criteria are met then the ED visit is deemed a drug episode. For each drug episode in addition to alcohol in combination, up to four substances may be recorded as drug mentions. Drug episodes are not synonymous with the number of individuals involved in the reported episodes. One person may make repeated visits to one or several EDs with each episode recorded independently.

The limitations of this system are that the data are only as good as the information recorded by the hospital ED staff and reflect only self-reported drug use by the patient without laboratory confirmation. DAWN does not provide a complete image of problems associated with drug use but only reflects the impact of drug use on hospital EDs in the U.S. and the sort of drug-related problems that bring patients into emergency departments.

The DAWN emergency department data showed statistically significant increases in mentions of methamphetamine/speed in Atlanta, Dallas, Los Angeles, Phoenix, San Diego, and Seattle between 1986 and 1988 (NIDA, 1989). During 1988 and 1989 the national level of methamphetamine/speed emergency room mentions held steady, a drop was experienced in 1990 with a steady increase from 1990 through 1993 (Figure 1). In 1993 10,052 episodes (preliminary estimates) involving the use of methamphetamine/speed were reported in the coterminous U.S. up from a low of 4,887 reported in 1991, a 106% increase (OAS, 1994b). A total of 466,897 drug-related emergency room episodes were recorded for 1993, cocaine accounted for 123,317 (26.4%) and heroin accounted for 62,965 (13.5%), with meth/speed involved in just over 2% of the episodes, ranking 12th among all drug-related episodes. From 1990 through 1993 national estimates of total drug-related ED episodes increased 26% from 371,208 to 466,897 respectively, and increased 8% between 1992 and 1993. Approximately 10% of the 1992 to 1993 increase is attributable to increases in meth/speed mentions (OAS, 1994b).

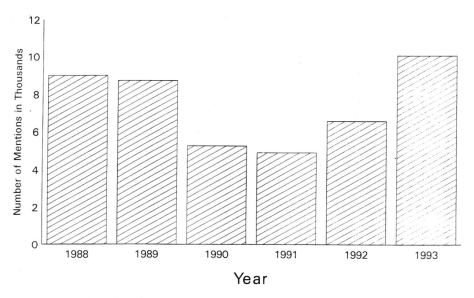

Figure 1   Estimated number of Methamphetamine/Speed Emergency Room Mentions in the Coterminous United States by Year: 1988–1993.
Source: SAMHSA, Drug Abuse Warning Network (April 1994 data file).
Note: The 1993 estimates are preliminary.

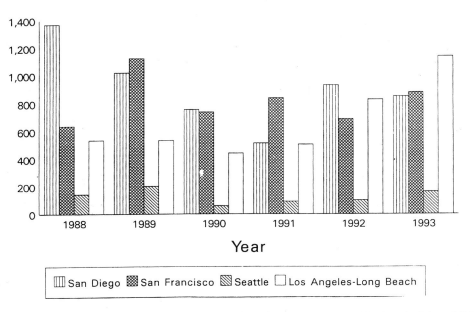

Figure 2   Estimated number of Methamphetamine/Speed Emergency Room Mentions in Selected U.S. Metropolitian Areas by Year: 1988–1993.
Source: SAMHSA, Drug Abuse Warning Network (April 1994 data file).
Note: The 1993 estimates are preliminary.

West coast U.S. cities including San Diego, San Francisco, Seattle, and Los Angeles-Long Beach accounted for over 30% of the total 1993 methamphetamine/speed ED mentions (1993 preliminary estimates). Over the six year period from 1988 through 1993 San Diego exhibited consistently high numbers of methamphetamine/speed ED mentions, leading all other cities during three years of this time period (Figure 2). Los Angeles led all MSAs in number of methamphetamine/speed mentions in 1993 with 1,140-accounting for 11% of total U.S. methamphetamine/speed mentions, followed by San Francisco, San Diego and Seattle with 879, 850 and 161 respectively (Table 1).

Table 1   Estimated number of methamphetamine/speed emergency room mentions in selected U.S. metropolitian areas by year: 1988–1993

U.S.	8992	8722	5236	4887	6563	10052
San Diego	1372	1021	758	515	931	850
San Francisco	639	1125	740	839	688	879
Seattle	142	201	59	90	99	161
Los Angeles-Long Beach	536	536	442	506	828	1140
Year	1988	1989	1990	1991	1992	1993

The profile of a typical methamphetamine user in 1993 is someone in the middle age range, male, and white (Source: SAMHSA, weighted preliminary 1993 estimates from the April 1994 data file). During 1993, 35% of meth/speed mentions occurred in the 18–25 year age range and 37% in the 26–34 age range. The ratio of males to females using meth/speed ranged from 5:1 in San Francisco to 1.7:1 in San Diego. The predominant motivation for use was dependence (34%), followed by recreational use (27%), followed by unknown (25%). The reason for ED contact for meth/speed mentions was unexpected reaction (37%), overdose (29%), and chronic effects (13%), with withdrawal, seeking detoxification, accident/injury, other, and unknown together comprising the remaining percentage. The route of administration reported for the DAWN mentions was 31% unknown, 27% sniffed or snorted, 22% injected, and 11% oral.

State treatment admission data

Several large nationally based treatment data systems exist. The emphasis within these data systems is on admission data concerning the most prevalent drugs of abuse, namely alcohol, marijuana, cocaine, and heroin. Data singular to methamphetamine were not readily available from these sources. State and city level admissions trends are reported for areas that have a significant methamphetamine problem.

In San Diego during 1993 amphetamine and methamphetamine primary admissions to publicly funded treatment programmes totalled 2,376, a 37% increase from 1992 (Haight, 1994). Methamphetamine was the most frequently reported nonalcohol primary drug of abuse among those entering drug treatment programmes during 1993, accounting for 41% of all nonalcohol treatment admissions. Numbers of methamphetamine admissions are rivalling alcohol admissions which historically have been most prevalent. The median age of methamphetamine users entering treatment was 28 in 1993, tending to be younger than cocaine or heroin users. The racial distribution of methamphetamine users entering treatment was 71% white, 5% African American and 17% Hispanic. An increase was seen in the number of methamphetamine treatment admissions reporting smoking as the preferred route of administration. In 1989 4% reported smoking as compared to 23% in 1993.

In San Francisco primary admissions for amphetamine abuse totalled 1357 increasing 17% from 1992 levels (Newmeyer, 1994). Amphetamine admissions accounted for just over 5% of the total non-alcohol admissions, behind heroin 67%, and cocaine 23%. The number and percent of amphetamine admissions has increased steadily each year since 1988 with 534 admissions (3.3%) reported in 1988 and 1357 (5.2%) reported in 1993.

Statewide methamphetamine treatment admissions in Hawaii have increased from 152 in 1991, to 268 in 1992, to an all-time high of 495 in 1993

(Wood, 1995). These data represent about 90% of the State-supported treatment facilities and do not include two large private facilities. In 1993, methamphetamine admissions accounted for 28% of the total admissions second only to marijuana admissions (excluding alcohol). The trend of treatment admissions continued to increase into the first half of 1994.

Several drug use indicators including treatment admissions point to escalations of methamphetamine use in Phoenix, Arizona (Dode and Dye, 1994). The number of detoxification admissions for methamphetamine increased by 114% between 1992 and 1993 and ranked second behind heroin among non-alcohol admissions. Admissions of methamphetamine users to treatment through criminal justice programmes rose from zero prior to 1992 to 30% in one programme, and 15% in another programme during 1993.

Amphetamine and methamphetamine admissions account for a small proportion of overall admissions in most other cities and States (NIDA, 1994). In Colorado amphetamine admissions comprised 5.6% of the total, a slight increase over 1992. In Texas, Seattle, and Los Angeles amphetamine and methamphetamine admissions account for 3%, and in Minneapolis 2%, of nonalcohol admissions.

DUF data

The Drug Use Forecasting (DUF) system is a monitoring system collaboratively administered by the National Institute of Justice and 24 booking facility sites across the nation. Interviews and urine drug tests for 10 illicit compounds are conducted at the time of booking of adult male, adult female, and juvenile arrestees, and represent drug use among those involved with the criminal justice system. For approximately 14 consecutive evenings each quarter local staff interview and obtain voluntary urine specimens from a sample of newly booked arrestees. At each site approximately 225 males are sampled and in some sites female arrestees and juvenile arrestees/detainees are also sampled. Response rates are 90% for the interview portion and 80% for the urine specimen portion of the system (NIJ, 1994a).

The DUF sample attempts to represent a sufficient distribution of arrest charges by limiting the number of male booked arrestees who are charged with the sale or possession of drugs (otherwise a majority of the sample would be made up of drug charge arrestees). Persons charged with drug charges are more likely to be using drugs at the time of arrest so this limitation tends to underestimate drug use in the male arrestee population. The DUF sample also generally excludes driving offences, emphasizing more serious crimes. In contrast, in order to obtain sufficient numbers of arrestees, all adult female and juvenile arrestees brought to the booking centre or detention facility during the data collection period are included in the DUF sample, regardless of the charge.

Urine specimens are tested for cocaine, opiates, marijuana, PCP, methadone, benzodiazepines, methaqualone, propoxyphene, barbiturates, and amphetamines. All amphetamine positive results are further tested to eliminate exposure to over-the-counter products. The testing detects drug use that occurred in the previous two to three days for most compounds. PCP and marijuana use may be detected as long as several weeks prior to the testing date.

In 1993 the DUF system collected data from 20,550 adult male booked arrestees in 23 sites (NIJ, 1994a). Data from 8,070 adult female booked arrestees were collected at 20 of these sites. Twelve DUF sites collected male juvenile arrestee/detainee data (NIJ, 1994b). At most sites during 1993 cocaine was the most prevalent drug among male arrestees, followed by marijuana (seven sites reported a rate of marijuana use higher than cocaine). Cocaine use among male adult arrestees ranged from a low of 19% in Omaha, Nebraska to a high of 66% in Manhattan, New York, with a median percentage of 43%. Marijuana use ranged from 21% in Manhattan to 42% in Omaha, with a median value of 28%. Opiate use ranged from a low of 1% in Fort Lauderdale, Florida to a high of 28% in Chicago, Illinois. Data from 20 sites revealed female arrestees to have marijuana in their urine a median of 16.5% of the time (range of 9% to 25%); and a range of opiate use from 3% to 23%. Results for juvenile arrestees/detainees nearly exclusively showed marijuana and cocaine use.

Overall, during 1993 in the majority of sites amphetamine use was very low or nonexistent. The predominant portion of amphetamine use was clustered in Western cities including San Diego, California; San Jose, California; Los Angeles, California; Phoenix, Arizona; and Portland, Oregon. The level of amphetamine abuse among adult male arrestees within these sites ranged from 36% in San Diego to 8% in Los Angeles, and 53% in San Diego to 10% in Los Angeles among female arrestees (NIJ, 1994a [Source: DUF 1993 data file]). San Diego had the largest prevalence of amphetamine use for all three user groups during 1993; males (36%), females (53%), and juvenile males (14%) were positive for amphetamine abuse. In San Diego, among male arrestees, amphetamine abuse followed marijuana and cocaine abuse at 36% compared to 40% and 37% respectively. Amphetamine abuse led all other drugs for females in San Diego. Phoenix had the second highest prevalence of amphetamine abuse with 16% of males and 26% of females testing positive. In all five western cities the percentage of female arrestees testing positive for amphetamines was higher than the male arrestee counterpart at the same site.

Emergence of Ice

During the mid and late 1980s, ice, a high potency, high purity and smokable form of d-methamphetamine hydrochloride was identified as a problem initially by Hawaiian law enforcement sources and later through Hawaiian drug treatment programmes. At the time of the emergence of ice the resident

Hawaiian population had limited experience with mainland forms of methamphetamine. Hawaiian users widely believed ice to be a 'new drug', and not related to other forms of speed. On the street this product which resembles rock candy in appearance was most commonly referred to as 'ice', 'crystal', 'shabu' (Japanese), or 'batu' (Filipino). In Hawaii the drug is almost exclusively smoked in a glass pipe. The inhalation of vapours leads to rapid absorption into the bloodstream and dissemination to the brain resulting in the immediate onset of effects, similar to what is experienced by intravenous administration (Chiang and Hawks, 1989).

The unique combination of characteristics of ice namely: high potency, high purity, and rapid onset of effects by smoking, resulted in an escalation of use among many abusers on the Island of Oahu (Miller and Tomas, 1989). The use pattern that emerged was one of binging and crashing, or continuous smoking in runs of 3 to 8 days followed by complete exhaustion, usually characterized by deep prolonged sleep. Many adverse social, psychological, and medical consequences were experienced by binge users including rapid addiction (Miller, 1991).

The presence of ice in Hawaii dates back to the late 1970s. During the early to mid 1980s ice use was limited to small ethnic gangs, but the outbreak beginning in mid 1980s and peaking in the late 1980s found use spreading to numerous ethnic minorities, the Pacific-Asian majority, Caucasians, both genders, people of all ages, and all socioeconomic classes (Miller, 1991).

Prior to 1990 all the ice entering Hawaii originated from Asian sources, namely Korea, Taiwan, and the Philippines (DEA, 1989). Ice distribution in Hawaii was an economic enterprise developed by organized crime networks in Japan and Korea with large corporate investors (Adamski, 1992; Schoenberger, 1992). Availability of ice in Hawaii was widespread through 1990. By 1991 the availability had decreased, price had skyrocketed and use indicators were declining (Wood, 1995). Large seizures of ice made by Chinese authorities in 1991 and 1992 confirm that illicit methamphetamine manufacture was also occurring in China. It is believed the Chinese contraband was smuggled into Japan, the Philippines, Hawaii, and the mainland U.S. during the early 1990s (NNICC, 1993). Current data are not available on the location and extent of ice manufacture within the United States.

Chemical Analogues

Synthesis of designer drugs or chemically related analogues to methamphetamine and amphetamine are emerging as new public health problems. Reports from ethnographers of a sharp increase of use of methylene deoxymethamphetamine (MDMA, XTC, Ecstasy) in association with the 'rave' scene have been received from San Francisco, Dallas, Houston, Miami, and Denver (NIDA, 1994; Kotarba, 1993 and Harrison, 1994). The rave scene is an increasingly popular form of dance and recreation predominantly frequented by young whites, but open to people of all ages, at clandestine locations (frequently abandoned warehouses), where high volume music and high tech entertainment is available. The use of hallucinogens, methamphetamine, or MDMA is often incorporated into the overall experience of the rave (ONDCP, 1995). MDMA is most commonly swallowed or snorted but can be smoked or injected. In addition to methamphetamine-like effects MDMA may cause sensory enhancements and distortions and mild visual hallucinations.

To date MDMA use has not been detected to any large degree on a national level through drug use indicator systems based on drug associated emergency room mentions, medical examiner reports, or within treatment data. Case reports and ethnographic information provides a glimpse of the problem but cannot be relied upon to represent the full scope and extent of this drug problem.

N-methylcathinone hydrochloride (methcathinone, 'cat', 'goob', 'sniff', 'star', 'wonder star') a structural and pharmacological analogue of methamphetamine is a potent and easily manufactured stimulant gaining popularity in the Midwest (Goldstone, 1993; DEA, 1994; Pinkert and Harwood, 1993). Cathinones occur naturally in the leaves of the Khat shrub *(catha edulis)* which are chewed in East Africa and southern Arabia for the mild stimulant effects. Methcathinone is typically snorted but can be smoked and injected. Symptoms and adverse effects similar to methamphetamine are reported for methcathinone.

Michigan treatment programmes report increasing numbers of methcathinone admissions, as many as 60 treatment admissions were reported statewide between October 1993 and March 1994 (Calkins and Hussain, 1994). Laboratories producing methcathinone were first identified in 1991 when five laboratory sites were seized in the Michigan Upper Peninsula. Methcathinone manufacturing is relatively simple from easily obtained materials, the technology is spreading to other nearby states throughout the Midwest and West (DEA, 1994).

Patterns of Youth Drug Abuse

The Monitoring the Future Study, also known widely as the National High School Senior Survey has been conducted each year since 1975 under a National Institute on Drug Abuse grant to the University of Michigan Institute for Social Research (Johnson *et al.*, 1991). The 1994 survey represents the 20th annual survey of high school seniors, data on 8th and 10th grade students have been collected since 1991. In 1994 a national probability sample of 15,929 high school seniors in 139 public and private schools nationwide were selected to be representative of all seniors in the continental US. The students completed self administered questionnaires during the Spring of the year. Questions from the MTF Study solicit responses on use of amphetamines referred to as 'uppers', 'ups', 'speed', 'bennies', 'dexies', 'pep pills', and 'diet pills' (HHS, 1994).

From 1982 to 1992 lifetime, past year, and past month use of stimulants (amphetamines) by high school seniors declined (Figure 3). This decline was consistent with an increase in anti-drug attitudes and beliefs in the harmfulness of drug use. Since 1992 there has been significant increases in lifetime, past year, and past month use of stimulants by high school seniors during both 1993 and 1994 (Figure 3). During 1991 through 1994 the study also showed a dramatic upturn in past year use of stimulants among 8th and 10th graders, paralleling the increase seen among seniors (Figure 4). Among senior students lifetime use increased for amphetamines from 13.9% to 15.7%, and increased for crystal methamphetamine (ice) from 2.9% to 3.4% over the 1992 to 1994 period (HHS, 1994). These estimates of drug use prevalence by the MTF Study may be underestimates due to the fact that the survey is conducted in secondary school classrooms and does not represent drug use by dropouts. Dropouts have been shown to have much higher drug use than seniors in the MTF Study (Gfroerer, 1993).

Since 1991 there has been a steady and accelerating decline in perceived risk of drug use, with only 65% in 1994 reporting a great risk associated with regular marijuana use as compared to 79% of seniors in 1991. Perceived risk of use of other drugs such as cocaine and LSD also declined. This decline in perceived risk of drug use is consistent with the increases in drug use demonstrated during the same time period. Perceived dangers and attitudes of peers toward drug use have been shown to predict future drug use.

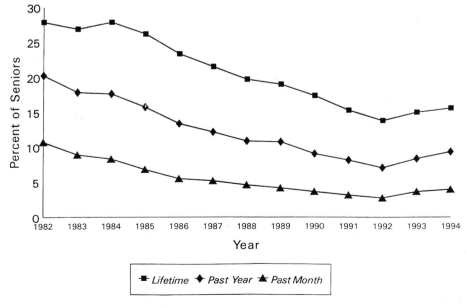

Figure 3   Estimated Prevalence of Lifetime, Past Year and Past Month Use of Stimulants Among High School Seniors: 1982–1994.
Source: The Monitoring the Future Study, University of Michigan.

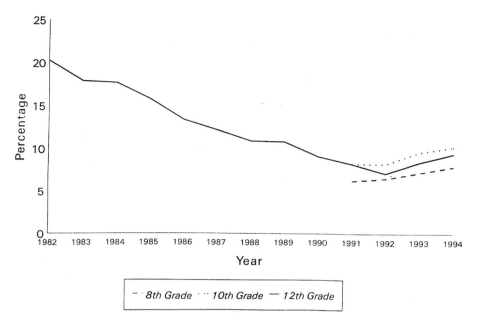

Figure 4 Estimated Prevalence of Past Year Use of Stimulants Among High School Seniors (1982–1994) and Eighth and Tenth Graders (1991–1994).
Source: The Monitoring the Future Study, University of Michigan.

CONCLUSION

In conclusion, methamphetamine abuse is endemic in West Coast US cities and Hawaii. From early use by housewives, students, businessmen, and truck drivers, methamphetamine continues to be a significant drug of abuse in the U.S. Morgan *et al.* (1994) in their study described current methamphetamine use to be firmly entrenched in disenfranchised communities, among troubled individuals and dysfunctional families, and spreading to new user groups. The favourable side-effects such as euphoria, increased energy levels, sexual enhancement, and weight loss makes methamphetamine appealing to diverse population sub-groups. With the potential for widespread dissemination, factors such as easy availability, low cost, long duration of effect, and multiple methods of administration may also serve to increase its acceptance in new groups and areas.

The potential for expanded methamphetamine use is particularly significant in light of increasing youth use of drugs (including amphetamines) changing attitudes toward drug use in general, the availability of new dosage forms, and new venues for use. Rave scenes, where both methamphetamine and its analogue MDMA are sold and experimented with, serve as sites for spread into younger age cohorts and higher socioeconomic groups than have historically abused methamphetamine. Ice, a smokable form of methamphetamine, continues to wreak havoc and devastation within low socio-economic status and working class Hawaiian neighbourhoods. Cat, an analogue, is gaining acceptance and use in the Midwest and the potential for new analogues presenting new threats to the public health is significant.

Methamphetamine poses current challenges to our public health and future legacies for our youth and promises to remain problematic in American society for years to come.

ACKNOWLEDGEMENT

A special acknowledgment to Arthur Hughes, National Institute on Drug Abuse for his valued assistance.

REFERENCES

Adamski, M. (1992) Yakuza Investors Sink Roots in Isles. *Honolulu Star Bulletin*, October 16.

Brecher, E.M. (1972) *Licit and Illicit Drugs*. Boston: Little Brown Publishers.

Bureau of Justice Statistics (BJS) (1992) *Drugs Crime and the Justice System — A National Report*. U.S. Department of Justice, U.S. Government Printing Office, Washington, D.C. (NJS-133652).

Caldwell, J. (1980) *Amphetamines and Related Stimulants: Chemical, Biological, Clinical, and Sociological Aspects*. Boca Raton, Florida: CRC Press, Inc.

Calkins, R.F. and Hussain K.L. (1994) Drug Abuse Trends in Detroit/Wayne Country, Michigan. In: *Epidemiologic Trends in Drug Abuse. Volume II: Proceedings Community Epidemiology Work Group June 1994*. Rockville, Maryland: National Institute on Drug Abuse. (NIH Pub. No. 94-3854).

Chiang, N. and Hawks, R. (1989) *Pyrolysis Studies: Cocaine, Phencyclidine, Heroin and Methamphetamine*. Technical Review Brief. Rockville, Maryland: National Institute on Drug Abuse.

Dode, I.L. and Dye C. (1994) Drug Abuse Trends in Phoenix and Arizona. In: *Epidemiologic Trends in Drug Abuse. Volume II: Proceedings Community Epidemiology Work Group June 1994*. Rockville, Maryland: National Institute on Drug Abuse. (NIH Pub. No. 94-3854).

Drug Enforcement Administration (1993) *Methcathinone (CAT) Drug Fact Sheet*. U.S. Department of Justice, Intelligence Division, Washington, D.C. (DEA-94007).

Drug Enforcement Administration (1994) *U.S. Drug Threat Assessment: 1993. Drug Intelligence Report*. U.S. Department of Justice, Washington, D.C. (DEA-93042).

Drug Enforcement Administration (1989) A Special Report on "Ice". In: *Epidemiologic Trends in Drug Abuse. Proceedings of the Community Epidemiology Work Group Decmber 1989.* Supt. of Docs., U.S. Govt. Print. Off., Washington, DC. (DHHS Pub. No. 721–757:20058).

Ellinwood, E.H. (1974) Epidemiology of Stimulant Abuse. In: E. Josephson and E. Carroll (eds.), *Drug Use.* Washington D.C.: Hemisphere Publishing Corporation.

Ellinwood, E.H. (1979) Amphetamines/Anorectics. In: R. DuPont, A. Goldstein and J. O'Donnell (eds.), *Handbook on Drug Abuse.* Washington D.C.: National Institute on Drug Abuse.

Fischman, M.W. (1990) History and Current Use of Methamphetamine in the United States. In: *Cocaine and Methamphetamine: Behavioral Toxicology, Clinical Psychiatry and Epidemiology.* Proceedings from Japan–U.S. Scientific Symposium '90 on Drug Dependence and Abuse. Tokyo, Japan.

Gfroerer, J. (1993) An Overview of the National Household Survey on Drug Abuse and Related Methodological Research. *Proceedings of the Survey Research Section of the American Statistical Association, Joint Statistical Meetings, August 1992.* Boston, Massachusetts.

Grinspoon, L. and Hedblom, P. (1975) *The Speed Culture, Amphetamine Use and Abuse in America.* Cambridge, Mass.: Harvard University Press,

Goldstone, M.S. (1993) "Cat": Methcathinone — A New Drug of Abuse. *JAMA,* **269**, pp. 2508.

Haight, M.A. (1994) Drug Abuse Trends in San Diego County. In: *Epidemiologic Trends in Drug Abuse. Volume II: Proceedings Community Epidemiology Work Group June 1994.* Rockville, Maryland: National Institute on Drug Abuse. (NIH Pub. No. 94-3854).

Harrison, L. (1994) Raving in Colorado — An Amateur's Field Notes. In: *Epidemiologic Trends in Drug Abuse. Volume II: Proceedings Community Epidemiology Work Group June 1994.* Rockville, Maryland: National Institute on Drug Abuse. (NIH Pub. No. 94-3854).

Health and Human Services. (1994*) HHS Releases High School Drug Abuse and "DAWN"* Surveys. U.S. Department of Health and Human Services Press Release, Monday, December 12.

Irvine, G. and Chin, L. (1991) The environmental impact and adverse health effects of the clandestine manufacture of methamphetamine. In: M.A. Miller and N.J. Kozel (eds.) *Methamphetamine Abuse: Epidemiologic Issues and Implications.* NIDA Research Monograph 115. Rockville MD: US Dept. Health and Human Services

Johnston, L.D., O'Malley, P.M. and Bachman, J.G. (1991) *Drug Use Among American High School Seniors, College Students and Young Adults, 1975–1990, Volume 1 — High School Seniors.* Rockville, Maryland: National Institute on Drug Abuse, (DHHS Pub. No. [ADM] 91-1813).

King, P.K. and Coleman, J.H. (1987) Stimulants and Narcotic Drugs. *Pediatric Clinics of North America,* **34**(2), pp. 349–362.

Kotarba, J.A. (1993) *The Rave Scene in Houston, Texas: An Ethnographic Analysis.* Austin, Texas: Texas Commission on Alcohol and Drug Abuse.

Lake, C. and Quirk, R. (1984) Stimulants and look-alike drugs. *Psychiatric Clinics North America,* **7**, pp. 689–701.

Lukas, S.E. (1985) *The Encyclopáedia of Psychoactive Drugs: Amphetamines: Danger in the Fast Lane.* New York: Chelsea House Publishers.

Mellinger, G.D., Balter, M.B. and Manheimer, D.I. (1971) Patterns of Psychotherapeutic Drug Use Among Adults in San Francisco. *Archives of General Psychiatry,* November, pp. 385–395.

Miller, M.A. (1991) Trends and Patterns of Methamphetamine Smoking in Hawaii. In: M.A. Miller and N.J. Kozel (eds.), *National Institute on Drug Abuse Research Monograph Series No. 115: Methamphetamine Abuse: Epidemiologic Issues and Implications* Washington D.C.: Supt. of Docs., U.S. Govt. Print. Off. (DHHS Pub. No. [ADM]91-1836).

Miller, M.A. and Tomas, J.M. (1989) Past and current methamphetamine epidemics. In Epidemiologic Trends in Drug Abuse: Proceedings of the Community Epidemiology Work Group December 1989. Washington, D.C.: Supt. of Docs., U.S. Govt. Print. Off. (DHHS Pub. No. 721-757:20058).

Morgan, P., Beck, J., Joe, K., McDonnell D. and Guiterrez R. (1994) *Ice and other Methamphetamine Use.* Final Report to the National Institute on Drug Abuse. National Institute of Health. U.S. Government Printing Office.

Morgan, J.P. and Kagan, D.V. (1978) The Impact on Street Amphetamine Quality of the 1970 Controlled substances Act. *Journal of Psychedelic Drugs,* **10**, pp. 303–317.

National Institute of Justice (NIJ) (1994a) *Drug Use Forecasting 1993 Annual Report on Adult Arrestees: Drugs and Crime in America's Cities.* U.S. Department of Justice, Washington, D.C.: National Institute of Justice.

National Institute of Justice (NIJ) (1994b) *Drug Use Forecasting 1993 Annual Report on Juvenile Arrestees/Detainees: Drugs and Crime in America's Cities.* U.S. Department of Justice, Washington, D.C.: National Institute of Justice.

National Institute on Drug Abuse. (1986) *Drug Abuse Trends and Research Issues. Proceedings of the Community Epidemiology Work Group December 1986.* Supt. of Docs. Washington, D.C.: U.S. Govt. Print. Off. (DHHS Pub. No. 181-332:60315).

National Institute on Drug Abuse. (1989) *Methamphetamine Abuse in the United States.* Supt. of Docs., Washington D.C.: U.S. Govt. Print. Off. (DHHS Pub. No. [ADM]89-1608).

National Institute on Drug Abuse. (1994) *Epidemiologic Trends in Drug Abuse. Volume 1: Highlights and Executive Summary: Community Epidemiology Work Group (June 1994)* Rockville, Maryland: National Institute on Drug Abuse, (NIH Pub. No. 94-3853).

National Narcotics Intelligence Consumers Committee. (1993) *The NNICC Report 1992.* Washington, DC: Department of Justice, Drug Enforcement Administration.

Newmeyer, J.A. (1994) Drug Use in the San Francisco Bay Area. In: *Epidemiologic Trends in Drug Abuse. Volume II: Proceedings Community Epidemiology Work Group June 1994.* Rockville, Maryland: National Institute on Drug Abuse. (NIH Pub. No. 94-3854).

Newmeyer, J.A. (1988) The Prevalence of Drug Use in San Francisco in 1987. *Journal of Psychoactive Drugs,* **20**(2), pp. 185–189.

Newmeyer, J.A. (1978) The epidemiology of the Use of Amphetamine and Related Substances. *Journal of Psychedelic Drugs,* **10**(4), pp. 293–302.

Office of Applied Studies. (1994a) *"Statistical Series: Annual Emergency Room Data 1992 Data from the Drug Abuse Warning Network (DAWN)."* Series 1, No. 12 — A. Rockville, Maryland: Substance Abuse and Mental Health Services Administration. (DHHS Pub. No. [SMA]94-2080).

Office of Applied Studies (1994b) *Preliminary Estimates from the Drug Abuse Warning Network — 1993, Preliminary Estimates of Drug-Related Emergency Department Episodes. Advance Report Number 8, December 1994.* Rockville, Maryland: Substance Abuse and Mental Health Services Administration.

Office of National Drug Control Policy. (1995) *Pulse Check — National Trends in Drug Abuse.* Washington, D.C.: Executive Office of the President.

Pinkert, D. and Harwood H.J. (1993) Khat (*Cathaedulis*): Background and Policy Questions. Prepared for National Institute on Drug Abuse (in draft). Rockville, Maryland: Drug Abuse Policy Center.

Pittel, S.M. and Hofer, R. (1970) The Transition to Amphetamine Abuse. In: E.H. Ellinwood and S. Cohen (eds.) *Current Concepts on Amphetamine Abuse* National Institute of Mental Health, Washington, D.C.: Supt. of Docs., U.S. Govt. Print. Off. (DHEW Pub. No. [HSM]72-9085).

Puder, K.S., Kagan, D.V. and Morgan, J.P. (1988) Illicit methamphetamine: analysis, synthesis, and availability. *American Journal Drug Alcohol Abuse,* **14**, pp. 463–473.

Schoenberger, K. (1992) "Yakuza Expand on Mainland." Honolulu Advertiser, January 5.

Smith, R. (1969) The World of the Haight-Ashbury Speed Freak. *Journal of Psychoactive Drugs,* **2**(2), pp. 77–83.

Smith, R.C. (1970) Compulsive Methamphetamine Abuse and Violence in the Haight-Ashbury District. In: E.H. Ellinwood and S. Cohen (eds.) *Current Concepts on Amphetamine Abuse* National Institute of Mental Health. Washington, D.C.: Supt. of Docs., U.S. Govt. Print. Off. (DHEW Pub. No. [HSM]72-908).

Spotts, J.V. and Spotts, C.A. (1980) *Use and Abuse of Amphetamine and Its Substitutes.* NIDA Research Issues 25. Washington, D.C.: National Institute on Drug Abuse.

Thompson, H.S. (1967) *The Hell's Angels.* New York: Ballantine.

Wood, D.W. (1995) Illicit Drug Use in Honolulu and the State of Hawaii. In: *Epidemiologic Trends in Drug Abuse.* Volume II: Proceedings of the Community Epidemiology Work Group. In press.

Wrede, A.F. and Murphy L.D. (1994) Recent Drug Abuse Trends in the Seattle-King County Area. In: *Epidemiologic Trends in Drug Abuse. Volume II: Proceedings Community Epidemiology Work Group June 1994.* Rockville, Maryland: National Institute on Drug Abuse. (NIH Pub. No. 94-3854).

7

The Legacy and the Paradox: Hidden Contexts of Methamphetamine Use in the United States

PATRICIA MORGAN and JEROME E. BECK

INTRODUCTION

Obscured by the spotlight shining on inner-city cocaine and crack use, methamphetamine is quietly marking its third decade as the illicit drug of choice for many Americans. Unlike cocaine, with its centralized foreign production and distribution, methamphetamine is usually manufactured in small amounts, by independent and local networks in isolated rural areas throughout the United States. Like cocaine, however, methamphetamine also has a long and varied history involving its own urban legacy beginning with the 1950s' era of widespread pharmaceutical amphetamine use (Graham, 1972; Carey and Mandel, 1968). It has been known to fuel licit labours and underground economies in rural and suburban locales. Although it remains firmly entrenched in the hearts and minds of blue-collar workers, the nature and extent of methamphetamine use outside these areas remains virtually unknown.

For most of the past quarter century, methamphetamine's legacy in the United States remained hidden behind a veil of misconception and indifference. Recent evidence suggests that this veil may be falling only to expose the scope and depth of our ignorance. As Miller (Chapter 6) has shown, this period of neglect underscores the need to have a comprehensive systematic understanding of the methamphetamine legacy (Currie, 1993; Flynn, 1993). This was also illustrated in the findings which emerged from a community-based exploratory study comparing methamphetamine use in San Francisco, San Diego and Honolulu (Morgan *et al.*, 1994). The study found that twin markers representing depth and diversity defined the range and prevalence of methamphetamine use. It also found evidence of an enigma or paradox shaping the consequences of methamphetamine experiences for many users.

Several rationales guided the selection of these comparative study sites (Morgan *et al.*, 1994). One major criterion was the widespread prevalence of methamphetamine across diverse communities in each area. Another was that users in each site favoured a different mode of use. Intravenous methamphetamine use was particularly common in San Francisco, as was intranasal in San Diego, and smoking in Honolulu. Finally, the historical contribution to the legacy provided another reason for choosing these particular sites. The major impact of methamphetamine use on the social environment in each area took place in different historical periods linking together forty years of methamphetamine experience in the United States.

Beginning with popular and legal pharmaceutical amphetamine, San Francisco linked the original street speed scene of the 1950s to the takeover of illicitly produced methamphetamine by outlaw biker clubs (Graham, 1972; Carey and Mandel, 1968). Miller notes in chapter 6 how, after World War II, widespread availability fuelled increasing popular demand for pharmaceutical amphetamine (Grinspoon and Bakalar, 1987). Many were attracted by therapeutic and utilitarian motives, while others preferred diverted ampoules of liquid amphetamine used with heroin by injecting drug-using members of the 'beat' counter-culture. In fact successful government elimination of these ampoules from the street in the mid 1960s resulted in the first illicitly manufactured powder methamphetamine as a better replacement than pills for injecting amphetamine users (Carey and Mandel, 1968; Grinspoon and Hedblom, 1975; Miller, this volume).

Two major user groups on the street — Bohemians and African American members of various counter-culture street scenes — began producing initial batches of what became known as 'bathtub crank'. A woman who was a central counter-culture speed dealer beginning in the 1950s, spoke about that early experience:

> *The first lab I knew of was in a flower shop and the crank was truly made in a bathtub. It was ... the first illegal lab in the city. I had to tell them to use wet blankets to cover the doors and windows so the smell wouldn't come out. The old Chinese opium smokers I knew taught me this trick.*

One of the original African American cooks claims to have had a diverse clientele during those early years, stating that during the mid 1960s his regular customers included:

> *... white folks in North Beach, black folks in the Hunter's Point projects, whites in the avenues, and down the Peninsula, black*

folks in Oakland and Richmond, and white bikers in San Francisco and the East Bay … I sold to everyone. (043)

The increasing popularity of speed within outlaw biker organizations was due in part to the better rush offered by the new powdered crank.[1] More than amphetamine pills, the quick uptake of powder methamphetamine fits especially well within their fast-paced, hard-living deviant lifestyles. Realizing the big money to be made from bathtub crank, biker clubs began using fear and intimidation and quickly dominated the manufacture, distribution and sales of crank in Northern California. Flooding the city with an abundance of poor quality methamphetamine, biker distribution networks attracted a more marginal deviant group of young users who became known as 'speed freaks'. In the late 1960s, their uncontrolled and grotesquely heavy use patterns caused a dramatic rise in methamphetamine-related health and criminal problems leading to the prevailing belief that 'speed kills' (Kramer *et al.*, 1967; Rawlin, 1968). This 'speed epidemic' drove away almost all middle-class and most of the former Bohemian and African American users, resulting in a dramatic loss of status for methamphetamine (Morgan *et al.*, 1994). Symbolizing a rare common rejection of both mainstream and counterculture, the 'speed freak' became the definitive image of a methamphetamine user after the late 1960s (Grinspoon and Bakalar, 1976; D. Smith, 1969; R. Smith, 1969).

Societal concern shifted to and stayed with the explosive re-emergence of cocaine. Thus, when a resurgence of methamphetamine popularity in San Diego ushered in a second era of use during the early 1980s, it was almost completely overshadowed by the Drug War over crack (Haight, 1993). In San Diego, for example, although outlaw biker groups began making and distributing a form of methamphetamine called 'Peanut Butter Crank' in the 1960s, it did not spread beyond biker networks. The limited popularity of methamphetamine waned in San Diego during the early 1970s as cocaine became the leading stimulant of choice. In the early 1980s, organized crime syndicates began manufacturing ephedrine-type methamphetamine in the eastern areas of San Diego County. Known as 'crystal meth' it attracted a diverse population of new users. Young, working-class whites took to this local, long acting and inexpensive speed throughout the eighties, so that eventually San Diego became known as the 'Bogota' of methamphetamine in the US. However, little attention on the national arena focused on increasing production and use of this 'poor man's cocaine' which quietly continued to spread among marginalized working-class residents of economically declining suburban communities (Hall and Broderick, 1991).

---

[1] For a comprehensive discussion of outlaw biker involvement in methamphetamine manufacture and distribution see Chapter 3 in Morgan *et al.*, 1994.

The most recent era began in the late 1980s as huge quantities of 'ice' landed in Hawaii from the Far East, bringing major drug use transformations throughout the State (Lerner, 1989; Wood and Carlson, 1991). The government's successful eradication campaign against marijuana (known as 'pakalolo' in Hawaii) had severe and unintended consequences. Pakalolo was the traditional drug of choice widely used, integrated into the local Hawaiian culture, and an important income supplement for many local kinship networks. The campaign drove up prices, drastically reduced availability and left locals without their traditional substance. Thus when a new, easy to use, smokeable product called 'Ice' entered the drug market, it was readily accepted as a substitute of sorts for pakalolo (Joe-Laidler and Morgan, Chapter 8; Dayton, 1994).

Most Hawaiians were unaware of its effects. They knew nothing about methamphetamine, or thought that it was a completely different drug from ice. Thus most locals involved with marijuana production or sales thought in the beginning that ice was going to be a lucrative substitute, and was quickly integrated into existing family or kinship pakalolo distribution networks. Almost every local family in some communities had at least one member who dealt, furthering the illusion that ice was just another type of 'homegrown' dope.

Sadly, local dealers described making a lot of money quickly, quitting their legitimate jobs, smoking up all their profits, and eventually losing their homes and their family. Widespread heavy consumption patterns in many communities led to increased crime and violence as local kinship networks began to unravel. The serious social and health problems (Morgan *et al.*, 1994; Whitney, 1995; Dayton, 1994) which emerged also fuelled fears of a potential crack-type methamphetamine epidemic on the mainland (Holmes, 1989; Jaffe, 1989; Zurer, 1989). However, public anxiety quickly evaporated when the ice menace failed to produce the feared 'speed epidemic'. By 1993, 'ice' had settled into its own niche in the islands. Although known to have damaged or destroyed whole families and communities, it continued to have a sizeable user population. During the early 1990s, with cocaine taking up the spotlight, methamphetamine once again slipped back into the shadow of public consciousness. Its legacy continued to be overlooked by a dominant perception still fixated on the 1960s image of the speed freak which accompanied a common belief, voiced by Eric Goode, that "the street speed scene is interesting today mainly for historical reasons" (1993: p. 244). It appears that the ability of crack and cocaine to define characteristics of U.S. drug policy is matched by an inability to recognize evidence of substantial methamphetamine use and its consequences. Using evidence from a comparative community-based study on methamphetamine, this chapter focuses on methamphetamine to compare contexts of use among diverse user groups emerging in three separate locations during three distinct historical eras. In the process, this analysis reveals surprisingly complex and intriguing characteristics (Morgan *et al.*, 1994; Lovett, 1994).

RESEARCH QUESTIONS AND DESIGN

This exploratory study examined and compared methamphetamine use among 450 moderate-to-heavy users living in San Francisco, San Diego and Honolulu between 1991 and 1994. Research incorporated both qualitative and quantitative data collection methods into a grounded theory approach appropriate for exploratory research into unknown and/or hidden populations established first by Glaser and Strauss (1967). An extended pilot phase located and identified preliminary target populations and a systematic sampling design was constructed that incorporated chain referral methods (Watters and Biernacki, 1989). Theoretical sampling and saturation was achieved through simultaneous data collection and analysis allowing for early identification of emerging issues and trends. Consequently, historical processes of use were charted and complex and multiple rationales, meanings and consequences were uncovered that framed patterns of use over time in each of the study sites.

In particular, we were able to observe how use patterns and problems evolved over time were shaped by diverse contextual influences. Many San Francisco respondents recounted significant changes in use patterns, problems, modes and motives. Shifts in patterns of manufacture and distribution were also drawn from the narratives of long-time users. In addition, we explored various rituals, rules and folklore guiding user expectations and experiences across time and place, and examined respondent experimentation and preferences for alternate routes of administration to assess potentially problematic modal transitions among different user groups.

The study revealed that methamphetamine possessed properties far beyond that of a 'second rate stimulant'. It revealed instead that heavy and continued use of methamphetamine could result in paradoxical effects. For example, those using this drug for productive purposes often discovered that methamphetamine became less a 'means to an end' and more an end in itself. Other users motivated by methamphetamine's ability to enhance sexuality, overcome depression, or increase social bonding, often found that it eventually produced the opposite effect. The data illustrate methamphetamine's ability to seduce the user into a spiral of escalating use and problematic consequences. Surprisingly, for other respondents the paradox was a positive experience. For these users, methamphetamine produced a calming or centreing effect that enhanced their ability to focus and

concentrate. The concept of drug 'career' was used as a construct to understand the meaning and significance of the drug over time in an individual
drug user.

SITE AND SAMPLE CHARACTERISTICS

Although the majority of respondents were under 40 years of age, significant
differences were found across sites. Over half of the Honolulu and San
Diego samples were under 30 years of age (56% and 53%) compared to less
than a third in San Francisco (31%). Conversely, over 29% of respondents in
San Francisco were over 40 years old, compared to less than 7% in San
Diego, and 15% in Honolulu. Whites accounted for over 55% of our sample
overall, representing three quarters of San Francisco and San Diego respondents. In Honolulu, Asian Pacific Islanders accounted for 78% of the sample.
Female users comprised almost a third of respondents equally across study
sites.

The San Francisco Bay Area

This site included the city and county of San Francisco, along with communities in Marin County to the north, and in Alameda, and Contra Costa counties
to the east, which encompassed a large geographical area of over 500 square
miles. This area is the source of an especially rich history of methamphetamine use, clearly seen in the diverse characteristics found among its respondents. They were from Latino, African American, Asian Pacific American
and Native American and Anglo European backgrounds and ranged in age
from 21 to 60. They included gay, bisexual and transgendered men and
women, of extremely varied occupations and incomes, living anywhere from
inner-city transient hotels and homeless shelters to hillside suburban homes
or wealthy apartments in exclusive neighbourhoods. In general, however,
the majority of our sample were from working class backgrounds and were
drawn from two major geographical areas: the City of San Francisco, and
East Bay communities located in the Western parts of Alameda and Contra
Costa Counties.

Respondents from the city of San Francisco were drawn from inner-city
areas such as the Tenderloin, Polk Street, and South of Market. These are
neighbourhoods typified by transient hotels, public housing, topless bars,
sex shops, punk rock clubs and small commercial enterprises. The varied
population in these areas include recently arrived Asian immigrants, low
level criminals and hustlers, the mentally ill, alcoholics, substance abusers,
assorted homeless living on government assistance, and sex workers of both
genders. In addition, there were some respondents from varied city residential neighbourhoods, who frequented the more 'respectable' dance clubs and

bars. Three major user groups were found in this central city location: long time inner city users, gay and bisexual users and counterculture youth users.

Those defined as *longtime inner city users* traced their methamphetamine careers back to the time of plentiful supplies of pharmaceuticals during the 1950s and 1960s. Since that time, most had led marginal lifestyles and were now found living in downtown neighbourhoods, alternating between jail, public assistance and periods of hustling and dealing drugs. They included *African American, Latino* and *Anglo* survivors of earlier methamphetamine eras. Compared to users in other sites they were the oldest and had used for the longest number of years (see Morgan *et al.*, 1994). Approximately a third of this group were *African American* long time users. They were an important part of San Francisco's original speed subculture and had played major roles as pioneers in the manufacture and distribution of the first illicit methamphetamine produced in California in the 1960s. These African Americans were older, compared to long time inner city users as a whole (averaging 45.3 years old) and also reported the lengthiest methamphetamine use histories, averaging over 20 years. These user groups, defined by a lengthy and common history, along with similar survival needs, marked these users in San Francisco more than others in the study, as representative of a more traditional subculture or user group.

Also found in San Francisco's urban neighbourhoods, were *gay and bisexual* respondents who represented over half of the total 71 gay and bisexual users interviewed in this study. Accounting for almost a third of San Francisco respondents, they represented a higher proportion of IV users compared to the overall gay and bisexual sample. They were from a number of ethnic backgrounds and included substantial numbers of *Latino* and *African American* gay and bisexual users. For gay or bisexual males methamphetamine use was inextricably entwined with their sexual behaviour. Many were employed as sex workers either as hustlers or as 'escorts'.

The third user type from central San Francisco were *counterculture youth* members of punk, grunge or other alternative scenes. Unlike more mainstream counterparts from the suburbs, they were full-time members of the street scene. Living in the Tenderloin, South of Market or Haight Street areas, they included a high proportion of women and IV users, often relying on petty crime, drug sales and various types of sex work to make a living. Others floated in and out of mainstream life, and would rotate from living off a boyfriend or girlfriend, crashing with friends or family to renting a room in a transient hotel. They tended to be under thirty years of age and were often found at rave scenes and other underground music locales.

The powerful legacy of methamphetamine defines the character of several communities found in sections of Contra Costa and Alameda counties East of San Francisco. These generally rundown and economically declining suburban communities include the towns of Richmond, Pinole, El Sobrante, San Pablo, along with parts of San Leandro, Hayward and Castro Valley. The city of Richmond has a sizeable African American population that came to work in the shipyards during the war and stayed to take on blue-collar jobs in the oil refineries and on the docks. The resident population in the other area comprises mostly Anglo blue-collar families who settled in the area after World War II to work in the now defunct steel and shipbuilding industries. There were two overlapping user types found in this area. The first, undereducated and underemployed, can be defined as *marginal lower-class Anglos*. Here, the use of methamphetamine was widespread across several generations of users who shared what Currie (1993) described as a "considerable local tradition and language" involving methamphetamine:

> *[It] goes back a long way in some of these families.... The kids have grown up with it, known about it all their lives, parents quite regular users, often for utilitarian reasons ... What did surprise me was the frequent stories of having been turned on to it by their parents. (CC #2)*

The strength of this legacy in these communities can be partially traced to its history as one of the earliest sites of methamphetamine production by outlaw biker groups in California. Today, *outlaw biker users* continue to play a major role in production in this area. The considerable overlap with Anglo working-class users underscores the notoriety of these communities as a particular domain of the Hell's Angels. Half of the forty respondents from this area reported some type of affiliation with *outlaw biker* groups. The overwhelming majority had criminal records and were heavily involved in the manufacture and distribution of methamphetamine.

The study also exposed significant methamphetamine use among *African American* residents of these East Bay Cities. As part of the same working class migration during the Second World War, the members of this community shared the same economic history and hardships as their Anglo neighbours. The younger generations also shared a preference for methamphetamine use and as residents of the methamphetamine heartland they were able to utilize longstanding Anglo distribution networks. Several of these respondents reported that they switched to smoking methamphetamine as a way of breaking a heavy crack habit.

The San Diego Area

Although this study site included segments of all five major districts in San Diego County, the target sampling design found the highest concentration of users primarily in three of these districts. The first was the South Bay District which included the coastal communities of Mission Beach, Ocean Beach, and Imperial Beach. Here, trendy and upper-middle class communities mixed with a number of lower-class 'beach' subcultures which included the traditional 'surfer bums', Punks, skateboarders, and a number of fearsome looking 'pseudo' bikers — united by the predominance of tattoos, and pierced body parts.

The inner city district included older neighbourhoods within central San Diego. These comprise residential areas made up of small clapboard houses inhabited largely by minority populations, especially Mexicans and Latinos. *Latino users* generally made their living by petty theft and/or dealing. All but one reported engaging in methamphetamine sales, mostly on a lower level. Many were members of gang organizations, some of which were reported to have connections with distribution networks in Mexico. More smokers (25%) were found among Latinos than other users in this site. This may be linked to the popularity of smoking methamphetamine in 'light bulbs'.[1] The neighbourhoods closer to downtown were made up of older rundown hotels and apartments, shelters for the homeless, and blocks of empty lots and boarded up abandoned buildings. Most of the inhabitants were living below the poverty line, and included homeless, mentally ill, older IV drug users, African American dealers and hustlers, and recent illegal immigrants.

The third major district encompasses East San Diego County, which is considered to be the heart of methamphetamine use and the domain of criminal methamphetamine manufacturers. According to a community consultant from this area:

> *The sparsely populated back country provides ample territory for cooking operations, isolationists and otherwise independent folk who have little love for government and cities. (cc #4)*

The urban landscape is made up of high density apartment complexes surrounded by auto repair garages, thrift shops, discount stores, along with welfare, homeless and other county service centres. These East County communities are home to *Anglo working class, welfare mothers* and *biker user types.* The marginal *Anglo working class* respondents from Eastern San Diego county possess similar characteristics but are generally younger and less experienced than their East San Francisco Bay Area counterparts. Respondents in these communities largely avoided injecting methamphetamine, and tended to choose smoking instead. A major user group was *welfare mothers.* These were female respondents on welfare found living in subsidized housing in poor suburban East County communities. Most married and/or had children during their late teens or early adult years and found that methamphetamine provided long lasting energy for managing children and household chores. Almost all were selling, dealing or distributing methamphetamine providing an economic supplement which also financed their continued use.

The Honolulu Area

Methamphetamine use in Honolulu was unique in several respects. There was little history of methamphetamine use among ice smokers. Many had not made a connection between the highly concentrated rock imported from the East which is smoked, with the crank and speed which were snorted or injected which they knew to be methamphetamine. For most respondents methamphetamine use was a very recent phenomenon. Less than 15% of this sample reported using methamphetamine for more than seven years. Most of these were Anglos who began using crystal methamphetamine on the mainland. Also unique to Honolulu was the central role of *Asian Pacific Americans* in the use of ice methamphetamine. Although ice in Hawaii is a problem seen in all ethnic groups, *Asian Pacific Americans* accounted for over three quarters of respondents in Honolulu and reflected the extensive ethnic diversity found among Asians in Hawaii. They included: Japanese, Chinese, Korean, Filipino, Native Hawaiian and Samoan with over a half self-identified as of mixed ethnicity. These ethnicities represented long-term residents in Honolulu and fit the ethnic proportion in the general population (see Joe, 1995). Some of these respondents were drawn from metropolitan Honolulu neighbourhoods with large Filipino, Samoan and Pacific Islander populations. Suburban areas on the south and Leeward coasts included mixed ethnic communities with large numbers of Filipino and Native Hawaiian residents. In each of these areas extended kinship networks commonly played prominent roles in the use and distribution of meth and other drugs (see Joe-Laidler and Morgan, this volume).

DOMAINS OF USE

Energy Enhancement

We found a greater tendency among Anglo working class respondents from California to use methamphetamine initially for increased energy on the job. This was commonly cited by those employed in occupations requiring intensive and/or prolonged hours of labour. Many claimed that speed helped them to survive and even enjoy otherwise tedious and/or, physically demanding jobs. One El Cajon man described how he was introduced to 'peanut butter crank' by his boss to increase productivity:

> *I think I was 18 and a senior in high school and I was working in a waterbed manufacturing place. This guy who ran it, the manager, used to … do the same job you did. He'd stand next to you and he'd … do it 100 times faster! This guy was wired out of his mind! The*

first thing he'd do in the morning was put a bunch of peanut butter crank in his coffee and then all day long, he'd be doing spoons of crank! Finally, he decided to up the production on the floor and he started giving me and my friend spoons of crank. I can remember, even after work, I'd go home and be wired. (205)

For other users methamphetamine eliminated the boredom associated with other types of mundane tasks. One 30 year-old woman described herself as a 'white tornado' ready to clean house for countless hours. "It got me wound up, I thought I was on top of the world. There was nothing I couldn't do when I was wired. I could clean everything! (070)" Welfare mother respondents, especially those from San Diego, commonly described how methamphetamine provided the means to undertake household tasks with renewed interest. One woman reported sessions lasting 48 hours or more.

I stayed up and did my bills, got my paperwork done, got my coupons organized, started projects I had been procrastinating on like filling photo albums and doing baby books. Just getting caught up on laundry and housework. I never stopped! (343)

Unfortunately, for most who first tried methamphetamine to improve their work capacity, increased and prolonged use had the opposite effect. Respondents reported becoming increasingly dysfunctional after prolonged use, especially after transitions to a stronger mode of use. For example one respondent described the difficulties encountered as a hair cutter when she switched from snorting to shooting meth, and bingeing for longer periods of time:

You do become dysfunctional. You shake real bad, that's kind of hard when you're cutting hair! ... After doing it for a couple of days, [you] definitely become slower. You think you're going fast but you're going slower. At first you're going real fast and then the more you stay on it, you start slowing up and then your hands start shaking and your vision gets blurry. (002)

Many working-class users who began using speed to increase energy at work developed problems from their meth use which caused them to lose their jobs. It was common for users to be fired by the same person who first introduced them to the drug at work. Those who began using to increase energy for weekend social and recreational activities, attempted extensive methamphetamine binges without interfering with work week responsibilities. The tendency for 'weekends' to encompass much more than two days became particularly evident when the drug's long lasting consequences eventually impaired work performance which was remedied by extending use into the work week.

Many eventually gravitated towards daily use of large amounts allowing only occasional brief periods of rest and recuperation. This was true across all sites and among all user types. In the 12 months prior to the interview, only 5% of respondents overall were able to maintain a daily sleep pattern while using. A typical 'use episode' involved three or more days without sleep for over two-thirds of our sample in San Francisco, 54% in San Diego, and 60% in Honolulu. Furthermore, almost one fifth of Honolulu respondents averaged seven days or more without sleep during a typical episode.

Performance

Even though prolonged bingeing often resulted in loss of employment, the episodes themselves continued to be filled with paradoxical patterns of activity where respondents typically spent their time 'tweaking' — that is, fixated for hours on the same activity of 'fixing', 'tinkering' or 'artistic crafting'. The pattern of taking things apart and putting them back together was so common in San Diego that respondents often referred to it as the McGyver Syndrome after a popular TV show where the hero created ingenious contraptions out of assorted material. In the case of our respondents, however, a common appliance more often ended up as an ingenious, if unintentional collection of assorted parts. One respondent described what happened when he tried to find a new way to heat up a light bulb for smoking methamphetamine:

> *At first ... I want some way to heat this light bulb up because I didn't want to use a lighter cause it turned everything black. I hated this black shit, so o.k. a little stove, or maybe the heating element of the coffee pot, and I would take this things apart and find out no, this doesn't work, so then you got a perfectly ruined coffee pot, you got this torn apart, that torn apart, you got friend around wondering 'Hey what the Hell is this guy doing, that thing worked yesterday'?. Just uncontrolled energy thinking you can do anything, or I can take this and turn it into that, I guess the McGyver effect. (296)*

For many, especially male users in San Diego, tweaking gave them license to tinker — to perform with a goal perhaps, but always free from deadlines. A San Diego woman claimed that speed gave her a lot of energy "... but it was going nowhere ... couldn't finish anything. I'd start a little of this, go to that, I'm moving real fast but I was getting nothing done." Thus, being busy while high on meth, had a paradoxical effect, or as one respondent described it.

> *... speed is a real funny name for the drug! The longer you do it, the slower you get! ... It's like watching the wheels of a car spinning*

so fast it starts to turn backwards or stand still. That's what speed does. (059)

Eventually, heavy prolonged bingeing patterns ended, to be replaced by the inevitable prolonged discomfort of the comedown which often lasted for days. Known as the 'Post Crystal Syndrome', one user in San Diego offered this very articulate description:

> *There's a certain pattern, ... your first day off you're okay because the stuff is still kicking in your system so you don't feel the high that you did but you don't feel the down that you're going to. On the second day, you become a zombie, some Haitian voodoo doctor's idea of a good human being! ... you're an eating and sleeping machine! You get what we call the "waking nods"! Third day is even worse, it's the absolute coma. The only time that you wake up are the times you want to eat! Fourth day, same thing! It's kind of a mimic of the second day, you're a zombie ... You have no motivation, you don't have a terrible desire to do the drug because you know it won't work on you! Fifth day, you start to wake up. ... you get a glimmer of your real self back and that's the time you start again! Go back out and find some and you do it and boom, you're right back up to where you were. (205)*

Across most dimensions of activity the initial desire for increased energy or performance circled in to form its own paradox where increased energy became increasingly unfocussed.

Sexuality and Sexual Performance

Although commonly believed to enhance sexuality and sexual performance, we found a range of opinions and experiences describing a more complex picture. Gay users as well as Asian Pacific American males in Honolulu stand out as the most enthusiastic devotees of 'meth sex', but for different reasons. Honolulu males spoke most often about methamphetamine in terms of durability. Gay and bisexual users, on the other hand, tended to speak about methamphetamine ability to release inhibitions. A gay male hustler described this effect from injecting the drug the first time he used meth.

> *There was a party going on and I heard about all these wonderful experiences about doing speed. Shooting it up and these sexual feelings that went with it. I wanted to try it. My friend fixed me up a point and I did it. The feeling and the rush was so incredible, intense. I was running around trying to have sex with everybody! (035)*

Many non gay IV users were equally enthusiastic. For them enhanced sexual pleasure was closely linked to the IV rush from methamphetamine. One San Diego user described every injection experience as a sexual one stating "... When I slam meth, I go off to that sexual drive high.... It increases ... euphoria in your head, your mind comes ... (324)" Another long-time female user from San Francisco who began injecting liquid ampoules in the mid 1960s, had no doubts about its sexual effects:

> *... when a woman does a hit of crank, a woman comes. Climaxes! Every woman who has ever done crank, that happens. That's why so many women like it. Unlike men, who climax every time they ball, that doesn't happen with women. It's something that nothing else does. (055)*

A number of respondents in each site experienced extremely heightened and prolonged sexual activity of marathon dimensions. A 30 year-old woman described never leaving her bedroom during a two-week marathon with her partner:

> *I had no idea it was two weeks! It was a lot of sex, listen to the stereo, more sex, do dope, talk, have more sex, for two weeks ... I could a went for more! My kids missed me! Days turned into nights and nights turned into days! (070)*

Many respondents, however, found that eventually methamphetamine use eliminated or impeded sexual desire. Males especially complained of pharmacological inhibition of orgasm and erectile difficulties resulting from heavy and prolonged use (Estep and MacDonald, 1993; Morgan *et al.*, 1994).

Social Contexts

Many respondents, especially 'local' Hawaiians, and Latinos in San Diego reported that methamphetamine gave them the opportunity to hang out with buddies, and made it easier for them to bond with their social network ... to be "part of the ritual". Respondents were rarely able to sustain use in recreational or social contexts. For most, what began as a social drug eventually led to solitude in which users would stay isolated for hours, days or weeks, often in a single room

> *At first, I wanted to go out and be with people. At the middle and towards the end ... I didn't want to be around anybody! I just wanted to be by myself. My best friend was my pipe, I was happy! It never took anything from me. I blamed everything on my friends, not the drug! (469)*

Over one half of our respondents reported that isolation eventually merged into paranoia, and described experiences which were remarkably similar across many different user groups. A common experience involved standing for hours peeking through a curtain, looking for the police who they believed were hiding in the bushes. Another common example:

> *I see things laying in bed, staring at the wall or ceiling. I look for shadows and get paranoid. Be peeking out my window every five minutes! While everybody else is asleep, I'm thinking somebody is going to steal my car or stuff like that. (248)*

Men, in particular, described how paranoia progressively led to increased irritability, anger or violence. Forty-four percent of male respondents reported violence due to methamphetamine use. Violence was highest (among both male and female) respondents in Hawaii — 44% of females in Honolulu reported violent behaviour, compared to 37% in San Diego and only 18% in San Francisco. A San Diego respondent speaks of the convergence of several effects from long-term heavy use by his friends.

> *Yeah, I've seen ... people who, pre-meth use, were ... normal people. Actually they were over-achievers and once ... introduced to the culture and really dove into it, turned into hermits that never rarely left their house ... I've seen major paranoia ... It's done some pretty remarkable things to fairly normal people. (254)*

Confidence, Clarity and Focus

A significant minority of respondents reported experiencing dramatic positive psychological effects linked to their use of methamphetamine. This seemed to be especially true for those who were hyperactive as children. Many were part of the era when the explosive increase in diagnoses of childhood hyperactivity was fuelled by the promotion of pharmaceutical amphetamine compound medicines, such as Ritalin, which were used to manage this disorder. Over 10% of San Francisco respondents and 5%–7% in our San Diego and Hawaii sites recalled being medically diagnosed as 'hyperactive' as children often resulting in their use of prescription stimulants at a very early age. In addition, much greater numbers of respondents in each site self-diagnosed themselves as hyperactive children. An intriguing and somewhat interrelated finding concerns those respondents reporting a history of asthma problems. These respondents also were exposed to various stimulant compounds, which were among the medications making up the armamentarium combating serious asthmatic attacks.

The most intriguing finding reveals that in all three sites, the respondents that reported histories of either asthma or hyperactivity uniformly stated that methamphetamine had a calming or centreing effect on their mood and/or behaviour. Although defined as a strong stimulant these respondents uniformly felt greater clarity and less 'speediness' with methamphetamine than they felt with other stimulants such as cocaine. Like other asthmatics in our sample this user describes the effect as 'calming'.

> *Instead of getting me up, because I'm asthmatic, it had an opposite effect … calmed me down and slowed me down…. I was able to sleep normally. It was when I mixed it with asthma medicine or cocaine freebase, then I'd get a mean rush! The mix of meth and cocaine would keep me up. … Sometimes I'd get a feeling of soberness, sometimes a feeling of strength or euphoria. It was never disoriented, it was always a feeling of clarity. (468)*

Methamphetamine had a similar effect on respondents with histories of depression at least during period of initial use. For many depression disappeared after initial use. As one user describes:

> *[it] brought me out of my depression. After the high was over with, I felt fine. The depression I had for years was gone! I felt beautiful and pretty. I felt like everything I should have been during the high … Not hungry. Energy. It felt wonderful. The best feeling I've ever felt. … Pretty, successful, makes you feel really beautiful. Like I can achieve what I want to achieve. … I could handle doing everything I had to do if I was on speed. It gave me that extra, needed touch. (094)*

Respondents in all sites reported that methamphetamine helped them to feel emotionally detached from the pain and struggle of their daily existence.

> *Sometimes, when I don't want to be depressed or melancholy, I know that I can get the euphoria and at the same time become detached in emotional ways, it really does occur. … in a way, it makes you a little bit, it does cut off emotion. It does make you hardened to emotions. (115)*

For many who began using the drug to decrease depression, loss of control and increasing dependency produced an effect where depression entered on the heels of massive guilt:

> *The things I was doing, the guilt; and I couldn't look at myself in the mirror no more. Cause I didn't want to see myself, knowing the things that I had done to my family and to others. So, ice made me didn't give a shit about myself anymore. Or anybody else! (403)*

Eventually however, over two-thirds of the total sample reported that depression was a serious consequence of prolonged heavy use. It was seen most among San Diego respondents and least among veteran users in San Francisco.

CONTROLLING THE PARADOX

The negative paradoxical effects which framed the experience for many of our methamphetamine users was not uniform, nor was it universal. A substantial proportion, particularly older, more experienced users, eventually managed to stabilize their use with diverse and multiple efforts that maximized benefits and minimized problems. Users employed a range of strategies in the hope that this would enable continued use of methamphetamine. Some attempted to follow particular rituals, while others made a conscious effort to live by a set of normative values and principles. These acted to govern those aspects of everyday life held to be important to a particular respondent. A very common example is found in a long time female user who established a set of rules governing her monthly methamphetamine high, which allowed her to safeguard her responsibilities to her children. She described a process which began when she received her monthly $688 welfare cheque.

> *When I buy speed at the beginning of the month, I buy me 1/16th.*
> *... I like to be high three days, ... If I'm high three days it's worth it.*
> *I don't feel like I'm cheating myself! ... ... I pay my rent first. ... I*
> *buy food ... Then I buy speed.... This was the understanding with*
> *my children, I'm high three days and don't bother me! [laughs] They*
> *don't. I cook and prepare food in the freezer. All they had to do was*
> *put it in the oven! I made sure they had money, I made sure I did*
> *everything I had to do for them. That was the understanding be-*
> *tween me and them. We never lost that. ... I took care of my kids.*
> *Always, no matter what. Ain't no such thing as I'm high and I ain't*
> *gonna take care of my kids, never hungry! Clean clothes and*
> *combed hair. Those always be my kids, my responsibility. (149)*

Another user constructed survival rules involving regular food and rest, especially during heavy binges.

> *Before morning, about 4:00, I'd lay down and rest. At least stop*
> *and think! I tried to eat a little bit all the time, especially drink some*
> *V8 juice and keep myself healthy enough to get high! That was very*
> *important to me, I understood and saw the affects of being able to*
> *stay a little healthy to get high still. I always utilized it as such.*
> *(293)*

'Control' and 'addiction' defined the context of rules and rituals among our respondents. Although 60% of the sample reported 'ever' feeling addicted to methamphetamine, only 48% stated they had lost control over their use. This discrepancy was more pronounced among women users who were more likely to report feeling addicted to their use of methamphetamine than men but less likely to report losing control over their use than men. The major exceptions were Honolulu male respondents with a slightly greater percentage reporting addiction than loss of control. Analysis of the qualitative data suggests a significant number of our respondents considered themselves to be 'controlled addicts'. Respondents often talked about addiction as if it were a normal consequence. However, there were several different interpretations which defined the basis of their addiction. Whether respondents saw their addiction as physical or psychological, they all had very strong feelings about being either in control or out of control.

An important finding was that women generally were described, by both male and female respondents, to be more likely to retain control over their use and of their lives while using methamphetamine. Qualitative data also revealed that women were more likely to stress the ways they managed to stay in control, while men were more likely to discuss how they had lost control. Women users often provided evidence on the importance of self control through numerous and dramatically different stories describing their ability to maintain control regardless of the mode or level of use. The establishment of set rules governing control were key factors among women from all study sites and user lifestyles. They often constructed rules to help minimize negative consequences by controlling the set and setting of their use.

> *If it's a hassle to get it, I won't. … I won't buy from just anybody! …*
> *I don't want to be with other people when I get high. Not in a room*
> *full of strangers. Also, I wait until I get home to shoot up. … I don't*
> *do anybody's hit. I get high with people I know and watch the*
> *amount I take. I never have felt out of control with my use. Because*
> *I have these rules, I don't even think about the rest. I've done it for a*
> *long time and know how to be safe and not get busted. I don't ever*
> *desperately need it! (027)*

Moreover, we found that the majority of women respondents used these rules of self-control to construct successful careers in the illicit methamphetamine economy (Morgan and Joe-Laidler, in press). For example, a woman who injected almost a gram daily also managed a highly successful high-level methamphetamine distribution enterprise. While raising her children in a very upper middle class environment she has been able to maintain a very controlled business enterprise by dealing only in pounds and limiting her sales activity to one hour per day. She described myriad self-made rules keeping her from slipping out of control.

I have this phobia of something controlling me! Don't get me wrong, this controls me but, I have some kind of hold on it and I refuse to give in. If I have been up two or three days and I feel like I'm getting detached, I don't want to let myself get to the point where it could get any further. You hear these horror stories all the time and I refuse to let myself get to that point. So, if there's any warning signs of any kind, I listen to them and I'll go lay down and go to sleep. If I need to eat then I'll eat. … I don't want to hallucinate, I don't want to be in la-la land where I have no control over what I'm seeing … I know when I get these little signs that it's time to go to bed, then I don't let it over power me. I never let it come before my rent or food! Ever since I started doing it, I made money on it so I can have my own personal stash, without it coming out of money that is already spent. (297)

Qualitative analyses of interview data from both sexes revealed that, although women were significantly more likely to maintain control over their lives and their use, they were also more likely to hold on to the illusion of control long after they lost it. This was especially true for women with histories of parental or spouse abuse and unsuccessful treatment experiences.

SUMMARY

Contrast and Similarity

We found surprising similarities linking particular user groups across the three study sites. We also found some interesting diversity within sites. For example, the overwhelming majority of our respondents came from traditional working class backgrounds. In the California sites, the marginal Anglo working class user type represents a large proportion of the study sample. In each area they lived in declining economic communities on the periphery of coastal urban cities. Eastern San Diego county respondents possessed similar characteristics but were also generally younger and less experienced than their San Francisco East Bay counterparts. Most of the Asian/Pacific American respondents in Honolulu lived in very similar working-class environments and suffered from almost identical economic marginality. Furthermore, although using for less period of time, it was common to find users in Honolulu from two or three generations smoking ice within the family.

A significant concern that emerged from respondent interviews were the many reports of seriously dysfunctional family histories. These include accounts of serious parental drug and alcohol problems, as well as physical and sexual abuse. The qualitative interviews of respondents' life histories revealed the ways in which these childhood experiences shaped later patterns and consequences of methamphetamine use. Growing up within extremely stressful, abusive, and often violent family environments was the most commonly reported background history across study sites and user populations. Moreover, the types of experience were surprisingly similar, and often were interconnected. The high proportion of respondents reporting parental alcohol and/or drug problems described how it provided the setting for an entire range of abusive behaviours. The majority of respondents who grew up with a substance-abusing parent spoke of living under extremely stressful, and often dangerous, conditions. In Honolulu especially, spouse and child abuse almost always accompanied a parent's heavy use of alcohol or drugs. Approximately one-third of the males stated that their fathers would beat their mothers after heavy drinking episodes, and that they themselves suffered from regular physical beatings. Approximately 40% of the females in Honolulu described living in extraordinarily violent homes with a third being physically abused by one or both parents, or sexually abused by their father or close male relative (See Joe, 1995).

Extremely abusive histories were also common among inner-city 'outlaw' women users in both California sites. Their background experience usually included sexual molestation by a family member. Running away from sexual abuse was the most common reason given for beginning their life on the streets. Most had made this transition before age 18, and several left home permanently as young adolescents. Although more serious abuses were found among these respondents in Honolulu and downtown San Francisco, the majority of respondents growing up in economically disenfranchised communities in all sites describe substance abuse, violence and sexual abuse as common experiences in their families and in their communities. We found abuse so pervasive in the childhood environments of poor and lower-class respondents that most grew up under the assumption that they had 'normal' upbringings. This might have created a particular conflict. Although they may not have felt stigmatized within their own community, they eventually realized that other more affluent communities lived under different values and norms. Faced with this potential conflict, many respondents felt less marginalized and more secure remaining in their home environment, knowing as adults they were living in a 'deviant' community. This was especially true among respondents in economically declining, and often more geographically isolated areas found in each site. Those who escaped from abusive homes were faced with traumatic and stressful lives on the street and tended to form tight social support networks drawn together by common abuse experiences and by similar needs and patterns of drug use. The 'outlaw' users in downtown San Francisco, for example, built long lasting support networks perhaps created in order to feel less marginalized.

A major commonality across sites concerned the large percentage of respondents who grew up in households involving significant parental drug and alcohol problems. Over half stated that one or both parents had serious alcohol problems. Moreover, 44% of respondents reported parental use of marijuana, 22% parental use of methamphetamine, and 20% parental use of cocaine. Among those reporting illicit drug use by parents, almost half stated that one or both parents had serious problems with use of an illicit drug. These were equally reported in all three sites. A trend common to the vast majority of these respondents was the tendency toward self-destructive behaviour including heavy drinking and drug use beginning at very young ages.

We found biker user groups differed significantly between sites. Biker networks were more organized in the San Francisco Bay Area, there were many older users, and younger biker users represented second and even third generation users within a family or organization. In San Diego, they were much less organized and tended to be younger. These were young emulators who represented the second era of use beginning in the early 1980s.

Methamphetamine Use in the Context of American Values

In 1962, as law enforcement began its campaign against illicit methamphetamine laboratories, the American Medical Association Council on Drugs issued a report claiming that there was little reason for concern associated with the 8–12 billion amphetamine pills produced annually. According to Edison (1978) the irony of such simultaneous condemnation and complacency was also connected to the frequent reluctance of Western cultures to control (meth)amphetamine production. Both stemmed from initial unrealistic expectations of the drug's positive attributes. In fact, he argues that the image of the (meth)amphetamine user is linked to the most prized American virtues:

> *intense activity, efficiency, persistence and drive, and the desire to excel,to break records, and to move with even greater speed. These are admirable behavior patterns that are not easily relinquished, even when a drug is required to achieve them (Edison, 1978: 609).*

We found that although the perception of the methamphetamine user is no longer positive, those traits are still connected to the drug by our users who reported every one of these "widely admired American traits" as important motivations for their early use of methamphetamine. The most common of these involved the drug's ability to improve endurance and function: that is, to accomplish tasks, to do so quickly, efficiently and in greater numbers with enthusiasm.

According to Grinspoon and Hedblom (1975) amphetamine seemed to fit ideally into the cultural mind set, because it was a drug "whose psychopharmacological properties accord with their ideas of behavior and performance". Given that these traits are highly valued in the work place, it becomes clear why so many of our respondents were introduced to methamphetamine on the job, often by their supervisors or employers. In addition, we found

Edison's (1978) assertion that the "unrealistic expectations" of the drug's attributes led to over consumption then crisis on a societal level offers a partial explanation for the paradoxical effect of methamphetamine. For our respondents, their initial positive experiences led to unrealistic expectations and overuse, which in most cases, evolved into problematic binge patterns and serious consequences.

Although socioeconomic characteristics of the user ran through many findings on patterns, motives and consequences, there were several interconnecting issues which establish the strength of class-based dynamics raised by the findings in this study. Among respondents with lower-working class backgrounds, we found a major commonality in strongly held values of a 'work ethic'. Respondents defined a range of activities and motivations which were remarkably close to the American traits described by Edison (1978). Methamphetamine's perceived ability to improve functioning on the job was seen as attainment of a worthy goal. In other words, the drug not only made tedious or strenuous jobs more enjoyable, it also helped them to value the experience.

Respondents continued to speak of a work ethic even after their drug use began to impede their work performance, causing many to lose their jobs. Paradoxically, our evidence suggests that the subjective meaning remained linked to this initial motivation, even though their activities could no longer be defined as productive. Although many perceived methamphetamine to increase their ability to function, the activities themselves changed as use evolved into heavier often bingeing episodes. Within this recreated reality they continued to engage in activities which they defined as functioning, but without control. Sadly, 'work ethics' often turned into 'tweaking ethics' where the ability to function was trapped on a treadmill.

Methamphetamine and U.S. Drug Policy

In many ways, findings from this study raised as many questions as answers. We found that the legacy of methamphetamine has been shaped partly by the drug policies, steeped in the cocaine culture which surrounds it, and partly by the strength of traditional sovereignty belonging to particular user groups. Across both of these is the yet unknown influence of the particular paradoxical effects peculiar to methamphetamine.

The perils of powders

The history of legal actions against amphetamine suggests that unintended consequences often become dominant forces in shaping methamphetamine availability. For example, the removal of liquid methamphetamine ampoules from the outpatient prescription market in 1963 had a significant impact on injectors accustomed to the purity of the product and its ease of administration. According to longtime respondents, this seemingly insignificant control effort created a demand for a new illicit enterprise — the illegal manufacturing of water-soluble powder methamphetamine. Clandestine laboratories mushroomed, producing increasing amounts of powder of uncontrolled standards and unreliable quality organized through closed networks of out-law biker clubs, a combination which only furthered the deviant notoriety of both the producer and the product. As law enforcement clamped down on biker manufacturing and distribution networks, driving them further under-ground, it also encouraged new and independent cooks and distribution networks to emerge, and 'crank' became even less controlled and more toxic. Successful government efforts to cut off the availability of essential chemicals for manufacturing P2P crank resulted in the emergence of the ephedrine reduction process of cooking methamphetamine (see Morgan *et al.*, 1994). This method used easier-to-buy precursors, and was easier to make, further encouraging the growth of many more small, local independent operations, with even more product variability, while further expanding the population of users. By the mid 1980s crystal manufacturing and its use had exploded throughout the western United States. In addition to the potential hazards posed by toxic byproducts or adulterants, the uncertain potency typically fosters overuse to ensure desired effects from products of widely varying and unpredictable potency (Chesher, 1991).

The continuing campaign against marijuana

The study also found that successful periodic campaigns designed to elimi-nate this 'evil herb', served to steer the user toward more dangerous sub-stances, including methamphetamine. Grinspoon and Hedblom (1975) note the factors that might have induced American society of the 1930s to greet the arrival of amphetamines as medical marvels while simultaneously con-demning the 'killer weed':

> *While marijuana was being brought to the public's attention as a menace capable of wreaking great havoc, amphetamines were in-troduced and promoted as perhaps the earliest technology-derived drug to provide "better living through chemistry." Amphetamines were products of modern technology; they came from the laborato-ries of great corporations, and, in the days before the growth of consumer skepticism, this lent them legitimacy; unlike the danger-ous foreign weed, they seemed to have reliable, safe, known proper-ties. And, of course, they had the backing of medical authority (Grinspoon and Hedblom, 1975: p. 289).*

Findings on the social consequences of ice in Honolulu demonstrated that the latest version of the American campaign against marijuana continues to have the same unfortunate consequences. As government authorities began the campaign to eradicate marijuana in the 1980s, a smokable drug known as 'batu' from the traditional home of Island Filipinos, began to be used in place of the increasingly rare and expensive pakalolo. However, batu was not a traditional intoxicant like pakalolo, it was a stimulant. As our interview data demonstrate, its popularization and widespread use had a number of unintended and harmful consequences for individuals as well as whole communities. Although the prevalence of ice use is not decreasing, there is a growing awareness among users that this is a dangerous substance, and a poor substitute for pakalolo.

Raves as the nexus for new user group expansion

This study revealed that many high risk behaviours were crossing boundaries into other social worlds. In San Francisco, for example, the club and Rave scenes have become a nexus for a wide array of user types, ranging from straight suburban heterosexuals to those in the fringe gay social worlds. These are central places for selling methamphetamines and for trying new and potentially dangerous experiences. The other major finding concerns the increasing diffusion of injection drug use at all three sites. This is occurring in groups that previously shunned it completely. Most notable are members of biker networks, and prisoners who turn to IV administration because of its more economical uptake. This is true even among prisoners in Honolulu. With its fast rush and cost-effective aspects, injection is more frequently seen as an alternative. This raises serious concerns since our findings suggest that users rarely move back into a slower mode once they begin injecting. In addition most IV using respondents admit to needle sharing activities during their drug use career.

Methamphetamine in the cocaine culture

Clearly, the major focus of US drug policy continues to be cocaine. Consequently, any discussion of methamphetamine tends to be in comparison to cocaine and in the language of the cocaine culture. The costs, physical properties, user groups, and effects are all articulated in this manner. The drug itself is most often referred to as the 'poor man's cocaine'. The articulated image then is one of an inferior product, one that mimics the effects of cocaine, but which does not quite match the quality of the cocaine high. The notion that the goal of a methamphetamine high may be different from cocaine seems lost to all but the drug's users. It is certainly not articulated by US drug policy makers.

CONCLUSION

It is clear from the results of this study that methamphetamine is not only firmly entrenched in some communities but is continuing to spread into new areas and populations. Importantly, it is doing so without a high media profile. Use continues to expand among the disenfranchised and marginalized populations that are most likely to sustain the methamphetamine legacy in the United States. Among those populations, paradoxical effects emerge with prolonged heavy bingeing which seductively transforms the hope for enhanced self esteem into the despair of increasing paranoia, isolation, and violence. Energy and increased productivity are transformed into a paralysis of obsessive and unfocused 'tweaking' behaviour.

The paradox effect takes on new meaning within multi-generational communities which incorporate the methamphetamine legacy into their own identity. Especially for these users, years of heavy and prolonged bingeing had not diminished their belief in methamphetamine's ability to renew energy, enhance self-image, and alleviate depression. Remarkably, many sustained this belief even after they realized that methamphetamine produced only the *illusion* and not the reality of their desired goal.

Two major structural conditions help to shape these individual dynamics: the characteristics of American Drug Policy and the economic conditions that are shrinking the blue collar labour market. Clearly, the battle lines of the American drug war extend beyond the cocaine culture, waged on hidden battlefields beyond the inner city. The growing economic disenfranchisement that is spreading across more varied working class communities affects both demand and supply mechanisms. Methamphetamine supplies increase when necessity pushes people into illicit manufacture and distribution as opportunities in the licit economy decline. In addition, battle-scarred veterans of the war against marijuana growing are pulled into methamphetamine production for many reasons. Compared with marijuana production, methamphetamine requires no more capital investment and skill, but has a potential for greater profit. It takes less space and time to produce, and so reduces the likelihood of detection. Very importantly, like marijuana, methamphetamine is a home-grown commodity embodying traditional American values of individualism and independence held by marijuana growers. And like marijuana in previous years, methamphetamine is also likely to move into the heartland of the country.

Similar structural conditions frame the emergence of new and expanded user groups ouside the inner city drugs scenes. The young, unskilled, marginalized and white working-class population, where methamphetamine is most entrenched, is rapidly increasing. They are being joined by working-class Asian Pacific Americans with similar demographic characteristics. The easy access to methamphetamine in many communities combines with structural conditions promoting use among these populations. Yet the very serious individual and social consequences described in this chapter ilustrate that the havoc caused by methamphtamine extends into whole communities. The future does not look bright.

ACKNOWLEDGEMENT

Research for this paper was supported by a grant to the Institute for Scientific Analysis from the National Institute on Drug Abuse (RO1-DA06853) awarded to Patricia Morgan, Ph.D. entitled "Ice and other Methamphetamine Use: An Exploratory Study. The data collected for this paper was helped by the collaborative efforts of the study research staff: Karen Ann Joe, Douglas McDonnell and Rachel Gutierrez.

NOTES

1. The practice of smoking methamphetamine in light bulbs was widespread in many San Diego County communities. It was most popular, but not limited to, Mexican and Latino populations. The basic procedure involved breaking off the metal base and removing the filament. The drug would then be melted in the bottom of the glass bulb and the fumes inhaled through a straw. The trick, according to our respondents was to keep from melting the lettering marking the wattage on the bottom of the bulb, because it generally made the smoker ill. We also found a correlation between the size of the habit and that of the light bulb. After a while of habitual smoking methamphetamine via a light bulb, the user often transitioned to a pipe similar to the ones used by Hawaiian ice smokers. (See Morgan, *et al.*, 1994)

REFERENCES

Carey, J.T. and Mandel, J. (1968) The Bay Area speed scene. *Journal of Health and Social Behavior,* **9**, pp. 164–174.

Chesher, G. (1991) Hazardous amphetamine use: the need to consider dosage" *Drug and Alcohol Review,* **10**, pp. 299–303.

Currie, E. (1993) *Reckoning: Drugs, the Cities and the American future.* New York: Hill and Wang.

Dayton, K. (1994) Prediction in '89 Pot Report is Pointed Out. Honolulu *Advertiser,* April 6.

Edison, G.R. (1978) The drug laws: are they effective and safe? *Journal of the American Medical Association,* **249**, no. 242578–2583.

Flynn, N. (1993) Epidemiology of AIDS in California. *Report to the California Statewide Epidemiology Work Group Meeting*, California Department of Alcohol and Drug Programs. Sacramento, CA.

Glaser, B. and Strauss, A. (1967) *The Discovery of Grounded Theory: Strategies for Qualitative Research.* Chicago: Aldine.

Goode, E. (1993) *Drugs in American Society* (4th Edition). New York: Alfred A. Knopf.

Graham, J.M. (1972) Amphetamine Politics on Capitol Hill. *Society,* **9**(3), pp. 14–23.

Grinspoon, L. and Bakalar, J.B. (1979) *Psychedelic Drugs Reconsidered.* New York: Basic Books.

Grinspoon, L. and Hedblom, P. (1975) *The Speed Culture: Amphetamine Use and Abuse in America.* Cambridge, MA: Harvard University Press.

Haight, M.A. (1993) Drug abuse trends in San Diego County. In: *Epidemiologic Trends in Drug Abuse.* Proceedings of the Community Epidemiology Work Group, National Institute on Drug Abuse, Rockville, MD: Government Printing Office.

Hall, J.N. and Broderick, P.M. (1991) Community networks for response to abuse outbreaks of methamphetamine and its analogs. In: M.A. Miller and N.J. Kozel (eds.), *Methamphetamine Abuse: Epidemiologic Issues and Implications*, National Institute on Drug Abuse, Research Monograph Series 11. Washington, D.C.: U.S. Government Printing Office.

Holmes, E. (1989) New Drug 'Ice' Called Worse Peril than Crack. San Francisco *Chronicle*, August 31.

Jaffe, J. (1989) The Re-Emergence of Methamphetamine. Paper presented before the Select Committee on Narcotics Abuse and Control, U.S. House of Representatives, October.

Joe, K. (1995) "Ice is Strong Enough for a Man But Made for a Woman". *Crime Law and Social Change*, **22**, pp. 269–289.

Kramer, J.C., Fischman, V.S. and Littlefield, D.C. (1967) Amphetamine Abuse. *Journal of American Medical Association,* **201**(5).

Lerner, M.A. "The Fire of 'Ice'." *Newsweek*, 37, pp. 7–9, November 27, 1989.

Lovett, A.R. (1994) "Speed: Wired in California." *Rolling Stone.* May 5, 1994 pp. 39–40.

Morgan, P. and Joe-Laidler, K., (1996) Uncharted Terrain: Contexts of Experience Among Women in the Illicit Drug Economy. *Women and Criminal Justice.* (In Press) 1996.

Morgan, P., Beck, J., Joe, K., McDonnell, D. and Guiterrez, R. (1994) *Ice and other Methamphetamine Use.* Final Report to the National Institute on Drug Abuse. National Institute of Health: U.S. Government Printing Office.

Rawlin, J.W. (1968) Street level abusage of amphetamines. In: J.R. Russo (Ed.) *Amphetamine Abuse.* Springfield, Ill.: Charles C. Thomas.

Smith, D.E. (1969) "Acid Heads vs. Speed Freaks: Conflict Between Drug Subcultures." *Clinical Pediatrics,* **8**, pp. 185–188.

Smith, R. (1969) The World of the Haight-Ashbury Speed Freak. *Journal of Psychoactive Drugs,* **2**(2), pp. 77–83.

Watters, J.K. and Biernacki, P. (1989) Targeted Sampling: Options for the Study of Hidden Populations. *Social Problems,* **36**(4).

Whitney, S. (1995) "Ice: The Prozac of the Poor". *Honolulu Monthly.* August.

Wood, D.W. and Carlson, C. (1991) "Trends in illicit drug use in Honolulu, Hawaii. In: Johnson Bassin and Shaw Inc. (eds.) *Epidemiological Trends in Drug Abuse*, Proceedings Community Epidemiology Work Group, December 1990. Washington D.C.: U.S. Government Printing Office.

Zurer, P.S. (1989) "Federal Officials Plot Strategy to Stop Methamphetamine Spread." *Chemical and Engineering News,* November 6.

8

Kinship and Community: The 'Ice' Crisis in Hawaii

KAREN A. JOE LAIDLER and PATRICIA MORGAN

INTRODUCTION

Situated off the west coast of the continental US in the Pacific Rim, Hawaii's eight main islands conjure up dreamy visions of paradise. The islands of this 50th State encompass over 6,400 square miles, and are home to slightly less than one million people. The majority of residents live and work in the city and county of Honolulu, which constitutes the entire island of Oahu. Oahu, along with the islands of Hawaii, Maui, Kauai, Lanai, and Molokai were originally plantation societies, however, by the 1950s, the pineapple and sugar industries had given way to tourism as the main economic base.

Hawaii has long been noted as the site for high quality 'pakalolo' (marijuana). Dozens of tee shirts, posters, baseball caps, key chains, and other memorabilia boast of the locally grown 'Kona gold'. In local social networks, pakalolo is perceived to be a harmless mild relaxant. In the mid 1980s, however, Hawaii drew national attention as the centre of a new drug epidemic. Law enforcement and health officials reported the emergence of a new destructive illicit drug on the streets, known locally as 'ice' or 'batu' (see Miller; Morgan and Beck, this volume). Media headlines predicted that ice would spread to the continental US, replace crack-cocaine, and become *the drug* of the 1990s (Joe, 1995). The attractiveness of ice (crystal methamphetamine) stemmed from the distinctive 'high' which was less edgy and longer lasting than crack. A limited number of reports on treatment and clinical populations indicated that use was prevalent among the state's Asian Pacific American

163

populations and among women who found the drug appealing for its appetite suppressant qualities (Miller and Tomas, 1989). Little else was known about ice.

Beginning in 1991 through 1994, we embarked on an ethnographic study to examine the crystal methamphetamine scene in California and Hawaii. During the course of our field observations and in-depth interviews with moderate to heavy users, we discovered significant differences in the distribution and use patterns in these locales. This chapter draws from this study and briefly describes the major trends in the use of crystal methamphetamine in Hawaii — its arrival, availability and sources. We then examine the distinctive networks of users and dealers in Hawaii's ice scene and explore the primary effects of these networks on the community.

EMERGENCE OF ICE IN HAWAII

Methamphetamine use in Hawaii is almost exclusively limited to ice. Ephedrine is the precursor used in its manufacture. According to the U.S. Federal Register, ice is a "mixture or substance containing d-methamphetamine HCl of at least 80% purity" (Federal Register, 1991). Ice derives its street name from its translucent, crystalline form, and is usually smoked in a glass pipe. One user described its appearance this way:

> *Looks kinda like rock salt, clear. Almost like rock candy. Some can be big, like a diamond, looks almost like diamonds! (Case 488)*

Ice is also referred to by two other terms. The most common is 'batu', an Ilocano word from the Philippines meaning 'rock', which is widely used among several ethnic populations of ice users in Hawaii. Also known in Hawaii, but less commonly used, is the Japanese term, 'shabu'. It is interesting to note that in the Philippines, ice is more commonly referred to by the Japanese term rather than by its Ilocano name.

Ice was developed and distributed completely independently from U.S. mainland methamphetamine networks, so for several years, users and some law enforcement officials assumed ice was an entirely different drug from methamphetamine. Although methamphetamine powder was available in the Honolulu area as early as the 1960s, its use was generally limited to transplanted haoles (caucasians) from the mainland, and included a small enclave of bikers on the Big Island (Hawaii). The predominant drugs of choice in Hawaii into the 1980s were marijuana and cocaine.

Unlike our California sites, Hawaii had little experience of other forms of methamphetamine, and Honolulu users distinguished ice from other methamphetamine products from the mainland. We discovered that many

respondents were confused about the link between methamphetamine powder and ice. Most knew nothing about methamphetamine, and those that
had heard of it thought that meth was a completely different drug. Some
users now believe that methamphetamine is a type of ice, rather than believ-
ing that ice is a type of methamphetamine. It is referred to as 'powdered ice'
or 'meth ice'.

Patterns of Availability and Price

The earliest reports of ice in Honolulu date back to the late 1970s, although
its use did not begin to rise until the mid eighties. By 1989 it had reached
epidemic proportions, and the news of a drug potentially more dangerous
than crack was in the headlines across the country (Essoyan, 1989; Holmes,
1989; Lerner, 1989; Zurer, 1989; Corwin, 1989; Tabor, 1989). Arrests for the
possession of ice were three times higher in 1989 than in 1987 (Hawaii Attorney General's Office, 1990). As one user stated, by 1990 there was widespread availability:

> *When I went in jail in 1987, it didn't seem it was that rampant. But
> when I came out at the beginning of 1990, it was everywhere! It
> was like an epidemic! Everywhere you turned, everybody was smok-
> ing it! Before I went in, I knew a few dealers and most people I
> knew didn't use it. The locals, they didn't even know where to get it!
> If you didn't have any connections, you could ask anybody who
> was into drugs and they'd know where to get it for you. (Case 519)*

By 1991, however, official and street reports suggested that the availability
and use of ice had begun to drop. The exact source of the drought could not
be established. Some users believed the drought was related to dealers' attempts to drive up market prices. Others believed that shipments were simply not coming in. By this time too, police had stepped up their efforts to
deal with the drug. Clearly, however, ice had 'dried up', and prices had
soared. According to the Honolulu police:

> *An ounce of crystal meth now costs nearly $21,000 on the street —
> nearly double the price of a year ago. The street price of ice tripled
> in the first half or so of 1990 (Honolulu Advertiser, 1991).*

Ice is generally packaged in 'papers' which sell for $25, $50 or $100. The
relationship between volume and price vary widely. Because it is purchased
by the paper rather than weight, there is great uncertainty about the cost per
gram. At times, a $50 paper buys one-eighth of a gram and a $100 paper a
quarter of a gram. More often, however, a paper buys only one-tenth of a
gram. Many respondents believe that in 1989 a $25 paper bought a quarter of

a gram. When the 1991 drought increased the price, the lack of experience of buying in grams resulted in widely differing accounts concerning price. One user complained when recalling different prices:

> *Out on the street, it's really expensive. It varies from week to week, even month to month, it depends on how much is around. ... 1986 one gram sold for $450. In 1987, that same gram sold for $600. Now, one gram currently goes for $200 to $250 per gram. (Case 519)*

By mid 1992, another major change occurred. Ice was more abundant and prices had declined. A number of respondents believed that the continued fluctuations were due to factors other than availability, in particular a buyer's personal connections and perceived socio-economic standing.

Factors Related to the Increasing Prevalence of Ice

According to our respondents and confirmed by discussions with various social agencies, at least two factors are related to the remarkable growth of ice in Honolulu. First, users were pushed away from pakalolo, their smokeable drug of choice, and pulled toward ice by a well organized marketing campaign by Asian distributors.

Second, in the 1980s, law enforcement agencies launched an intensive pakalolo eradication campaign which resulted in the destruction of large and small crop productions and transformed the illicit drug economy. This eradication effort drove up prices, drastically reduced availability and left local residents without their customary, and many would say, relatively benign smoke. Also very importantly, many local residents derived either part or all of their livelihood from marijuana production. Robbed of this needed income, many experienced considerable economic hardship. Thus when a new, easy to use, smokeable product entered the drug market, one which at first seemed to be non-threatening to youthful novitiates, it was readily accepted as a product to be exploited. Initial users were often likely to think of it as a substitute of sorts for pakalolo (Dayton, 1994).

The Sources of Ice

Our own fieldwork, as well as government data, suggests that ice is primarily produced in, and distributed from, the Far East, especially the Philippines, Korea, Taiwan, and Japan (Adamski, 1992; Glauberman, 1992). There is also some evidence that mainland China is involved as a source of ephedrine. More recent but less well documented evidence suggests the existence of distribution networks involving the U.S. mainland, Canada and Mexico.

Several sources suggested that ice distribution in Hawaii was an economic enterprise developed by organized crime networks in Japan and Korea involving large corporate investors (Adamski, 1992; Seto, 1991; Schoenberger, 1992).

Manufacturing began in the Far East which had a free flow of ephedrine. Comments from knowledgeable Honolulu respondents indicate that Korean manufacturers may have been the first to begin large-scale production in the mid 1980s. They then transferred their base either to Taiwan or the Phillipines after heavy pressure from Korean law enforcement agencies (Glauberman, 1992). Before that time, however, some of our respondents claim that ice was distributed, and possibly manufactured in the Philippines. According to most accounts, there seems to be a particular link between the Koreans and the Filipinos. One Honolulu respondent offered this assessment:

> *Most people think it's the Filipinos, [in control] but the Koreans give 'em to the Filipinos cause the Filipinos don't talk too much! … the Filipinos keep their mouth shut! The Koreans don't get into the labor part, they won't take the risks, they just play the big man and distribute. The Filipinos do the dirty work. The stuff comes from Korea, so the only way they can get it is from Koreans … I used to think it was coming from the Philippines. But that was dirty stuff, shabu stuff. It ain't happening. (Case 521)*

USING, DEALING AND EXTENDED KINSHIP NETWORKS

User Networks

As Morgan and Beck (this volume) indicate, the ice users in our study represent the state's ethnic diversity. Over 75% of our respondents identified themselves as being of Asian Pacific American ethnic descent. Over half of them reported a multi-ethnic background. This pattern reflects the historical blending of the state's population, and is in sharp contrast to our respondents in California who overwhelmingly were Caucasian and, to a lesser extent, African American and Latino.

Unlike the experiences of our Californian respondents, we found that extended kinship networks in Hawaii had a more significant role in initiating and supporting continued use of ice and other drugs among many of our Asian Pacific American respondents (Joe, 1995). This pattern was clear for both males and females.

The setting for initial and continued use among males almost always occurred in a male peer group setting. This peer group often included a mix of cousins, neighbourhood friends and/or co-workers.

> *My cousins saw me partying and turned me on to meth. They been using meth all their lives, they're like 42 now…. They turned me on with meth, just lines at first. I was 14. We were in a garage. You don't take meth in a house, you take it in a garage! (Case 430)*

This overlap between relatives and friends is, in part, a reflection of the centrality of kinship ties and the enclosed geographical boundaries of an island society.

> *It was at my friend's house. At that time, right along that same time, we started doing coke and stuff. And so the brother [of my friend] brought that [ice]. I mean, he came — he was just down from the Big Island just this one time, and then we were just about to crack some lines, and he said, 'Here, try these.' And then we were, you know, fucking curiosity. (Case 427)*

Among the women, there were more diverse sources by which they were were initiated to ice. Several had tried ice with a small group of girlfriends, while others were introduced to ice by a relative, typically a cousin or in-law. In these cases, the initial experience was often linked to trust and camaraderie (Joe, 1995). These women continued to use in the same networks, and found these familial connections to be a reliable and trustworthy source for their supplies. One 34 year old woman recalls:

> *The very first time was in '89. I was living with my friend, O. My sister in-law was with him. They close to my family. She was doing ice that day. She say come, come to the house. They always see me working and they say come, 'relax! You'll feel good, no be scared!*
>
> *After that, I did 'em couple weeks after that. She [cousin] used to be home, maybe I hit one or two ... I moved to Nankuli with my family ... The whole house is doing it. Everywhere you go, get out the pipe! ... I started buying from one of my cousins. I used to always burn myself cause I was trying to learn how the hell to do this thing without wasting 'em. My cousin used to see me do that so she taught me ... I stayed with her for three months. They were big time dealers. They was selling big quantities of it. I help her clean up the house, a big, big house. My auntie's house. Because I would help her clean and cook, she always used to give me free stash. (Case 411)*

Several younger women indicated that male dealers, who had motives other than a new potential customer, mediated their first experience with ice. Another source was through their partner. Their encounters were typically associated with sexual enhancement (Joe 1995).

> *My first experience was with my husband, he introduced me to it. He showed me how to smoke it ... God, what sex we had! Go! Go! Go! ... Our sex was always good, high or not. It gave me more courage, it made me braver. (Case 445)*

Women were not the only ones who found ice improving their sex lives. Many men also believed that ice provided them with 'men of steel' qualities, including sexual virility.

Dealing Networks

Our research revealed several major types of dealing networks in the Honolulu site which differed from those in California. One of the most common in Hawaii were *hotel dealers* who had a direct supply source and dealt in ounces. Buying and selling were typically connected to kinship and neighbourhood ties. According to one respondent:

> *He was Filipino, a local. Born and raised here. He was a Waialua boy. He was getting out of hand with the money, flashing his money and jewelry … I started calling him Mr. T. because his gold, his diamonds, he was really choke! He had chains on his neck that he'd wear like Mr. T. It got to the point that business was going so good for him that he was flashy! If you knew him and the work he did, you'd wonder where is he getting all his money? On every finger was a ring. A Rolex watch … He started dealing out of Aiea. He never stayed in an apartment more than 6 months. He'd lease a place and deal there and live there. He never brought the dealing home to his wife and family. He had a couple of right-hand men who stayed with him. He had computers there, everything. He'd move it around every time he moved. (Case 542)*

In the heady months of easy availability and enthusiastic customers, such flashy behaviour was not uncommon. For most of these *hotel dealers*, their success was shortlived. In the case above, this person also continued working at a naval shipyard where he eventually attracted the wrong attention, and was arrested.

Similarly, *neighbourhood dealer* transactions usually took place within the context of familial and long time local connections. Many respondents indicated that most neighbourhoods on the island were extremely tightly knit, and consequently, obtaining ice is 'all a matter of who you know'. Neighbourhood dealers were most often Native Hawaiian, Samoan or Filipinos who are from the most economically marginalized groups and communities on the island. Typically they were former pakalolo sellers who initially thought ice was going to be a lucrative substitute and began dealing to supplement the family income and at the same time, have a bit of smoke left over after sales. In contrast to the hotel dealers, neighbourhood dealers conducted their business from their homes, and sometimes integrated various kin into the enterprise. One 42 year old Filipino male recounts the process by which his nephew introduced him to the business and his offsprings' subsequent involvement in dealing.

*At first I knew nothing about dealing. My nephew showed me how.
I got my own scale and started from there. He taught me and I
perfected it in my own way. My 50 cent papers was bigger than
anyone on the island! That's why I was a success ... At home, I was
always the MAN. I had what they wanted. I was arrogant cause I
knew I had what they wanted and I played games with them. Out
in public, I was low key.*

*In the beginning, I had confidence cause I was making money. I
got shaked down twice and nothing happened. I was confident
cause I was making so much money and I couldn't believe it! [The
police] knocked on the door and my son answered and let them in.
They saw scales on the counter and paraphernalia on the counter.
They questioned me and my son and we denied that we were dealing. Then they left. (Case 461)*

Dealing provided them with immediate popularity, an enhanced self-image,
and lifted them above the mundane and unrewarding lives of poverty and
hard work. Many of these dealers, like the father above, describe the early
days of the business with a sense of pride, especially around their children.

*I got the feeling when he was working, he was a big man. He
brought people home from work to introduce them to me. My
daughter was in high school and her friends were using and
wanted to meet me. (Case 461)*

Eventually, however, his use increased to the point where he could not do
business, where pride and confidence were replaced by compulsive use,
then guilt and denial. He ended up losing the business, his wife, his home,
and his children.

A neighbourhood 'auntie' recalls a similar story about when she began
dealing, almost immediately after her step-son introduced her to ice:

*I didn't even have a pipe then! I didn't know where to get one.
Sometimes I'd spend maybe $300 a day on ICE. Buying it and shar-
ing it with them. When his supplier came over one day to my house
and introduced himself to me, that's when I went into dealing ... I
liked the high. Also I went into dealing. So, in order to deal, I had to
stay up. That meant that I'd have free smoke. That was my main
purpose in dealing, to be able to smoke free, and make a little bit of
money for myself. Then it got into more and more and more customers and more demands. It got to be crazy! A lot of people who
know a dealer, they tend to sponge off the dealer or see what favors
they can get. They wanted ice, food, everything from me! People
started taking advantage and I stopped dealing finally. Then all of*

my so called 'good friends' seemed to become my enemies because I wasn't there … to give them the dope that they wanted anymore. (Case 449)

Familial and neighbourhood bonds were few or non-existent among *hustler dealers*. In these networks, dealing ice is one of a number of scams and illegal activities. These respondents of varied ethnicities led a very marginal existence and were often homeless. Some were sex workers, living and plying their trade in either the downtown red-light district or Waikiki areas. Almost no one in this group was making any money from dealing ice. Rather, they were dealing primarily for stash and could barely keep up. A male respondent in Honolulu described this cycle:

I'm surviving by getting enough for me, I'm buying by the oz. and selling by the 1/2 gram or 1/4 gram. I'm dealing. I'm turning $1000 into $3000. I'm doing it once a week but I'm using also. I'm paying some of my bills, not all of them. I'm drinking hard. I'm buying everybody in the bar drinks! … I couldn't keep it up anymore, then I got homeless. I put everything in storage and met a guy in a bar. He was the 'hot-shot' kid, the biggest dealer in porno in California! … We opened up our own film distribution company: make our own films, film at home, edit our own stuff and party. Fuck around, do all the things that we like to do! We got funding and a big house and played at the beach. I'm still dealing ice, I'd weigh it out … and stay up. If something happened, I wouldn't miss it. I was feeling good about nothing and depressed. Everything at this point in time is false. I don't like anybody, I don't trust anybody. (Case 453)

Distribution Networks

Dealer networks in Honolulu went beyond familial connections. It was built upon a partnership between a group of Hawaiians, Samoans and Filipinos, and structured to distribute the flow of ice from the Philippines into local communities on the island. This larger network was forged from established ties of brotherhood among those who have been historically the most disenfranchised groups on the islands. A Filipino dealer outlined how this partnership began, organized around 'The Hawaiian Brothers' when ice first began flowing into the islands.

They had gatherings to advertise the ice. It was mostly Filipino immigrants who spoke bad English and you had to smoke ice. There was a leader, we called him the 'Contributor' and he gave funding. He supports it with money. I've known the leader for a long time, he's back in jail, has no money but everybody goes to him. … it

> *started with a few guys and then it became bigger. Nationalities stick together, so everybody was solid at that time. The person at the top started advertising and using the Hawaiian Brothers got big. (Case 523)*

Several respondents described how these networks began to unravel as tensions and paranoia escalated with the increasing use of ice within these communities. Eventually a violent homicide fractured the network into smaller groups.

> *This guy shot somebody, so the flow of the drugs got slowed up. Everybody started breaking out into some small groups. Everybody was paranoid, it was a hard time to get some. I was holding on to a lot of shit when he got busted, in 1987, about 10 people were holding his stuff. (Case 523)*

As a consequence, territorial competition increased and cooperation among dealer networks began to disintegrate. This required some action in order to maintain an equitable marketplace.

> *I didn't stop using and I knew plenty guys in the Hawaiian syndicate ... the local guys. They paid taxes to 'Papa' and he used to take in about $200,000 a month. The 'Waianae Connection' would make us pay taxes to them for certain things. It was territorial. The local guys used to rip off other dealers and they'd retaliate. [like paying protection?] Yes. This connection gave plenty benefits for dealing with him. That's basically how it is. (Case 523)*

According to this respondent, under this new structure the connections among the groups remain friendly.

Although most users and dealers claim that most ice is from the Philippines and Korea, opinion varies widely about the exact sources and distribution routes. Periodically, large ice seizures at the docks, or busts involving Korean or Japanese (Yakuza) gangsters reinforce this belief. For many of our Honolulu respondents, knowledge of where ice actually originates is limited to these news accounts. For example:

> *Next door to us was an apartment building and the guy there got busted. It was the largest bust they had here. He had $10,000 cash in his car! He turned over on the Koreans. Our understanding was that ice was either coming from the Philippines or thru Korea. That's where this guy got it. Our people were mostly local who were middle men. We never went with any of the big guys. (Case 518)*

Occasionally, co-worker and familial connections provide a direct source for developing those international links and local distribution. A major distributor in Honolulu, became involved after seeing the advantages connected to his employment at the city harbor. The key was his co-worker who was also the brother of an international ice distributor.

> *When I was young and got the job at the Harbor, his brother used to run a ship with gambling and stuff. He's my friend. The trust was there. How we did it. It used to look like a family visit. I'd have my son and my old lady walk up with me. I'd come home with a shit load of stuff to take to people and sell. Some for me too. I was trusted. (521)*

Both users and dealers from the downtown red light district often exist outside dealing networks. Mainland transplants and locals who have 'bottomed out' and are homeless, dominate this scene. They have few, if any, reliable or established connections for buying and selling.

> *Most of my friends were local and most of them were Hawaiian/ Samoan. But I know they got ice from Filipinos. We sometimes got it from a couple Black friends. (Case 518)*

Because of their lack of established connections, the quality and purity of ice sold in this area was highly variable. Sellers in the downtown area were also more likely to sell bogus product. One male sex industry worker claimed that as a haole he never got 'good deals' on ice, and often got sold bogus product.

> *Purity is a big thing, you get a lot of crap! You have to be really careful. People sell styrofoam, shit like that! I can't imagine what shooting that will do to you! Probably nothing good! Yeah, we got a lot of crap. That's basically why we quit. It just got to be ridiculous. We were trying to screw each other over and playing games we promised we wouldn't play! (Case 529)*

We found, however, that mixed ethnic 'locals' relying on downtown dealer networks had similar problems.

One aftermath of the ice goldrush era is that some individuals got on the dealing bandwagon and developed alternative sources. Some started making trips to the West Coast, buying meth at mainland prices, bringing it back, and attempting, in various ways, to turn it into ice and make a little profit. Consequently, ephemeral dealer networks sprang up, resulting in a saturated ice market and no quality control.

A number of respondents indicated that ice was also being locally manufactured and there were reports of small labs on Oahu. One respondent with extensive dealing experience made the link between Koreans and local manufacture.

> ... *as far as I know, he was the only distributor. He had two other people above him, which was the person he was getting it from and the person he was getting it from was the cook. The stuff that we had, had its own chemist. [The chemist was here in Hawaii?] ... I'd say, if he was here at one time, he only stayed for 3 months at the longest. He would move his laboratory every 3 or 4 months to a different location. (Case 542)*

Reports of locally produced ice still continue. When asked if he knew if there were laboratories on the Island, one respondent replied:

> *I never ask questions, no! I never cared to ask. I have no idea. I think a lot of it was synthetically produced. Sometimes there was such a difference in the taste. The stuff that was synthetic seemed to be more white. This is my assumption. It wasn't bitter, it had more of a vanilla extract taste to it. Yeah. It was more white. Where it came from, you don't ask questions like that because that will get you in BAD trouble! Physically, bad troubles! Yeah. You just consider everything you get manna from heaven! I know a lot of it was probably out in the country. Waimanalo-side, more than Waianae-side. I suspect a lot of it was [manufactured here] because there's Hawaiian housing out there and they're well protected. They're protector-owned out there, yeah. I strongly believe that. (Case 527)*

Considering the limited knowledge that Honolulu ice users have about methamphetamine in general, it seems most likely that these reported laboratories are, in fact, supplies of powder methamphetamine brought in from the mainland and then turned into ice crystals by locals or recent haole arrivals in Hawaii.

CONSEQUENCES OF ICE ON KINSHIP AND COMMUNITY

Thus far, we have shown some of the distinctive ways in which kinship ties operate in Hawaii's ice scene. While extended familial networks played a significant role for many of the users we interviewed in Hawaii, this is not to suggest that this was the case for all. Some respondents reported that they tried to conceal their use and their dealing from immediate and extended family members, hoping to avoid bringing shame and embarrassment to themselves or their loved ones. In other cases, respondents had cut themselves off long ago from any familial connections. In these cases, they had an especially violent and abusive childhood, and left home at an early age to start their own family (Joe, 1995). Importantly, the effects of ice on family relationships and the community have been felt by nearly all of our respondents.

Effects on Family

Family problems resulting from using and dealing crystal methamphetamines was significantly more prevalent among our respondents from Hawaii than in California. In Honolulu, 60% of the males and 61% of the females reported problems with their family and loved ones (See Morgan *et al.*, 1994).

For many of the Honolulu respondents, several negative consequences merged to produce a devastating effect on their families. Males often described the downward spiral of their relationships:

> *Later in my addiction, I started to get abusive, more abusive than ever! Cause of the paranoia, I couldn't handle it. My wife was trying to help me quit but I didn't listen. The greed and my addiction got the best of me. My life with my family started to deteriorate. My son started doing his own thing cause he seen me doing my own thing. I was too busy to notice that my family life was falling apart. It deteriorated slowly. I wasn't paying attention to my family, I was just concentrating on my using. She would come home from work and I'd still be smoking. When she got up to get dressed for work in the morning, I'd still was up smoking ... When she did voice opinions later, it was too late. I was too far into the addiction and making money. Twice after that, she tried to get me into treatment. I never went. (Case 461)*

Another male user described how his heavy ice use led first, to the loss of his job, and followed quickly by the loss of his family.

> *I lost jobs, I lost my family, lost my house ... I stayed partying and didn't go to work. I never used to call in case I was high and I'd lose the job. I lost my family cause I never used to come home. My wife got mad and tossed me my clothes out the door ... She told me she had enough of my shit and that I wasn't giving a shit about her and the kids. I was mostly getting high and drinking ... On paydays she would come down and pick up my check. She'd give me $40 or $50 from my check to party with. I figured it was okay to party and not come home cause she had the check. But she never liked the idea that I never called her up to tell her where I was*

staying or what I was doing ... On my days off I took of with the guys and partied instead of being with the kids. (Case 517)

Women also experienced the disintegration of the family, but the experience was qualitatively different from their male counterparts. One woman recalled how her and her husband's use and 'business' gradually resulted in violence:

His attitude towards me changed [when he started dealing]. We used to do a lot of family things. Go to the beach, go fishing, camping, take the kids on Saturdays or Sundays somewhere. That changed. He'd stay home all the time, waiting for a sale. He wouldn't take us out as a family anymore. He wouldn't go grocery shopping anymore. A dealer doesn't spend much time with their families, I found that out. That's when our problems started. I was feeling a lack of his attention and love ... I had affairs ... At that point my husband started getting abusive. We used to freebase cocaine together and he never got abusive. It was the batu that made him really edgy ... I used to fight back when he hit me. I got tired of taking his punches. So I turned him in. (Case 445)

After selling their house, she found herself living on the streets. At present, she relies on various friends for temporary shelter as her relationship with her own family has been extremely strained from her ice use. Given the absence of a home, one of her former husbands has taken custody of her children.

Effects on Community: Societal Disenfranchisement

One respondent who lived in California before moving to Honolulu felt strongly that ice had a significantly more negative impact on the social networks in the community than it did in California communities.

Ice costs are so high ... they use it for the power here. It's a power play. Whoever has got the most is in the lead! It's kind of a game people play. It really gets disgusting when you're spending every dime you have for ice and some of the things you do for it, to deal with people's power plays! A lot of people get hurt, ripped off, things taken from them that mean a lot to them. Over here, there's no loyalty. No brotherhood, everybody rats each other off, they all steal from each other for the ice. I know brothers who steal from each other for the ice. Then a week later, they're all friends again. Everybody I met here that did ice, nobody worked! But they all paid for this drug! There was no loyalty, no dreams. They're all like dead here ... I can see myself falling into the same category as they are. No life, no dreams, the only thing that matters is ice. (Case 530)

Another respondent from Honolulu provided an even more intensely grim portrait.

> *A lot of the violence going on in Hawaii, people hurting their families, I know if you interviewed those people, that have murdered people on that shit, people they supposedly loved, they'd tell you about ice stories. Real bad, they probably didn't realize what they were doing. It's happened a lot over here, lately. I think somebody should talk to those folks, find out what ice they were doing. I guarantee that every time we see that on TV, we all think it was somebody fucked up on ice! The rage is just fucking, flipped-out rages, man. The people I meet on it that deal it or do it, they're real scary, they have real dead eyes! I don't think they feel anything for anybody! (Case 529)*

An important finding emerging from this study concerned the effect on individuals and communities of the scarcity of marijuana due to the official eradication campaigns. Users often reported that this was a major contribution to the increase in the use of meth, especially in Honolulu. In many communities it had a devastating effect. As one respondent explained:

> *The ice use on the Waianae Coast is greater than a lot of other places in the State! This is like a central distribution center for ice. It's a known fact among the drug addicts and users on the island. It's easier to get than weed! It's not much more expensive than weed, either! The amount of people here that use ice is increasing because people who couldn't find weed were starting to find ice easier! Plenty guys I know use ice because they can't get pot! I'd rather see them smoking pakalolo cause they were mellow, nice people. On ice, they change into robbing houses and carrying guns in less than one month. Things they never did on weed. (Case 468)*

CONCLUSION

In many ways, pre-existing drug use practices among Asian Pacific Americans set the stage for the introduction of ice into Hawaii. Earlier studies have documented the role of alcohol in relation to indigenous intoxicating beverages, the eradication of those traditional beverages, and the simultaneous promotion of western types of alcohol beverages, and institution of native specific alcohol control regulations (Keaulana and Whitney, 1990). On the surface, Native Hawaiians and other Asian Pacific Island residents in

Hawaii accepted this substitution. However, there is a possibility that eradication of traditional alcoholic intoxicants was quietly replaced by pakalolo grown by local residents in family yards and fields.

As government authorities began the campaign to eradicate marijuana in the 1980s, a smokable drug known as 'batu' from the Philippines began to be used in place of the increasingly rare and expensive pakalolo. However, batu was not a traditional intoxicant like awa or pakalolo, it was a stimulant. As our interview data demonstrate, its popularization and widespread use had a number of unintended and harmful consequences for individuals, their families and local communities. Although the prevalence of ice use remains unabated, there is a growing awareness among users that this is a dangerous substance, and a common realization that it is a poor substitute for pakalolo.

REFERENCES

Adamski, M. (1992) Yakuza Investors Sink Roots in Isles. Honolulu Star Bulletin, October 16.

Corwin, M. (1989) Potent Form of Speed Could Be Drug of '90s. Los Angeles Times, October 8.

Dayton, K. (1994) Prediction in '89 Pot Report is Pointed Out. Honolulu Advertiser, April 6.

Essoyan, S. (1989) Use of Highly Addictive 'Ice' Growing in Hawaii. Los Angeles Times, October 17.

Federal Register (1991) Amendments to the Sentencing Guidelines for United States Courts. Vol. 56, No. 95, May 16.

Glauberman, S. (1992) Anti-Drug Program Teams with Two Korean Officers. Honolulu Advertiser, October 6.

Hawaii Attorney General's Office (1990) Crime in Hawaii 1989. State of Hawaii.

Holmes, E. (1989) New Drug 'Ice' Called Worse Peril than Crack. San Francisco Chronicle, August 31.

Joe, K. (1995) Ice is strong enough for a man but made for a woman: A social cultural analysis of crystal methamphetamine use among Asian Pacific Americans. *Crime, Law and Social Change*, **22**, pp. 269–289.

Keaulana, K.A. and Whitney, S. (1990) ka wai kau mai o Maleka — Water from America. Contemporary Drug Problems. Summer.

Lerner, M.A. (1989) The Fire of 'Ice'. Newsweek, November 27.

Miller, M.A. and Tomas, J.M. (1989) Past and current methamphetamine epidemics. In: Epidemiologic Trends in Drug Abuse: Proceedings of the Community Epidemiology Work Group December 1989. Washing, D.C.: Supt. of Docs., U.S. Govt. Printing Office (DHHS Pub. No. 7210757:20058).

Morgan, P. *et al.* (1994) Ice and Other Methamphetamine Use: An Exploratory Study, Final Report to the National Institute on Drug Abuse. San Francisco, CA: Institute for Scientific Analysis.

Schoenberger, K. (1992) Yakuza Expand on Mainland. Honolulu Advertiser, January 5.

Seto, B. (1991) $11 Million of 'Ice' Seized. Honolulu Star Bulletin, November 8.

Tabor, M. (1989) 'Ice' in an island Paradise. The Boston Globe, December 8.

Zurer, P.S. (1989) Federal Officials Plot Strategy to Stop Methamphetamine Spread. Chemical and Engineering News, November 6.

9

The Methamphetamine — HIV Connection in Northern California

RACHEL ANDERSON and NEIL FLYNN

INTRODUCTION

In this chapter we will draw upon several of the University of California, Davis' studies to describe the epidemiology, demography, profiles of methamphetamine users and their subcultures, adverse consequences of methamphetamine use (in particular Human Immunodeficiency Virus Type 1 [HIV-1] infection). We will also comment on possible strategies for reducing the harm to individuals and society related to methamphetamine use in this region. The studies were conducted by the HIV Prevention Studies Program at the University of California, Davis (UCD-HPS) between 1987 and 1995 in Sacramento County, California.

Sacramento County is the capital of the state of California and is located approximately 90 miles northeast of San Francisco. It is situated at the northern end of California's great central valley, covers approximately 1,000 square miles, and has a population of 1.2 million. It is ethnically diverse, according to the 1990 census data; 69% of the population are Caucasian, 12% are Latino, 9% are African American, 9% are Asian/Pacific Islander, and less than one percent are Native American.

UCD-HPS and Dr. John Newmeyer of the Haight Ashbury Free Clinic in San Francisco collaborated in 1995 to more accurately estimate the overall number of drug injectors in the county and, specifically, to estimate the number of local methamphetamine injectors. The methodology of this estimation was based on a combination of various data sources (Newmeyer,

1991): the "back calculation" method used to estimate the IDU impact on the AIDS epidemic (Aldrich, 1990; Kaplan, 1994), emergency room data, coroner data, information from street outreach workers, drug treatment programmes admission data, and census data. This project estimated that there are 7,000 regular, daily injectors of methamphetamine in Sacramento. Estimates for the number of heroin and cocaine injectors were 7,000 and 700, respectively, for comparison (Newmeyer, 1995). There are also a significant number of methamphetamine injectors who do not inject every time they use the drug or who only use (mainly by injection) methamphetamines occasionally. Therefore, these occasional injectors would be expected to appear in the indicator data (which reflect problematic use situations) used to make population estimates.

After tobacco, alcohol, and marijuana, methamphetamine (often referred to as crank, CR, wire, meth, crystal, and speed) is the predominant drug of use/misuse in this geographic region. By contrast, only 10% of entrants into local drug treatment programmes between July 1, 1994 and June 30, 1995 entered for primarily methamphetamine-related problems, compared to 47% for primarily opiate-related problems (Nisenbaum, 1995). Methamphetamines are readily available throughout the county, are relatively low in cost (approximately US$30 for a 'gram' compared to $100 for a 'gram' of powder cocaine and $120 for a 'gram' of heroin), and their use carries less social stigma than opiates or cocaine, but more stigma than marijuana or alcohol use. A regular methamphetamine user in Northern California may spend only 1/3 as much for her/his drug as a regular heroin or cocaine user. Sacramento County is one of the larger producers of methamphetamines in the United States (SEWG, 1993). Methamphetamines are so readily available and simple to produce that we have termed them the 'bathtub gin of the nineties', a reference to homemade alcoholic beverages produced during the period of alcohol prohibition in the United States (1920–1933). Local methamphetamine production is also associated with production of environmentally significant quantities of toxic waste materials, a problem that has received relatively little attention in the scientific community (Brown, 1994).

Most methamphetamine users in this area are heterosexual, sexually active, are well-integrated into society, continue to hold jobs, and interact socially and sexually with the non-drug-using population. A significant proportion of local methamphetamine users are injectors (50% of arrestees who tested positive for methamphetamines in the Drug Use Forecasting study in 1993 reported a history of injection). They are a diverse group of people, who represent a cross-section of society.

In addition to the direct drug effects and legal consequences of methamphetamine use, injectors have a much greater risk of acquisition of HIV and other bloodborne viral infections, which can, and does, tremendously complicate these problems.

METHODS

In this section we will describe several studies conducted by UCD-HPS, on which this chapter is based. In the results section we will weave the results of these studies into an overview of methamphetamine use in Northern California. All studies were reviewed and approved by the UCD Human Subjects Review Committee (UCD's Institutional Review Board) before studies were implemented.

Quantitative Studies

The first study[1] was conducted among injectors and their sexual partners in various drug treatment programmes (DTP) in Sacramento County from 1987 to 1991. Programme entrants who agreed to participate (they were given US$25 for participation) were administered a detailed Knowledge, Attitude, and Behaviour (KAB) questionnaire and were tested for HIV-1 antibodies with enzyme-linked immunosorbent assay (ELISA) and Western blot (N = 1,269). For purposes of comparison in this chapter, opiate injectors (N = 421) were defined as those who named an opiate as their drug of choice and reported never injecting cocaine (in the late 1980s it was rare to find an injector who injected heroin and methamphetamines). Stimulant injectors (N = 118) were defined as those who named a central nervous system stimulant as their drug of choice and were not opiate dependent at the time of interview. Seventy-six percent (N = 90) of these stimulant injectors named methamphetamines as their drug of choice.

Because methamphetamine users represented less than 10% of the in-treatment population, and because they had a significantly higher risk for HIV acquisition and transmission among in-treatment IDU, we were led to investigate illicit drug injectors that were not in treatment. Out-of-treatment injectors were surveyed in 1992[2] and 1994[3]. Current injectors (illicit drug injection in the 12 months prior to interview) who reported no drug treatment experience in the year prior to interview were recruited by street outreach workers in areas of the county known to have a high incidence of drug use, administered a KAB questionnaire, and tested on site for HIV-1 antibodies with finger-stick blotter tests, using Western blot confirmation. Participants were paid $25 for their time and information. In these studies, drug of choice was defined as the drug injected most frequently in the past year.

---

[1] Funded by the California Universitywide AIDS Research Programme (UARP) and the United State's Public Health Services' National Institute on Drug Abuse (NIDA).
[2] Funded by NIDA.
[3] Funded by the California State Office of AIDS.

A study of individuals arrested in Sacramento County for non-drug-related felonies (crimes such as burglary, rape, murder) was conducted by UCD-HPS in 1993. This study, called the Drug Use Forecasting (DUF) Study[4], was conducted in collaboration with the University of California, Los Angeles Drug Abuse Research Center. Within 48 hours of their arrest, arrestees who volunteered were administered a questionnaire and asked to give a urine sample to be analyzed for illicit drugs. The questionnaire contained questions about drug use, sexual behaviour, and criminal history, as well as demographic information. Participants were given candy bars (the only allowable form of payment in the jail) for their time and information. All urinalysis results and questionnaire information were kept confidential and were unavailable to custody staff.

Qualitative Studies

In July 1994, a video study was initiated[5]. UCD-HPS research staff videotaped groups of injectors during injection sessions, conducted short KAB interviews after the filming, and wrote out their observations of the activity. Injectors were recruited by street outreach workers and paid $50 for their participation in this study. Identifying features such as faces and tattoos were not recorded in the videos. The goal of this study was to examine, in detail, the techniques of drug injection and to focus particularly on the elements of injection behaviour which carry a potential risk of HIV and blood-borne virus transmission. To date 15 (of an anticipated 20) injection groups have been videotaped and interviewed.

UCD-HPS programme staff have monitored the local needle and syringe exchange programme since its inception in February, 1994. This is an underground (illegal) exchange programme that provides the HIV Prevention Studies Programme with limited demographic and qualitative data. The Sacramento Area Needle Exchange (SANE) is a pager-operated, mobile exchange with no fixed sites. It is a one-for-one exchange with no upper limit. Exchanges are conducted in Sacramento County and in four counties that border Sacramento on the north, west, and east. Many of the IDU networks that are served designate a representative to exchange for that network (in the time period mentioned above, 41% of exchanges involved IDU exchanging for others). Some of these designated exchangers (DE) represent networks that are geographically distant (some exchanges are conducted as far away as 50 miles), customers (DE are drug dealers), professionals who do not want to be identified (i.e. government workers, teachers, etc.), HIV-infected IDU too ill to travel, and 'paranoid' methamphetamine injectors. The DE are trained in HIV prevention strategies and needle and syringe exchange protocol. This protocol allows a

---

[4] Funded by the National Institute of Justice.
[5] Funded by UARP.

very small, illegal programme to serve a large geographic area, IDU not willing to be identified at a site, a significant number of young IDU, and more IDU than a traditional fixed-site exchange could. It also provides a venue for IDU to become involved in HIV prevention activity in their community. From July 1, 1994 to June 30, 1995 the Sacramento Area Needle Exchange (SANE) exchanged 52,194 needles and syringes during 817 exchanges.

In collaboration with the Center for AIDS Prevention Studies at the University of California, San Francisco, UCD-HPS conducted focus groups with current injection drug users (IDU) in February, 1995, to assess the feasibility of drug user organizations in Sacramento County. Similar focus groups were conducted in August of 1993, assessing the impact of the change in the "national bleach message" (Haverkos, 1994). Participants were recruited by street outreach workers and paid $25 for their assistance with these focus groups. During the course of these groups qualitative information was obtained concerning the amphetamine-injecting subculture of IDU.

In the summer of 1995, a study of Sacramento teenagers was conducted to inform the designers of a national HIV risk-reduction marketing campaign targeted at adolescents[6]. UCD-HPS programme staff carried out the 'formative' research for this youth survey and intervention project, which involved conducting focus groups and individual interviews with adolescents (ages 14–18) and their parents. Participants were recruited from designated areas of the county with the highest rates of sexually transmitted diseases among the target population, and were paid $25 for their contributions to the project. They were asked to discuss HIV risk, knowledge, sexual and drug use risk behaviours, HIV information sources and social and community norms. Interviews were conducted, transcribed and studied by a team of project staff and community service providers over the summer of 1995.

Although data in the above mentioned studies excluded men who reported engaging in sexual activity with other men, two additional studies currently being conducted in the Psychology Department at UC Davis (under the direction of Dr. Greg Herek) offer some indications about methamphetamine use among gay and bisexual men in the Sacramento Valley. The first of these studies is a large scale community survey looking at the incidence of hate crimes based on sexual orientation in the Sacramento area[7]. Over 2,583 lesbians, gay men, and bisexuals completed the instrument as of November 17, 1995. Of all respondents, 2.3% self-reported using methamphetamines within 7 days of completing the survey. Gay and bisexual men (3.8%) were more likely to report using this drug than were lesbians and bisexual women (0.5%). The mode of methamphetamine intake was not recorded in the survey.

---

[6] Funded by the Centers for Disease Control and the Academy for Educational Development.
[7] Funded by the National Institute on Mental Health (NIMH).

The second study concerns the HIV risk reduction and coping in a cohort of 309 gay and bisexual men (recruited as of November 17, 1995)[8]. Participants in this longitudinal face-to-face interview were selected according to identity categories proposed by Herek and Glunt (1995). Methamphetamine use in the past 12 months was reported by 14.3% of these men. So far, 8.8% of respondents have reported ever using injectable recreational drugs and 5.2% reported needle sharing behaviours. Out of these, 14.8% reported injection drug use in the past 12 months (1.3% of the total sample). Two respondents in this cohort (.6%) report needle sharing behaviours in the past 12 months[9]. The data discussed in the rest of this chapter characterize heterosexual drug injectors only. See Table 1 for gender and ethnic composition of heterosexual study populations.

RESULTS

Scope of the Methamphetamine Problem

Methamphetamines are one of the most predominant illicit drugs of use/misuse in Northern California. It is estimated that there are 7,000 daily injectors of methamphetamines and an unknown number of occasional methamphetamine injectors in Sacramento County. In the DUF study, 71% of the participants tested positive for any illicit drug. More than half of these (51%) tested positive for methamphetamines, compared to 40% positive for marijuana, 32% positive for cocaine, and only 7% positive for opiates (this included licit and illicit opiates). Additionally, two-thirds (67%) of participants in the local syringe exchange programme reported methamphetamine injection compared to 40% who reported heroin injection, and only 15% who reported cocaine injection.

Who are Methamphetamine Injectors in our Region?

In general, these studies showed that methamphetamine users are a diverse group of people, comprising several subcultures. However, if there was such a thing as a "typical" methamphetamine injector (MI) in our region, it would be a male caucasian, aged 18–40 years, periodically employed, domestically unstable, single, with no children living in his residence, previously incarcerated, socially and sexually very interactive ('out and about and ready to play'). In addition to this 'typical' injector, we identified as relatively distinct subgroups: 'bikers', middle class 'white collar' workers, tradespeople and labourers, young injectors (teenagers), college students, homeless, previously

---

[8] Funded by NIMH.
[9] The authors thank Dr. Eric Glunt for these data.

non-drug-using women introduced to the drug in their early twenties by a male sexual partner, women of colour, and an emerging group of Latino methamphetamine users and manufacturers.

Methamphetamine is definitely the stimulant drug of choice in our region among younger people. Among 14–18 year old adolescents who use drugs (25%) other than alcohol and marijuana, methamphetamine was used most commonly (54% of those who had used illicit drugs). For those in drug treatment programmes 42% of stimulant injectors were under the age of 30, as compared to only 18% of heroin injectors. Among incarcerated young people under the age of 25, half were positive for an illegal drug, and 44% of these were positive for methamphetamine, 24% for cocaine, and 5% for opiates.

While males are the majority of methamphetamine injectors, women are also significantly involved with this drug. Caucasian women outnumber women of colour, but we suspect this is changing based on changing demographics of our syringe exchangers and DUF studies. Among women in the DUF study positive for an illegal drug, half were positive for methamphetamine, of whom 25% were women of colour. In this study there was a small subset of women (mostly 30–45 years of age) who reported no significant drug use prior to the age of 20, initiation into methamphetamine use in their early twenties (usually by a male sexual partner), and a rapid increase to sustained, problematic methamphetamine use. Street outreach workers and research staff have speculated that this phenomenon may be related to the perception in the user of improved confidence, competence, and effectiveness in both the sexual and social spheres of life, which may be particularly attractive to women who perceive themselves as powerless and ineffectual. We also noted that some young women began their methamphetamine use for weight control, and feared that cessation of use would lead to weight gain.

Another significant subgroup, contacted through the syringe exchange programme, use methamphetamine to increase alertness and stamina. These people were college students, postal workers, state government employees, and those who work in agriculture and manufacturing (Grinspoon and Hedblom, 1975).

Our studies have convinced us that methamphetamine injectors are not accessible in large numbers for harm prevention and risk-reduction education in our drug treatment programmes. Among 1,269 drug injectors interviewed in local treatment programmes only 90 were methamphetamine injectors. Furthermore, 86% of arrestees in the DUF study who tested positive for methamphetamine had never been in a drug treatment programme. Similarly 97% of MI interviewed in the out-of-treatment study in 1992 had never been in a drug treatment programme. Conversely, MI are accessible through jail in-reach, street outreach, and syringe exchange (Donmall and Millar, 1995; CDC, 1989). In our in-treatment study, 80% of the MI had been incarcerated previously. More then a quarter (27%) of out-of-treatment MI interviewed in 1994 had been arrested in the year prior to interview.

Methamphetamine users in our studies tend not to use other injectable drugs, whereas opiate or cocaine injectors report injecting methamphetamine. For example, one-third of opiate-positive inmates in the DUF study reported that they had used methamphetamine in the 30 days prior to interview, and 20% reported that they had felt dependent on methamphetamine at some time in their lives. Only 40% of these individuals reported that they had never tried methamphetamine. The majority (89%) of opiate-positive IDU and over half (58%) of cocaine-positive IDU reported a history of methamphetamine injection, whereas, methamphetamine-positive IDU reported no history of injecting opiates or cocaine. In the syringe exchange, 45% of exchanges were conducted with IDU who reported injecting only methamphetamine. We interpret these data to suggest that methamphetamines, when readily and cheaply available, are attractive drugs to a wide variety of injectors. Also, as we will discuss later, because methamphetamine injectors are several times more likely than opiate injectors to acquire HIV-1 infection, the cross-over use of methamphetamine by these heroin injectors may place them at higher risk for HIV exposure.

Injection Risk Behaviour

Methamphetamine injectors engage in more high-risk injection behaviours, with greater frequency, than do heroin injectors. MI in the in-treatment study were more than twice as likely as heroin IDU to name multiple syringe sources (36% versus 17%) and were half as likely as heroin IDU to report pharmacies as their primary source for syringes (14% versus 28%). Methamphetamine injectors were much more likely to report that they shared needles and syringes than were heroin injectors (p < .05) and somewhat less likely to report disinfecting their shared paraphernalia every time they injected (38% versus 43%). Most alarming, the methamphetamine injectors in this study reported sharing injection equipment with an average of 11 strangers and 8 casual sexual partners compared to 3.4 strangers and 2.6 casual sexual partners for heroin injectors in the year prior to interview. Similarly, two thirds of methamphetamine injectors in the DUF study reported a history of syringe sharing. Disturbingly, 96% of HIV-infected IDU in the first out-of-treatment study reported sharing needles and syringes in the past year and only 6% reported regularly disinfecting these shared syringes.

Notably, significantly more methamphetamine injectors (77%) than heroin injectors (11%) interviewed in drug treatment programmes reported no injection in the year prior to interview (p < .01). This suggests that there are large numbers of 'binge'[10] or occasional injectors of methamphetamine who may not self-identify as injectors and, therefore, not consider themselves at risk

---

[10] 'Binge' is a period of days or weeks of consistent use of significant amounts of drug, followed by a period of no use.

for bloodborne infections, and ignore infection prevention messages targeted at IDU. Also, these data suggest that there are windows of opportunity for disease prevention intervention with methamphetamine injectors when they are not using the drug.

Sexual Risk Behaviour

The sexual behaviours of methamphetamine injectors also place them at high risk for acquiring and transmitting HIV. More than half (55%) of methamphetamine injectors interviewed in the Sacramento County Main Jail reported having more than one sexual partner in the year prior to interview and 16% reported more than five sexual partners in the same time period. Similarly, methamphetamine injectors interviewed in drug treatment programmes reported significantly more types of high-risk sexual behaviours with significantly greater frequency than that reported by heroin injectors (p < .01). Disturbingly, more than two thirds of each group reported no condom use whatsoever. Half of MI in drug treatment (compared to 30% for heroin injectors) reported engaging in sexual activity under the influence of alcohol in the year prior to interview (p < .01) an average of 61 times and 35 times respectively (p < .05). The MI reported an average of 16 sexual partners in the past year compared to 12 for heroin injectors. More than half (52%) of female MI in drug treatment stated that they had participated in receptive anal intercourse in the last year as opposed to only one quarter of heroin injecting women in drug treatment (p < .05). MI also reported more sexual interaction with non-injectors than did heroin injectors.

Adverse Health Consequences of Methamphetamine Injection

Problematic drug use, and problematic drug control policies often overshadow perhaps the most destructive and harmful aspect of methamphetamine injection, that of infectious diseases that accompany its use. We in the U.S. have tended to focus on the drugs themselves, and criminal activity associated with their use, to the relative exclusion of even more serious health consequences of use.

The most talked-about health consequence of methamphetamine injection in our region is infection with HIV. Whether this is actually the most significant health consequence is not yet clear. It may be that, ultimately, the morbidity and mortality of other infectious complications such as viral hepatitis, and HTLV I and II infection may surpass those of HIV infection. In either case, we must begin to discuss infectious complications of methamphetamine injection with as much vigor as we do drug effects and social costs. They are not separable — there is little profit in addressing the direct effects and social costs of the drug if injectors acquire a disease which will kill them at a relatively early age, and which can be passed on to their sexual partners and children.

Human immunodeficiency virus infection

Our in-treatment and out-of-treatment studies all show that methamphetamine injectors are at a significantly greater risk of acquiring HIV-1 and other blood borne viruses than are opiate injectors in Northern California (Table 2). Similar findings were observed in Seattle, Washington, in the Pacific Northwest of the United States (Harris, 1993) and in the United Kingdom (Klee, 1992a, 1992b, 1993). This association between injection of a central nervous system stimulant and HIV-1 was also seen with cocaine injection in San Francisco (Chaisson, 1989). What accounts for this increased risk of HIV-1 infection among stimulant injectors?

In our studies to date gender (male), ethnicity (African-American), age (younger age), and needle and syringe sharing are also independently associated with higher probability of HIV-1 infection, when controlled for drug of choice ($p < 0.05$). Disturbingly, both of the out-of-treatment studies showed that young injectors, under the age of 25 years, were significantly more likely to be infected with HIV-1 than were those 30 years and older (Table 3). In the 1992 out-of-treatment study a significant difference was also found between injectors living in the downtown area of Sacramento (lower risk) and those living in the outlying areas ($p < .01$). It is important to note that most of the drug treatment service providers are located in the downtown area and public transportation from the outlying areas to downtown is time consuming and inefficient. Are these injectors at risk because they are injecting methamphetamine or because they are young or because they reside in areas of high risk? Unfortunately, our studies to date have not had sufficient statistical power to answer these questions.

In contrast to the situation in California, Kirsten Kall's studies in Sweden have found the opposite result — heroin injectors have a significantly higher seroprevalence of HIV-1 than do methamphetamine injectors (Kall, 1995). This intriguing paradox demands further investigation and explanation. What is it about the heroin-injecting culture in Sweden and the methamphetamine-injecting cultures in Northern California, the US Pacific Northwest, and the United Kingdom that puts them at higher risk for HIV-1 infection?

There are several alternative possibilities. It may be a simple probabilistic feature common to both cultures, such as the number of high-risk injections, injection practices (e.g., frontloading, backloading, disinfection practices) or the size of the syringe-sharing group. Or there may be underlying cultural phenomena common to both which result in increased risk, for example, the processes by which new injectors learn shooting techniques, or lifetime patterns of drug use.

Methamphetamine users who do not inject their drugs may also be at high risk for acquiring HIV-1. California methamphetamine users entering drug treatment programmes in 1988 reported on their primary routes of ingestion: 57% reported that they snorted; 29% injected; and 14% either smoked or took the drugs orally (Nisenbaum, 1995). Our information from our qualitative research is that MI associate frequently with non-injectors. Injectors will snort or smoke when in the company of users who do not inject or when needles and syringes are unavailable (this situation is common because possession of a syringe in California without a prescription is against the law). Methamphetamines stimulate sexual behaviour, so sexual contact between injectors and noninjectors occurs frequently in this setting. Therefore, MI are a likely bridge for HIV-1 and other infectious disease transmission to the non-injecting, methamphetamine-using population.

Many HIV-infected individuals in our area are, or have been, members of the local methamphetamine-using population. The Center for AIDS Research, Education, and Services (CARES) in Sacramento provides medical services to over 1,200 HIV-infected individuals. In 1989 when the Center served 400 patients, we examined 280 of the active medical charts (patient seen within the past six months) at this facility and found 62% (173) of the patients reported current (62) or past (111) drug use. Fifty-four percent (93) of these drug users reported a stimulant as their drug of choice and 9% named an opiate; 63% reported that they did not inject their drugs. The proportion of people with HIV/AIDS who have a history of methamphetamine use appears only to have increased since then. These findings suggests there is a significant, noninjecting, methamphetamine-using population in our area that is sexually interactive with members of the HIV-infected methamphetamine-using population. The uninfected methamphetamine users are engaging in behaviours that put them at high risk for acquisition of HIV. Our data also show that MI engage in sexual activity with noninjectors more frequently than do opiate injectors. The MI population is potentially a major conduit for the spread of the AIDS virus to the non-drug-using heterosexual population in our community.

Other infectious diseases associated with methamphetamine use

A subsample (N = 585) of participants in the in-treatment study (N = 1,269) was also tested for hepatitis B virus (HBV), hepatitis C virus (HCV), and human T-lymphotropic viruses I and II (HTLV I/II) infection (Zeldis 1992). Evidence of prior HBV infection was found in 71% of the population and HCV antibody was found in 72%. The prevalence of HBV was statistically higher in Latinos than in either Caucasians or African Americans (p < .01). Twelve percent of IDU were positive for HTLV I/II, with a statistically greater prevalence in people of color (p < .0001). The presence of each viral marker, except hepatitis B surface antigen antibody, correlated with duration of injection drug use. Age also correlated independently, though less strongly, with the likelihood of antibody to all markers except hepatitis B surface antigen antibody. The rate of HTLV I/II is higher in injectors more than 50 years old than in younger persons, even when corrected for similar length of injection history.

Although heroin injectors had a higher prevalence of both Hepatitis B and C than did methamphetamine injectors, this difference may be due to the greater average duration of injection drug use for heroin injectors (12.6 years) than for methamphetamine injectors (7.2 years).

Serological evidence of co-infection with more than one virus was common. Overall, 57% were found to be co-infected with HBV and HCV; 9% showed evidence of co-infection with all three viruses (hepatitis B, hepatitis C, and HTLV I/II). By far, the greatest co-infection prevalence is seen between hepatitis B and C, where 81% of the 417 anti-HBc reactive IDU were also anti-HCV reactive and 80% of the 421 reactive for anti-HCV were also anti-HBc reactive. Additionally, 100% of the 70 anti-HTVL I/II reactive injectors were also reactive for either anti-HBc (14%), anti-HCV (9%), or both (77%).

In the long run, chronic hepatitis B or C virus activity often leads to severe liver disease and death. Hepatitis C in particular appears to result in liver cirrhosis in nearly one quarter of all infected individuals, while about 2–3% of those infected with hepatitis B develop cirrhosis. From our serosurveys, then, we can estimate that up to 19% of IDU in our region will develop cirrhosis leading to death. At this point in time, this is nearly double the proportion who will develop AIDS. This morbidity and mortality may be reduced somewhat by newer treatments for chronic hepatitis C infection, but the impact will still be great.

Other adverse health consequences

There is also potential for additional health problems caused by the toxic residues dumped into the environment by methamphetamine producers. Many of the chemicals used to make methamphetamine are believed to cause cancer, and some are believed to affect the respiratory system. Some recipes for methamphetamine manufacture use cyanide salts that can be converted into cyanide gas (the same gas that is used in California's gas chamber). However, law enforcement and health experts are not sure what kind of health effects there will be. Officials have begun to study the problem of retention of these toxic materials in walls, floors, carpeting, etc., in houses and motel rooms in which methamphetamines are produced. There are also potential risks due to uptake of these substances in plants, soil, and groundwater. As yet, effective clean up strategies have not been developed (Brown, 1994).

Other serious health problems will arise for MI who regularly drink alcohol and smoke cigarettes. In the DUF sample, over half (52%) of the arrestees who tested positive for methamphetamine reported alcohol use in the 30 days prior to interview. Half of these individuals reported drinking alcohol on 15 or more days in the previous month, yet only 20% of these people felt that they were dependent on alcohol at the time of the interview.

Almost three quarters (73%) of those arrestees who were positive for methamphetamine reported regular cigarette smoking in the 30 days prior to interview. Ninety-five percent of these individuals reported smoking cigarettes on more than 20 days in the month prior to interview and yet, only 28% of these smokers felt dependent on tobacco at the time of interview. Clearly there are some perceptual problems regarding problematic use of *licit* drugs.

DISCUSSION

Methamphetamine is a popular stimulant drug of use/misuse in northern California. It is growing in popularity, inexpensive, and readily available (partly due to easy, local production). Methamphetamine is a drug used by young people (teenagers and young adults), tradespeople and labourers (both industrial and agricultural), and 'middle class' professionals. It is increasingly favoured by young women and women of colour and there is an emerging group of Latino users and manufacturers. Methamphetamine users in this region are a diverse group of people, who represent a cross-section of society. They are predominantly sexually-active heterosexuals, well integrated into society, who regularly interact socially and sexually with the non-drug-using population of Sacramento. A significant portion of methamphetamine users in this region are injection drug users (may be as high as 40%).

Methamphetamine use is associated with an increase in sexual desire and activity and, therefore, with an increased risk of sexually transmitted diseases. Methamphetamine injection is related to a high risk of infection with HIV in this region, the US Pacific Northwest, and the UK. Other potentially fatal viral infections (HBV, HCV, HTLV I/II) are also transmitted frequently among methamphetamine injectors. Possible reasons for this increased risk of infectious disease transmission and acquisition include: high risk injection behaviour (sharing injection equipment, not disinfecting shared equipment, obtaining needle and syringes from questionable sources, etc.) and high risk sexual activity (multiple sexual partners, receptive anal intercourse, trading sex for money or drugs, etc.). However, there is a paradox between the US findings and those of Kirsten Kall in Sweden where heroin injectors have the highest rates of HIV infection. Again we ask if there may be underlying cultural phenomena common to both cultures (Sweden's heroin injectors and methamphetamine injectors in the US and UK) that result in increased risk of disease?

Methamphetamine injectors in Sacramento County are not attracted to drug treatment (they represent only 10% of the population) because of lack of treatment availability and lack of substitution therapy (such as methadone for heroin injectors). Therefore, other venues must be used in order to contact methamphetamine IDU for HIV risk-reduction training. More effective means to access MI are frequent jail in-reach, syringe exchange, and street outreach. We have found street outreach to be a particularly effective tool when the street outreach workers are indigenous to the area and familiar with the various subcultures that exist within the methamphetamine scene.

Other strategies for harm reduction include involving current IDU in the planning, designing, and implementation of interventions, such as facilitating the formation of drug user organizations and IDU access to media. One local cable television station has agreed to provide training for local users and a weekly 1/2 hour time slot for drug users to produce their own television show (which will include risk-reduction training). A proven method of accessing out-of-treatment IDU and slowing the spread of HIV is a high-volume needle and syringe exchange programme. However, this is difficult to achieve in Sacramento as the governor of California has vetoed three attempts by the state legislature to change the law and allow legal syringe exchange programmes to operate in California. Changing the focus of risk-reduction messages from individual behaviour to community norms, by targeting social networks of drug users rather than individual injectors, may make an impact on the spread of disease. We believe that changes can be made in community norms regarding sexual and drug use behaviours just as community norms have been changed in California regarding smoking tobacco, albeit with a higher degree of difficulty. If 'peer pressure' can be used to support harm minimisation strategies, the spread of HIV can be slowed. One tactic that has been suggested for this strategy is 'narrowcasting'. This involves small posters with harm reduction messages targeted to a specific population (such as MI) placed in the bathrooms of public places (i.e. bars, coffee shops, etc.) known to be frequented by the target group. A multicomponent community intervention, designed in collaboration with Dr. Ross Gibson of the Center for AIDS Prevention Studies at the University of California, San Francisco, comprising all the strategies mentioned above and a few others will be implemented in Sacramento in the spring of 1996. The intervention will be evaluated for effectiveness and degree of penetration into the community by surveys of drug users in the intervention city, Sacramento, and a comparison city, San Diego (California), before, during, and after implementation.

Table 1   Sample size, gender, ethnicity of UCD-HPS studies

Study	Number	Female	Male Percentages	C	AA	L
In Treatment, 1987–91	1,269	44	56	70	8	19
Out of Treatment, 1992	546	37	63	48	21	23
Out of Treatment, 1994	500	34	66	49	33	9
DUF, 1993	1,134	33	67	40	31	14
Video, 1994–5	75	35	65	39	41	10
Needle Exchange, 1994–5	817	40	60	57	19	17
IDU focus groups, 1993–5	60	NA	NA	NA	NA	NA
Youth Survey, 1995	166	55	45	43	17	18

Note: C — Caucasian, AA — African American, L — Latino

Table 2   Prevalence of HIV among UCD-HPS populations, stratified by drug of choice.

Study	HIV+ Op IDU	HIV+ MI	p	OR	CI
In-treatment	.5%	3%	<.05	7.7	1.2, 50
Out-of-treatment 92	4%	11%	<.02	3.4	1.1, 10
Out-of-treatment 94	5%	9%	ns		

Table 3   Prevalence of HIV among IDU stratified by age

Study	IDU<25	IDU>25	p	OR	CI
Out-of-treatment 92*	29%	7%	<.001	5.6	2.8, 11.3
Out-of-treatment 94+	16%	7%	<.05		

*Chi square, + Fischer's exact

We know the patterns of drug use and transmission of HIV and bloodborne viral infections in our community. There are effective means for reducing transmission of HIV and we know how to access IDU at risk. However, the political climate in California and elsewhere in the US is not conducive to implementing these strategies. Whether we will be able to implement them to a degree that will significantly reduce transmission of fatal viral infections will be known in the next two to three years. If we fail, these infections will result in early death for many injecting drug users, perhaps as many as 25% of them presently living in Sacramento.

REFERENCES

Aldrich, M., *et al.* (1990) A spreadsheet for AIDS: estimating heterosexual injection drug user population size AIDS statistics in San Francisco. *Journal of Psychoactive Drugs,* **22**(3), pp. 343–9.

Brown, M. (1994) Meth labs leave toxic trail: Costly cleanup problems remain after many drug busts. *The Sacramento Bee,* May 9.

Bureau of Narcotic Enforcement (BNE) (1993) *Report to California Statewide Epidemiology Work Group.*

Centers for Disease Control (1989) Coordinated community programmes for HIV prevention among intravenous drug users — California, Massachusetts. *MMWR,* **38**, pp. 369–74.

Chaisson, R. E., Bacchetti, P., Osmond, D., Brodie, B., Sande, M.A. and Moss, A.R. (1989) Cocaine use and HIV infection in intravenous drug users in San Francisco. *JAMA,* **261**(4), pp. 561–5.

Donmall, M. and Millar, T. (1995) Do syringe exchange schemes attract different clients from services providing treatment? Paper presented at the VI International Conference on the Reduction of Drug Related Harm, Florence, Italy.

Grinspoon, L. and Hedblom, P. (1975) *The Speed Culture: Amphetamine Use and Abuse in America.* Cambridge M.A.: Harvard University Press.

Harris, N., Fields, M.J. and Gordon D.C. (1993) Risk factors for HIV infection among injection drug users: Results of blinded surveys in drug treatment centers, King County, Washington 1988–1991. *Journal of AIDS,* **6**(11), pp. 1275–82.

Haverkos, H. and Jones, T.S. (1994) Reports on NIDA/CSAT/CDC Workshop on the use of bleach for the decontamination of drug injection equipment. *Journal of AIDS,* **7**(7), pp. 741–76.

Herek, G. and Glunt, E. (1995) Identity and community among gay and bisexual men in the AIDS era: preliminary findings from the Sacramento Men's Health Study. In G.M. Herek and B. Greene (eds.) *AIDS, Identity, and Community: The HIV Epidemic and Lesbians.* Thousand Oaks, California: Sage.

Kall, K. (1995) *Sexual behaviour of incarcerated intravenous drug users in Stockholm in relation to human immunodeficiency virus (HIV) and hepatitis B virus (HBV) transmission.* Stockholm: The Karolinska Institute, Institution of Clinical Neuroscience.

Kaplan, E.H. and Brandeau, M.L. (eds.) (1994) *Modeling the AIDS Epidemic: Planning, Policy, and Prediction.* New York: Raven Press.

Klee, H. (1992a) Sexual risk among amphetamine misusers: Prospects for change. In: P. Davies and G. Hart (eds.) *AIDS: Rights, Risk, and Reason.* London: Falmer Press.

Klee, H. (1992b) A new target for behavioural research — amphetamine misuse. *British Journal of Addiction,* **87**(3), pp. 439–46.

Klee, H. (1993) The sexual behaviour of injecting women: Heroin and amphetamine using women compared. *Addiction,* **88**, pp. 1055–62.

Newmeyer, J. (1991) The Barefoot Epidemiologist: "What Works" in Drug Abuse Prevalence Estimation. *Published Proceedings of the National Institute of Drug Abuse's Community Epidemiology Work Group (CEWG),* Rockville, MD.

Newmeyer, J. (1995) *MidCity Numbers,* August, **8**(5), p. 4.

Nisenbaum, S. (1995) Personal communication, California Department of Alcohol and Drug Programmes.

Zeldis, J.B., Jain, S., Kuramot, J.K., Richard, C., Sazama, K., Holland, P. and Flynn, N. (1992) Seroepidemiology of viral infections among intravenous drug users in northern California. *West Journal of Medicine,* **156**(1), pp. 30–5.

Introduction to Section 3: Japan and Sweden

Japan and Sweden are the two nations that are traditionally most associated with the use of amphetamine. Whereas other countries have experienced occasional epidemics and developed problems with other drugs, with them amphetamine and methamphetamine are the preferred and persistently problematic drugs.

The countries are similar in other ways too. They have developed legislation and initiated law enforcement policies that are particularly severe. Both would claim some containment of the problem through these means and both attribute a considerable proportion of their difficulties to the policies, or lack of them, of neighbouring countries.

It is interesting to place them in close juxtaposition, not only to highlight similarities, but to note the differences between them: in their cultures; their political, military and economic history; their attitudes and experience of other drugs. One feels that if the use of amphetamine by Japan and Sweden were better understood, this would throw some light on the patterns of use observed elsewhere in the world. However the identification of critical correspondences remains elusive and difficult.

10

Methamphetamine Abuse in Japan: Its 45 Year History and the Current Situation

HIROSHI SUWAKI, SUSUMU FUKUI and
KYOHEI KONUMA

INTRODUCTION

Japan has suffered almost 45 years of methamphetamine abuse. Epidemic has become closer to endemic, since we have found abusers in every prefecture throughout Japan for the past 15 years.

The history of methamphetamine abuse in Japan is instructive because it reveals the emergence of three entirely different patterns of behaviour toward a potentially dependence-inducing substance. The relationships between the drug and society are quite different from one period to another. We have learned much from its history, but it is still difficult to overcome the extensive spread of abuse (Suwaki and Bjorksten, 1983; Suwaki, 1991; Fukui *et al.*, 1994).

This chapter describes the history of Japanese methamphetamine abuse which can be divided into four periods: Calm period; Period of the First Epidemic; Period of diversification to other substances, and Period of the Second Epidemic. Each period differs in the magnitude of abuse, the social context and attitudes, and the underlying dynamic relationships with other substances of abuse. We shall focus attention on the relationship between the drug and the attitudes of Japanese society. Subsequently we shall consider more recent developments in methamphetamine abuse in Japan including supply, cost, counter-measures and demographic and social backgrounds. Finally the psychiatric implications of methamphetamine abuse, the nature of psychiatric populations and patterns of abuse and psychosis over time will be explored.

THE HISTORY OF METHAMPHETAMINE ABUSE IN JAPAN

Like many other countries, national epidemiological data from household surveys on substance abuse are unavailable in Japan. However, the number of arrests for substance control law violations are one of the indicators which reveal the magnitude of the problem. Figure 1 shows the number of arrests for violations against various substance control laws from 1950 to 1993 (Ministry of Health and Welfare, 1994). In the case of organic solvents, persons under the age of 20 who are admitted to treatment or correctional institutions are also included in the data until 1988, when data collection methods of the National Police Agency changed and the figures no longer included such individuals. The following description of methamphetamine abuse history is largely based on the data shown in this figure.

The Calm Period Prior to 1945

Prior to 1945, substance abuse was not a problem in Japan, with the exception of alcoholism. However, incidental abuse of opiates and cocaine did occur. Most opiate abusers were from outside Japan, whereas most cocaine abusers consisted of a small number of medical doctors. The estimated total number of abusers was about 400. Thus, substance abuse was neither a social nor a medical problem in that period.

While amphetamine was reported to be synthesized by Edeleano, in 1887, methamphetamine was first synthesized by a Japanese pharmacologist, Dr. Nagayoshi Nagai in 1893 from alkaloid ephedrine which also had been

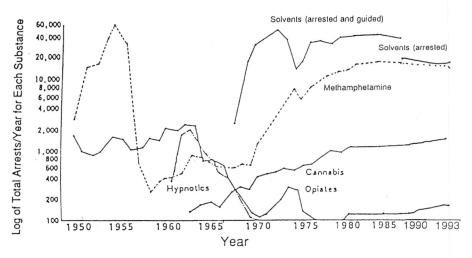

Figure 1   Arrests for drug statute violations excluding alcohol.
Source: Ministry of Health and Welfare, Bureau of Pharmaceutical Affairs (1994).

isolated from mao (Ephedra sinica) by Dr. Nagai himself. However, until the 1940s methamphetamine did not attract much attention from society as a pharmaceutical product.

During World War II, methamphetamine was used mainly for Japanese military objectives. At times, soldiers were forced to consume methamphetamine to enhance their fighting spirits and to keep them awake while engaged in nocturnal battles. Also, in order to increase efficiency and productivity in military support industries, workers were coerced into using methamphetamine.

In 1941, pharmacies began to sell methamphetamine over the counter under commercial names such as Philopon and Sedrin. However, methamphetamine abuse was not a social issue at that time. Japan had a strong military power with a totalitarian society, in which people shared the same objectives as military leaders. Under such circumstances, people did not think of its use in terms of potential harm or drug dependence. Most Japanese were ignorant of the hazardous properties of methamphetamine, and no laws controlling its sale or distribution existed at that time.

The Period of The First Epidemic (1945–1957)

After the war, pharmaceutical manufacturers began over-the-counter sales of methamphetamine, advertising the product with the slogan, "Fight sleepiness and enhance vitality." Methamphetamine from army stocks also became available on the black market. Thus, people were supplied with methamphetamine in abundance but had no awareness of its dangerous effects. The methamphetamine abuse epidemic spread rapidly in a society which was discouraged and depressed by the war. The younger generation was particularly eager to experience the euphoric and mood-elevating effects of the drug.

The first incidents of methamphetamine abuse were seen in the Kansai area centering on Osaka and Kobe, in 1946. The number of abusers rapidly increased and spread to rural areas throughout the country. Writers, journalists, artists, entertainers, factory workers and even students used methamphetamine to enhance their efficiency while working or studying overnight. Juvenile delinquent groups that stayed out all night also used methamphetamine as a stimulant and for pleasure. By 1948 5% of individuals between the ages of 16 and 25 years are believed to have abused methamphetamine.

We believe the reasons for the rapid increase in methamphetamine abuse at that time are as follows: an aimless, nihilistic and confused postwar social environment; an unlimited supply of methamphetamine to the market-place without any understanding of the dangerous effects of its abuse and dependence; the demands of a younger generation, that had lost their purpose in life, for the euphoric effect of methamphetamine. These three factors; social environment, availability, and population vulnerability brought about the epidemic of methamphetamine abuse.

Although the Stimulants Control Law was enacted with strict enforcement in 1951, active illicit manufacturing, smuggling, and sales by the underworld continued to supply a large amount of methamphetamine, resulting in an unprecedented epidemic of abuse.[1]

During the later stage of this period, a shift in the population of abusers occurred to include antisocial and alienated people, such as gang members and the unemployed, rather than ordinary citizens.

At the same time, injectable methamphetamine became available as an alternative to tablets. Taken intravenously, the acute stimulant effect of methamphetamine on the central nervous system is enhanced greatly. Methamphetamine abusers began to take the drug intravenously by prefer-ence, which led to an increase in the number of homicides and other crimes under the pharmacological influence of methamphetamine. Methamphet-amine injection abuse rapidly increased the problems related to social order. During the peak period of 1954, the number of methamphetamine abusers is estimated to have reached 550,000, including 55,000 who were suffering from Methamphetamine-induced psychosis.

In 1954, a Kyoko-chan homicide incident (a youth with methamphetamine abuse murdered a 10-year-old girl under influence of the drug) triggered a public outcry that pressed for an amendment of the Stimulants Control Law. This amendment led to stricter enforcement of the law. After this peak in 1954, methamphetamine abuse declined rapidly. Contributing factors for this in-cluded: severe critical public opinion against methamphetamine abuse; the strict application of punishment under the Stimulants Control Law; the adop-tion of treatment of chronic addicts under an involuntary admission pro-gramme based on amendments to the Mental Health Act; economic recovery and improved living standards, that perhaps reduced the desire for the eu-phoric effects of the drug; and a blockade of the illicit manufacturing bases (the supply sources of methamphetamine) located within Japan by the police.

The Period of Diversification to Other Substances (1957–1969)

Between 1957 and 1969, rapid industrialization moved Japanese society into a period of high economic growth. In this period, the number of drug-related arrests was less than 1000 annually (see Figure 1). The problem of methamphe-tamine abuse was no longer an issue in society or in the medical professions.

However, other substances of abuse were introduced into Japanese society one after another. Interestingly, in this stage of substance abuse history, people who started to abuse drugs were distributed across several age groups.

---

[1] Interestingly, cocaine was not included in the Stimulants Control Law but was included later in the Narcotics Control Law (1953). Amphetamine and methylphenidate, which along with methamphetamine are the main drugs targeted by the Stimulants Control Law, but have rarely been abused in Japan.

Teenagers began to take hypnotics and analgesics between 1960 and 1975. Then their preference shifted to organic solvents in 1967. This spread at a very high rate throughout the country and has continued unabated. Older people prefered tranquilizers such as meprobamate and chlordiazepoxide. Heroin abuse also began in the Kansai area and gradually spread elsewhere. Co-ordinated government action began in 1962 with the organization of the Ministers' Council for Narcotics Counter-measures, and in 1963 with amendments to the Narcotic Control Law which increased the penalties for narcotics violations. These measures, combined with vigorous enforcement, were successful and heroin abuse had declined by 1970.

Even in this period, methamphetamine was being manufactured illegally by organized criminals in Kansai area, and it was abused in illicit gambling parties and sleepless vigils there. Japanese organized gangs originated during the 1960s in the Kansai area, and methamphetamine became part of their culture and lifestyle. This precipitated the second methamphetamine epidemic. Previous efforts at control had not eradicated abuse since abuse levels during this period were still considerable.

The Period of The Second Epidemic (1970-Present)

Between 1970 and 1974, methamphetamine abuse swept across Japan from the Kansai area, but was limited to a core group of organized criminals and the people within their sphere of influence. The number of arrests increased rapidly from less than 1,000 in 1970 to a high of 8,510 in 1973. During this period, 60% of those arrested for violations of the Stimulants Control Law were organized criminals. In addition to this core group, individuals in contact with these criminals (such as the unemployed, workers in restaurant and liquor bar industries, bar hostesses and social escorts) became involved in the abuse of methamphetamine.

As methamphetamine abuse spread, there was an associated increase in the number of cases of methamphetamine induced psychosis. To cope with this situation, amendments were made to the Stimulants Control Law in 1973 to introduce penal provisions that were equivalent to those of the Narcotics Control Law. Unfortunately, the effectiveness of these amendments proved to be limited.

From 1975 until 1981, a group of methamphetamine abusers who were in some way associated with organized crime expanded, and also involved construction workers and truck drivers. Blue-collar workers, daily-paid labourers, shop assistants, students, housewives, and other citizens from the ordinary social strata who came in close contact with this second group of methamphetamine abusers also became involved. Thus the abuse penetrated whole populations at this stage of epidemic. The number of arrests for drugs violations exceeded 10,000 in 1976, and continued to increase by 20–30% each year to reach a figure of 22,000 in 1981.

During the course of this epidemic many people suffered from methamphetamine-induced psychosis. A large number of cases with aggressive behaviour and prominent psychiatric symptoms presented troublesome problems to mental hospitals. Although the exact number of hospitalized patients was unknown, a one-day survey conducted on June 30, 1981, by the Ministry of Health on the number of hospitalized methamphetamine dependents, suggested 3000–4000 hospitalization cases.

With an increase in the incidence of violent crimes committed under the drug's influence, coupled with the problems caused by its smuggling and illicit sales by organized criminals, methamphetamine abuse had again developed into a serious social problem.

The Fukagawa incident in 1981, when two housewives and two children were murdered by a methamphetamine abuser in Fukagawa, Tokyo, unleashed a flood of strongly critical public opinion. In general, Japanese society, perhaps like many other societies, is often reluctant to introduce changes in policy, even if the problems are severe, until such an incident sparks off deep sympathy. In the face of such reactions the Japanese government pushed through a number of more punitive policies. With marked law enforcement and other measures to eradicate methamphetamine, combined with public campaigns against abuse, some changes occurred. The number of arrests peaked at 24,372 in 1984 and then decreased to 15,267 in 1990. The number of violent crimes committed under the effects of methamphetamine had increased dramatically between 1975 and 1981, with 553 arrests registered in 1980. However, after the Fukagawa incident, the number rapidly decreased, with only 108 arrests in 1990. The number of individuals who were hospitalized for methamphetamine-induced psychosis also declined.

THE SITUATIONAL CONTEXT OF THE CURRENT EPIDEMIC

Rapid changes accompanying the high economic growth in 1960s brought benefits to the Japanese people. However, they also brought about a distortion of the social structure, for example: changes in the industrial infrastructure; rapid urbanization; hedonistic trends, and increased materialistic values rather than spiritual ones, thus producing a social background conducive to methamphetamine and organic solvent abuse. School drop-outs formed antisocial groups that commonly abused these substances.

For the past decade, the numbers of arrests for methamphetamine and solvent-related violations have plateaud, and may be declining (see Figure 1). On the other hand, the numbers of arrests for heroin, cocaine and cannabis-related violations are steady. In 1993, the number of arrests for Cannabis Control Law violations was 2,055, a 25.4% increase on the previous year; heroin-related arrests numbered 111 and cocaine-related arrests 126, respectively (Ministry of Health and Welfare, 1994).

The nationalities of those arrested now include many non-Japanese. In 353 arrests for Morphine and Other Psychotropic Drugs Control Law violations in 1993, 178 (50.4%) were non-Japanese, of whom 63 were Malaysians and 37 were from South American countries. In 132 arrests for Opium Control Law violations, 64 (48.5%) were non-Japanese, and 60 of them were Iranians. In 2,055 arrests for Cannabis Control Law violations, 322 (15.7%) were non-Japanese. Thus Japan may again be entering a period of change, one which is more internationally oriented. We must be wary of the spread of drugs such as heroin, cocaine and marijuana and continue to monitor dynamic patterns in drug misuse with the help of information from abroad. We also need international collaboration for combating drug violations and for preventive countermeasures.

Sources of Supply of Methamphetamine

In 1966, Japan entered a high economic growth phase until the 'Nixon Shock' in 1971, followed by the 'Oil Shock' in 1973, brought about a global economic slump that affected, in particular, construction and service industries in Japan. Organized gangs suffered financial strain, having relied heavily on these industries as a source of income, and turned to the illicit sale and smuggling of methamphetamine. High profits could be generated from such activities and methamphetamine was available in large supply. The gangs made efforts to maintain supplies through their well-regulated illicit imports, their control over smuggling routes and through diverse and organized drug dealing over extensive regions. The involvement of organized gangs is believed to be the greatest factor contributing to the current epidemic.

In 1993, 41.4% of the total number of 15,495 methamphetamine-related arrests had some relationship with organized gangs. The amount of methamphetamine seized by the police in 1993 was 96.8 kg, decreasing by 41.8% from the previous year. Almost all the illicit products of methamphetamine were from abroad, mainly from Taiwan and mainland China (Ministry of Health and Welfare, 1994).

In Japanese medical society, methamphetamine can be prescribed for the treatment of narcolepsy, depression and the hyperactivity of 'minimum brain syndrome' in children. Physicians are obliged to report their use of the drug in detail. However, there are few physicians now who prescribe methamphetamine for medical purposes.

The Cost of Methamphetamine on the Black Market

The price of illicit methamphetamine differs between regions and dealers. It is quite difficult to ascertain the exact price and the following are the prices obtained from the arrests in 1993: 3–30 dollars yen for 0.03–0.05 gr of methamphetamine in one shot; 50–300 dollars for 1 gr methamphetamine in 10 gr–100 gr unit methamphetamine dealing; 20–100 dollars for 1 gr methamphetamine in 1000 gr unit methamphetamine dealing. In late 1993, the prices of methamphetamine rose by two or three fold on those in the previous year, because smugglers using the main route from Taiwan were arrested and availability was more limited in many areas in Japan (Ministry of Health and Welfare, 1994).

Counter Measures Against Methamphetamine Abuse

In contrast to the first epidemic, present day amphetamine abuse is much more criminal, and counter-measures tend to be legal rather than medical. In 1981, the Ministry of Health and Welfare issued an unusual policy statement which urged hospitals to accept more methamphetamine abusers, which indicated that even the medical profession tended to view their behaviours as more criminal than medical. Today there are a few self-help groups such as NA (Narcotics Anonymous) and DARC (Drug Abuse Rehabilitation Center) for methamphetamine and other drug abusers in Japan but few outpatient treatment programmes. Educational efforts continue and it is hoped that they are attenuating the incidence of methamphetamine abuse, which, fortunately, has declined a little recently.

Currently, law enforcement agencies continue to combat the importation and distribution of methamphetamine by imposing strict sentences for drug violations. The medical management of methamphetamine abusers includes hospital care with special attention to the social readjustment to drug-free lifestyles after discharge. However the increase in long-term heavy users is causing problems, often they present with psychotic symptoms, are difficult to treat, and their readmission rates are high.

THE DEMOGRAPHIC AND SOCIAL BACKGROUNDS OF METHAMPHETAMINE ABUSERS

Gender

In 1993, out of the total number of 15,495 drug-related arrests 81.4% were male and 18.4% female. Of the 233 methamphetamine abusers investigated by Fukui and his colleagues (Wada and Fukui, 1990; Fukui, 1994), in 21 psychiatric hospitals in 1988, 196 (84.1%) were males, 34 (14.6%) were females, and 3 (1.3%) were unstated. The number of males greatly exceeded that of females, but as abuse spread into the general population, the percentage of female abusers has gradually increased.

Age

Age-group distributions of people arrested on methamphetamine abuse and related charges showed that 20 to 39 year-olds made up the dominant age group during the second period of abuse, which commenced in 1970. As abuse became more widespread in the general population, increases in the number of arrests of individuals aged 40–59 and of those aged 19 and under were observed, highlighting the spread of abuse across all age groups.

After the Fukagawa incident in 1981, arrests of minors aged 19 and under for methamphetamine abuse crimes slowly declined. However, the number of arrests of people aged 40 years and over tended to rise. Thus, the history of arrests suggests that the period of abuse for a given individual had been prolonged.

According to a hospital survey carried out in 1976, methamphetamine dependents in their twenties and thirties comprised 93.3% of the patients. The surveys of 1981 and 1982 showed that the percentage of dependent individuals in their twenties and thirties decreased, while the percentage of those in their forties and those over fifty increased. In the surveys of 1987, 1989, and 1991, a decrease in the percentage of methamphetamine-dependent individuals in their twenties and thirties was noted, as was an increase in the percentage of those in their forties and those over fifty (Shimizu and Fukui, 1994).

In 1993, the age distribution of methamphetamine-related arrests showed that 6088 (39.2%) were 20–29 years of age; 3790 (24.5%) were 30–39 years; 3,256 (21.0%) were 40–49 years; 986 (6.4%) were in the age-group 19 and under (Ministry of Health and Welfare, 1994).

Nationality

The distribution of nationalities of those arrested on methamphetamine charges in 1993 were: 14,818 Japanese (95.6%) and 677 non-Japanese (4.4%). Among non-Japanese arrests, there were 330 South Koreans; 220 Filipinos; 63 North Koreans; 17 Taiwanees; 9 Thailanders; 8 Americans; 5 Iranians and 15 Persons from Hong Kong (Ministry of Health and Welfare, 1994).

Occupation

The distribution of occupations of persons arrested for methamphetamine-related violations in 1993 were: 7,524 (48.6%) unemployed persons (not including students and housewives); 2,404 (15.5%) construction workers; 674 (4.3%) transportation workers; and 620 (4%) bar and restaurant workers (Ministry of Health and Welfare, 1994). Similar occupational distributions have been found for the last twenty years — unemployed people always being 40%–50% of the total arrests and construction, transportation and bar and restaurant workers are the top three occupations.

Education

Analyzing the educational background of the methamphetamine abuse subjects in a survey of psychiatric hospitals, Fukui and colleagues (1994) showed that 50% had completed Junior High School, and an additional 26% consisted of Senior High School dropouts, indicating that 76% of the abusers had completed their education only as far as the compulsory level. This is contrary to common academic expectations since over 90% of the general population go to senior high schools. The complicated family background of abusers and their delinquent behaviours may have made them unable to complete their high school education.

Criminality

Methamphetamine abuse is closely associated with criminal activity in Japan, and prisons contain 10 times more methamphetamine abusers than do hospitals, although many of them are casual users. According to a survey of Kochi Prefectural Prison (Suwaki *et al.*, 1985), 105 of 405 male prisoners (26.1%) were convicted under Stimulants Control Law violations, and 222 prisoners (55.1%) admitted using methamphetamine. In addition, prisoners generally were younger than hospital patients; 61.9% were 20 to 29 years old, and 25.2% were 30 to 29 years old.

In the same study Suwaki and colleagues (1985) found, of the 394 persons under probation to Kochi Probation Office, 130 (33.0%) were methamphetamine abusers and 129 (32.7%) solvent abusers, indicating the serious nature of substance abuse problems in prisons and probation.

Of the 233 abusers in psychiatric hospitals, 104 (44.6%) were in criminal reform centres for violations of the Stimulants Control Law and 71 subjects (30.5%) were imprisoned (Fukui *et al.*, 1994).

PATTERNS OF ABUSE AND PSYCHIATRIC IMPLICATIONS

Substance Abuse Trends in Psychiatric Hospitals

Table 1 shows the number and percentage of psychiatric patients with various types of substance abuse from 1976 to 1993 (Shimizu and Fukui, 1994). Patients who are treated in psychiatric hospitals tend to have a longer history of abuse and have become drug dependent.

An epidemic of a given substance is reflected a few years later in admissions to psychiatric hospitals, because of the increase in the substance-related mental health problems and associated complications. The number of patients surveyed in 1976 and 1981 were relatively small, but we can roughly trace the trends of substance abuse in recent years. After 1981, the proportion of methamphetamine abusers among all abusers has been almost constant at around 40%, and is followed closely by solvent abusers (34–42%). These are the two most common substances of abuse in psychiatric hospital populations. Cough syrups containing codeine, ephedrine and caffeine

Table 1 Psychiatric, patients of substance abuse with the exception of alcohol (value in percentages)

Substance of Abuse \ Year	1976	1981	1982	1987	1989	1991	1993
Methamphetamine	31.3	40.3	42.7	39.2	40.8	35.3	41.9
Solvents	17.7	41.5	38.9	34.2	38.7	40.7	33.9
Hypnotics	13.5	6.0	5.4	9.6	5.5	6.9	10.4
Antianxiety drugs	9.4	1.2	2.0	2.4	1.9	2.7	1.9
Analgesics	25.0	7.1	9.6	9.5	7.0	6.5	4.7
Cough Syrups	—	—	0.7	3.4	3.9	3.4	4.4
Cannabis	—	—	—	0.1	0.8	1.3	1.5
Cocaine	—	—	—		0.2	0.2	0.3
Morphines	1.0	0.4	—	—	—	—	—
No of patients surveyed	96*	571	803	881	915	938	933

*inpatients only
Source: Shimizu and Fukui (1994)

appeared as a drug of abuse in 1982, but this has been limited to the Tokyo Metropolitan area, since they are quite expensive. The pharmaceutical companies have now changed the contents of the syrups. One case of cannabis dependence was reported in 1987, 8 in 1989, and 14 in 1993, and is only gradually increasing. However, the number of hospital patients is likely to be fewer than the actual number of abusers in society. Cases of cocaine and morphine (heroin) abuse are extremely rare in Japanese society.

Longitudinal Patterns of Substance Abuse and Polydrug Abuse

Substance abusers are often viewed by physicians as abusing only one main substance, and other substances of abuse are likely to be disregarded. Once a patient is diagnosed with alcoholism or methamphetamine dependence, physicians tend to focus on that diagnosis. Data from hospitals and police are also classified on the basis of restricted identification of the substance of abuse. However, in the authors' clinic, we often treat young patients who change their drug of abuse from organic solvents to methamphetamine, and middle aged methamphetamine abusers who simultaneously consume a large quantity of alcohol.

In considering such a situation, Suwaki and colleagues (1990) attempted to clarify patterns of substance abuse, covering all substances of abuse including alcohol. Subjects in their study were 225 patients with substance abuse problems who visited psychiatric hospitals from December 1987 to December 1988. Table 2 shows their sequential patterns of substance abuse. Subjects were categorized into four types and seven subtypes, based on the sequential pattern of abuse, that is, the initial substance of abuse and its continuation, shift to, or combination with other substances. In Type 1

Table 2   Pattern of substance abuse in psychiatric patients in Japan

Type	Subtype	Number of Patients (N = 225)
1. Alcohol	1a. Alcohol alone	91
	1b. Alcohol with tranquilizers, analgesics	52
2. Solvents Initiated	2a. Solvents alone	7
	2b. Solvents with alcohol, tranquilizers and analgesica	19
	2c. Solvents with amphetamines (alcohol, tranquilizers, analgesics)	26
3. Amphetamine	3a. Amphetamines alone or with tranquilizers and analgesicas	7
	3b. Amphetamines with alcohol (tranquilizers, analgesics)	21
4.	Not including alcohol, solvents or amphetamines	2

Source: Suwaki *et al.*, 1990

alcoholism, alcohol is consumed for a long period as a single substance of abuse. Many Type 1 abusers also had a cigarette smoking habit, but cigarette smoking is not used as a criterion for deciding pattern of abuse, because in a preliminary study of 57 patients, 53 (93.0%) had a smoking habit. Type 1b abusers consumed tranquilizers, hypnotics, or analgesics in later stages. Many of them initiated their use through physicians' prescriptions when they visited hospitals or clinics. Type 2 abuse involves organic solvents and is usually initiated at younger ages. This type is further subdivided into Type 2a, exclusively solvents; 2b, solvents with alcohol, hypnotics, or analgesics; and 2c, solvents with methamphetamine. The latter two types constitute a core group of polydrug abusers in Japan. Type 3 is the pattern of methamphetamine abuse without use of any organic solvents and is subdivided into 3a, without alcohol, and 3b, with alcohol. Most Type 3b patients used alcohol and methamphetamine at the same time. Type 4 abuse does not include alcohol, organic solvents, or methamphetamine. Regarding the age of initial use, the youngest case began the abuse of organic solvents at the age of 12 years, and most of the Type 2 cases began their abuse before the age of 20. Most of the Type 3 methamphetamine abuse cases began their abuse before 30 years of age. Type 1 cases also initiated their abuse relatively younger than expected, between 20 and 39 years of age.

Methamphetamine Abuse

The following descriptions of initial and persistent use of methamphetamine are based on the study of 233 methamphetamine dependents in psychiatric hospitals conducted by Fukui and colleagues (Wada and Fukui, 1990; Fukui *et al.*, 1994).

Initial use of methamphetamine

Many abusers began to use methamphetamine at some time between the age of 15 and 25 years. First-time use of methamphetamine among abusers was predominantly in the late adolescent years or in the early twenties. The main motive for first use was temptation (54.5%) or curiosity (42.5%), although most of the subjects had been motivated by a combination of both. Usually these youngsters were coaxed by their friends, although some were mildly curious. When asked who had been a key person in their first use of methamphetamine, the subjects cited friends and acquaintances more often than illegal dealers. Male abusers, mostly influenced by their male friends (37.8%), started using methamphetamine for pleasure-seeking or to avoid sleepiness and fatigue when gambling with their friends. However, most female abusers were encouraged by their husbands or boyfriends to use the drug for a heightened sexual response. In response to questions on the occupation of the person who had introduced them to methamphetamine, more than half the subjects replied that the person had been connected to gangs in some way.

Persisting use of methamphetamine

Many subjects resorted to continuous methamphetamine abuse because it produced a pleasant feeling (39.1%), to prevent sleepiness (28.3%), and to avoid fatigue (17.2%). From the first use of methamphetamine to continued abuse, contact with friends and acquaintances who used methamphetamine seemed necessary to sustain their involvement with the drug.

The subjects were mostly long-term abusers. Only 3.4% of them had been involved in methamphetamine abuse for less than 1 year, 15.4% of them for less than 5 years. In contrast, 78.2% had been chronic methamphetamine abusers for more than 5 years. In previous investigations, the percentage of individuals abusing methamphetamine for less than 1 year was 37% in 1978, decreasing to 28% in 1982. In 1987, the percentage of them declined to 4.1%. The sharp decline in the percentage of short-term abusers and the increase in abusers with an abuse history of over 5 years is noticeable. This trend coincides well with increases in the numbers of abusers in the older age groups.

Public disapproval and stringent controls contributed to a gradual decrease in the number of arrests for methamphetamine-related crimes and the number of individuals aged 19 and under. However, long-term abusers in their forties and over still continue their abuse. The survival of these long-term abusers may explain why the current epidemic has not seen a sharp decline similar to the one that occurred at the end of the first epidemic in 1957.

Methamphetamine psychosis

Of 331 methamphetamine-related patients who presented to psychiatric hospitals in 1991, 255 (77.0%) were in a hallucinatory-delusional state. However, 139 (42.0%) of them had not used methamphetamine since their last psychotic episode. These individuals sought treatment at the hospitals because of a prolongation or recurrence of methamphetamine induced psychosis (Shimizu and Fukui, 1994). The results support observations of methamphetamine psychoses that persist in excess of one month and sometimes recur after several years, or can be reactivated by insomnia, stress, or alcohol intake. The results also suggest that the probability of such prolonged psychotic symptoms increases when the methamphetamine abuse period exceeds 5 years.

Kato has classified sequelae of methamphetamine-induced mental disorders into two categories: a residual syndrome in which chronic symptoms have continued after abstinence and a relapse phenomenon in which symptoms that had disappeared, such as hallucinations and delusions, have promptly returned on the re-use of methamphetamine or in situations of psychological stress (Kato, 1987; Konuma, 1994).

Residual syndromes

The major residual syndromes are hypochondriacal and often involve fatigue, insomnia and anxiety over a long period of time. They sometimes accompany psychotic symptoms such as hallucinations and delusions.

The typical residual syndrome is not stationary but undergoes periodic remissions and recurrences. Usually, it improves gradually with treatment. However, as the hallucinatory paranoid state improves, emotional disturbances and amotivational states can emerge as predominant symptoms. Also, the aggravation of depressive and hypersensitive states by insomnia and stress occasionally may lead to auditory hallucinations.

The relapse phenomenon

Sato and colleagues have reported cases that showed recurrence of psychotic symptoms within 1 week (in some cases almost instantaneously) after the re-use of relatively small amounts of methamphetamine (Sato *et al.*, 1983). Subsequent clinical studies have demonstrated that a relapse into a hallucinatory paranoid state can be triggered by alcohol ingestion or psychological stress without the re-use of methamphetamine. They interpret this relapse phenomenon biologically, suggesting that methamphetamine administration increases the sensitivity of the brain to the drug (reverse tolerance). Since reverse tolerance remains in the brain over a long period after abstinence, the brain can still react sensitively to a small amount of methamphetamine.

Based on the concept of methamphetamine psychosis described above, relatively long-term use of antipsychotic drugs such as haloperidol is recommended for treatment of methamphetamine induced psychosis in Japan. In Europe and the United States, however, where chronic amphetamine psychosis is not well recognized, short-term use of antipsychotic drugs is considered to be enough (Schukit, 1989).

CONCLUSION

Japan has experienced two major epidemics of methamphetamine abuse, the magnitude of which cannot be compared with that of any other country in the world. Japan now seems to be at a crucial point in its drug history and perhaps on the brink of entering into a period of multiple substance abuse that includes heroin, cocaine and marijuana. There is also greater international collaboration and exchange of information is urgently needed to combat substance abuse problems.

REFERENCES

Fukui, S. Wads, K. and Iyo, M. (1994) Epidemiology of methamphetamine abuse in Japan and its social implications. In: A.K. Cho and D.S. Segal (eds.) *Amphetamine and Its Analogs — Psychopharmacology, Toxicology and Abuse.* San Diego: Academic Press.

Kato, N. (1987) Residual syndrome and relapse in patients with methamphetamine related mental disorders. In: Study Team on Drug Abuse Reporting System (eds.) *Information of Psychoactive Substance. Series No. 2, Amphetamines.* Chiba, Japan. (In Japanese).

Konuma, K. (1994) Use and abuse of amphetamines in Japan. In: A.K. Cho and D.S. Segal (eds.) *Amphetamine and Its Analogs — Psychopharmacology, Toxicology and Abuse.* San Diego: Academic Press.

Ministry of Health and Welfare, Bureau of Pharmaceutical Affairs (1994) *General Conditions of Administration of Stimulants and Narcotics in 1993.* Tokyo: Ministry of Health and Welfare.

Sato, M., Chen, C.C., Akiyama, S., *et al.* (1983) Acute exacerbation of paranoid state after long-term abstinence in patients with previous methamphetamine psychosis. *Biological Psychiatry,* **18**, pp. 429–440.

Schukit, M.A. (1989) *Drug and Alcohol Abuse: A Clinical Guide to Diagnosis and Treatment,* 3rd Edition. New York: Plenum Medical.

Shimuzu, J. and Fukui, S. (1994) A survey of drug-related psychiatric disorders in psychiatric hospitals. In S. Fukui (ed.) *The 1993 Report of Studies on Socio-medical and Psychiatric Features of Drug Dependence.* (In Japanese).

Suwaki, H. and Bjorksten, O.J.W. (1983) Substance abuse trends in Japan. *Public Health Reviews,* **11**(3), pp. 199–222.

Suwaki, H., Yoshida, T. and Ohara, H. (1985) A survey of methamphetamine abusers in prison, probation office, and mental hospitals in the Kochi Prefecture. *Social Psychiatry,* **8**(2), pp. 144–150. (Japanese Journal).

Suwaki, H., Horri, S., Fujimoto, A. *et al.,* (1990) A study of substance abuse patterns with special reference to multiple use problems in Japan. In: *1989*

Report of Studies on Etiological Factors and Pathological Conditions of Drug Dependence. Tokyo: Ministry of Health and Welfare. (In Japanese).

Suwaki, H. (1991) Methamphetamine abuse in Japan. In: M.A. Miller and N.J. Kozel (eds.) *Methamphetamine Abuse: Epidemiologic Issues and Implications, NIDA Research Monograph 115.* Rockville: National Institute on Drug Abuse.

Wada. K. and Fukui, S. (1990). Relationship between years of methamphetamine use and symptoms of methamphetamine psychosis. *Alcohol and Drug Dependence,* **25**(3), pp. 143–158. (Japanese Journal).

11

Amphetamine Abuse in Sweden

KERSTIN KÄLL

BACKGROUND

Sweden is one of the three European countries that most recently (January 1, 1995) became members of the European Community. Located on the Scandinavian peninsula it is the fourth largest country in Europe but the population is only about 8.5 million people, with the highest density in the south of Sweden. The capital, Stockholm, is the largest city with slightly above 1.5 million inhabitants within its county. Gothenburgh and Malmö, both south of Stockholm, follow next in size. Sweden has vast resources of iron ore and timber, and mining, steel and forest industries form the basis of the economy. Thanks to the geographical location, a policy of nonalignment in peace and neutrality in war and a great deal of luck, Sweden was able to stay outside both of the World Wars, with subsequent economic advantages resulting in a large economic growth, particularly after World War II. This coincided with a long period of Social Democratic government which was characterized by a number of social reforms including old-age pensions, child allowances, health insurance and educational reform. To accomplish this 'welfare state', taxes on income, business etc., were raised to quite a high level. Unemployment was kept at a low level, until the last few years when it has rapidly increased to typical European levels. The population of Sweden is relatively homogenous in language, ethnic stock and religion (although Swedes in general are not very religious), but waves of refugees in the last decade have given rise to ethnic conflicts. Sweden utilizes a personal identity code for citizen registration, which facilitates authority control of people and allows for reliable statistical information about the population, but also causes problems with invasion of privacy.

AMPHETAMINE IN SWEDEN

Due to the relative prosperity in Sweden after World War II, when the rest of Europe was more or less starving it was the only country where obesity was a health problem in the general population. Perhaps this is one reason why amphetamines, at this time often used for weight reduction, were more abundant in Sweden than in other European countries. However, Sweden had a serious post-war drug problem earlier than other European countries and the main drugs of abuse were amphetamine and related substances. Among injecting drug abusers amphetamine is still the most popular drug, although heroin has slowly gained ground. When heroin smokers are included, heroin now accounts for 50% of heavy drug abusers in Stockholm (Ågren *et al.*, 1993). In other parts of the country amphetamine is still the most popular drug.

Historical Review

Nils Bejerot, in the Swedish version of his thesis, included a calendar of the development of drug abuse, legislation and administrative measures in Sweden until 1970 (Bejerot, 1975b). Where no other reference is mentioned this is the source of the following brief historical review of amphetamine abuse in Sweden.

Amphetamine was introduced in Sweden shortly after it was introduced into clinical practice by Prinzmetal and Bloomberg in 1935 and it was sold without prescription until 1939. The first report of abuse was in 1944 (Goldberg, 1944) and the same year the amphetamines were incorporated under existing legislation on narcotic drugs[1] in Sweden.

About the time of the end of World War II a new type of amphetamine abuse emerged in Stockholm centred around a narrow clique of authors, musicians, artists and bohemians. Bejerot chose to call these abusers 'epidemic' as opposed to 'auto-established' (meaning that a person with access to narcotic drugs, e.g. medical staff, has started abusing by administering these to him/herself) and 'iatrogenic' cases, which are the cases initiated by doctors prescribing e.g. tranquilizers, sleeping pills or pain relievers to patients, who are later unable to stop taking the drugs and subsequently start to abuse them.

---

[1] 'Narcotic drug' in Sweden is any drug scheduled under the Swedish Narcotic Offence Act, which is the domestic Swedish legislation corresponding to the UN 1961 and 1971 Drug Conventions

The latter two he grouped into a category of 'single' or 'therapeutic' cases (the third main category introduced by Bejerot was 'endemic' abuse, e.g., alcoholism in the Western world) (Bejerot, 1968). Previously noted cases had been mainly of the therapeutic type. Some of these new amphetamine abusers were alcoholics who initially used amphetamine to cure their hangovers and later switched from alcohol to amphetamine as their favourite drug (p. 257). Bejerot pointed out several important differences between therapeutic and epidemic abuse, e.g., male predominance and younger age at initiation for epidemic abuse, much higher prevalence of criminality in epidemic than in therapeutic abuse, concealment of abuse typical in therapeutic but not in epidemic abuse and, most importantly, a social contagiousness in epidemic abuse which is not present in therapeutic cases.

Until this time only oral abuse of amphetamine was reported but one of the central figures of this primary clique, a poet well-known at the time, has reported that he first injected amphetamine in 1949. This bohemian core of the amphetamine epidemic probably consisted of a few dozen people at this time, but it soon broke into criminally active youth in Stockholm, and field social workers in Stockholm began to be concerned about the spread of amphetamine among young people in the early 50s. By 1954 drug peddling was quite extensive, and most of the drugs came from prescriptions received from unsuspecting doctors. The first sentence for illegal dealing with central stimulants was delivered in 1954.

Field workers reported to the Child Welfare Committee about their observations of drug abuse among young people in Stockholm. This was not taken very seriously by the Committee and the field workers undertook an investigation of their own. Their report in 1954 showed that at least 300 of the youths with whom they had contact had tried at least one narcotic drug, and about 50 were exhibiting distinct signs of abuse. The most popular drugs were cannabis, central stimulants (e.g., amphetamine) and sleeping pills. As a result of the report the National Board of Health initiated research of their own. Among other things they investigated police confiscation of drugs and concluded that the illegal dealing with drugs was not a serious problem at this time. This view was probably mistaken. The low level of confiscation was more likely a result of the very limited police efforts in the field of drug trafficking at this time. Before 1955 there were no police staff working full time in this field. The investigators concluded that persons abusing drugs received their drugs from unsuspecting doctors and the only action of the Board was to distribute a letter to the doctors in Sweden recommending them to be more careful in prescribing drugs popular among abusers (Bergvall, 1988).

In 1955 phenmetrazine (which is pharmacologically very similar to amphetamine) was registered in Sweden for weight reduction and its centrally stimulating effects were soon observed by abusers, and as amphetamine was becoming harder to obtain many abusers swiched to phenmetrazine.

Intravenous abuse of central stimulants was still unusual, but in 1956 a number of the regular abusers turned to this mode of administration and in the same year the first cases of central stimulant abuse of epidemic type were reported from Gothenburg, the second largest city in Sweden.

In 1958 amphetamine was classed as a narcotic drug as was phenmetrazine in the following year and metylphenidate, also resembling amphetamine in its effects, in 1960. These were the three most popular substances among the Swedish abusers. In 1960 large scale illegal import of central stimulants was first documented. The most popular drug at this time, phenmetrazine, was easily obtainable in southern Europe. One 22 year old man, not a drug abuser himself, was, for example, accused by a witness in a trial in 1960 of having brought in at least 40,000 tablets from Spain (Bergvall, 1988).

The bulk of the abused drugs still originated from prescriptions from doctors, however, which was acknowledged by the National Board of Health in a new statement in 1960 describing these activities in some detail. According to the Board, drug abusers preferentially turned to older doctors, often retired from medical practice, sometimes living in the countryside, and very often only a telephone call was needed to obtain a prescription. However, the Board only issued sharp criticism of the doctors for not checking the identity of the patients nor seeing them personally to judge their actual need for the drugs. Not until 1962 did the Board impose strong restrictions on the prescribing by telephone of narcotic drugs (maximum five tablets and no preparations for injection). This put a stop to this source but the street market for narcotic drugs had already been established and by now there were other channels available to replace telephone prescriptions.

At a symposium on the abuse of central stimulants in Stockholm in 1968 Rylander related his experience from the Clinic of Forensic Psychiatry in Stockholm, of which he was the head (Rylander, 1969). All prisoners in need of psychiatric treatment or observation were referred to this clinic. He had noticed a sharp increase of injectors of central stimulants, mostly phenmetrazine, beginning in 1964 when he had treated twenty three. In 1967 the number was eighty. The doses injected ranged from about 200 to 1000 mg per injection, 4–5 times a day.

Drugs Policy

Beginning in 1964 a debate about government strategy on drugs was initiated. The traditionally restrictive policy was questioned and a more liberal policy advocated. Referring to an experiment with liberal prescription of heroin to half a dozen Canadian immigrant opiate abusers in England by a psychiatrist, Lady Frankau (reported by the Brain commission in 1961 as not very successful), it was suggested that a similar experiment should be started in Stockholm (Bergvall, 1988). Following a large media campaign in favour of a liberalisation of drug policy an experiment with legal prescription of central stimulants and opiates for injection to abusers was initiated in April 1965. The idea behind the experiment was to relieve the drug abusers of the need to commit crime to acquire drugs of sometimes questionable quality by supplying them with the drugs they wanted. The aim was that the drugs should be prescribed in decreasing doses and that the abusers would thus be cured of their addiction. It did not work, for several reasons. Many of the drug abusers who enrolled were criminally active before they started to take drugs and they continued to be so when they obtained their drugs on prescription. Furthermore, the idea of decreasing doses was based on a heroin detoxification model, which was inappropriate since central stimulants do not normally give severe physical abstinence reactions. Most important, this model did not take into account the epidemic nature of drug abuse in Stockholm at this time, where one of the important aspects was the contagiousness of the abuse. The experiment has been vividly described by Bejerot (Bejerot, 1968, 1970). In short, at least half a million doses of opiates and three and a half million doses of central stimulants were prescribed to 156 patients. In addition to these there were several 'satellite' patients, who received their drugs from the 'legal' patients. The experiment was eventually stopped in May 1967 mainly in response to the death of a young girl from an overdose of morphine and amphetamine, legally prescribed to another person. A total of at least seven patients with some connection to the experiment died during this period.

The number of epidemic drug abusers was rapidly increasing before this experiment began, and it continued to increase at a rapid pace while it lasted, although it is difficult to show to what extent the experiment in itself contributed to this increase (Kühlhorn, 1994). The mere existence of this kind of 'generous' prescription of narcotic drugs indicated a liberal attitude toward drug abuse. This and the publicity it received were probably factors as important as the experiment itself for the rapid spread of drug abuse at this time.

Nils Bejerot was one of the strongest opponents to the experiment with legal prescription of drugs to drug abusers and when he failed to stop it, he initiated a study of drug injection at the Remand Prison in Stockholm in 1965. A nurse inspected the arms of all arrestees, noted injection marks, and asked questions about their drug abuse (e.g. year of first injection). This study is still running and the results have recently been analyzed (Kühlhorn, 1994).

The disastrous outcome of experimenting with legal prescriptions discredited the idea of legalizing the distribution of narcotic drugs to drug abusers in Swedish drug policy for a long time. In the following years debate focused instead on the levels of the drug distribution market that should be targeted in the battle against illegal drugs. Traditionally, police and customs had concentrated on the import and wholesale levels and this was successful at first, since only a few people were involved. The main source of imported amphetamine at this time was the Netherlands and when the main dealer from the mid 1960s, Karl Pauksch, was arrested in 1972, the effect was a marked

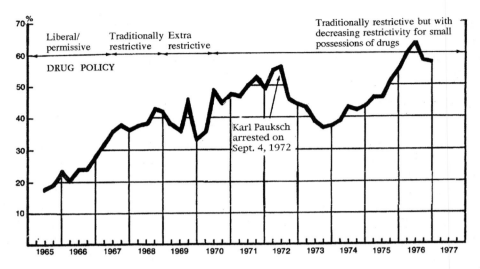

Figure 1 *Percentage male injecting drug abusers Swedish men (15–44 years old) arrested in Stockholm 1965–1976.* (printed with permission from Mrs Carol Bejerot, widow of professor Nils Bejerot)

decrease in the proportion of injecting drug abusers in Bejerot's injection mark study (Bejerot, 1975a). See Figure 1.

Soon, however, it became evident that high level dealers were easily replaced due to the extremely lucrative nature of this business. Another strategy was then advocated, namely to concentrate efforts on stopping drugs at the street level. The argument behind this strategy was that the consumer, the drug abuser on the street, is the only irreplaceable link in the drug distribution chain. Eventually this strategy was accepted and between 1977 and 1980 the Swedish parliament initiated changes in law enforcement in this direction (Kühlhorn, 1994). The effect of these changes was that the police organized special street groups with the focus on the street peddling of drugs. All possession of drugs, even small quantities, was prohibited. As a result drug abuse became much more uncomfortable and hazardous. The number of people who started to inject drugs (as measured by the injection mark study) decreased markedly during this period. In 1988 the consumption of illegal drugs was also criminalized, but this law was hardly used until 1993 when the law was changed so that urinalysis was allowed on reasonable suspicion of drug consumption. Prior to this change it was very difficult to prove drug consumption in court unless the actual consumption had been observed. The main argument in support of criminalization of drug consumption was the psychological impact on young people of a clear condemnation by society of any use of illicit drugs. The effects have not yet been evaluated, and the number of drug tests taken vary a great deal between different police districts.

The Narcotic Drugs Act in Sweden is based on the international conventions which Sweden has ratified and came into force in 1968. It has been amended several times in the direction of greater restrictions and emphasis on prevention. The maximum penalty for severe drug offences is now ten years imprisonment. The majority of indictments (about 70% in 1991) are, however, minor drug offences, that carry a maximum of six months' imprisonment (Swedish National Institute of Public Health, 1993).

Popular Movements

One important contributor to the development of this new drug policy was the pressure from organizations against illegal drugs that had developed from the 'grass roots' in response to the epidemic of drug abuse. The first organized movement was a client oriented group (Swedish Association for Help and Assistance to Drug Abusers, abbreviated RFHL in Swedish) that initially strongly advocated legal prescription of drugs to drug abusers, but changed direction following the failure of legal prescribing and which has since focused mainly on promoting drug treatment. The second group was more oriented towards drug policy (National Association for a Drug Free Society, RNS in Swedish) and it organized meetings, demonstrations and drug education. It was closely linked to a third group that organized parents of drug abusers (Swedish Parents Anti-Narcotics Association, FMN in Swedish). The two latter groups, as well as the Organization Against Drugs and Alcohol, were strong proponents of a restrictive drug policy.

The Size of the Present Drug Abusing Population in Sweden

An estimate of the drug abusing population in Sweden was made in 1992 using a case-finding method and a capture-recapture mathematical model on the overlapping of populations reported from different sources, mainly the social services, the criminal justice system, police, courts and detoxification units (Olsson *et al.*, 1993). The estimated number of heavy drug abusers (defined as persons who have either injected drugs or otherwise used drugs daily or almost daily during the last year) in Sweden was 17,000. In 1979 the estimate, using roughly the same methods, was 12,000. The age profile had however changed and the number of heavy drug abusers under the age of 25 years had gone down by more than 60%, again pointing to a decline in the initiation into heavy drug use.

The total number of heavy drug abusers actually reported in the above mentioned study was 9,103, 93% of whom injected drugs. Eighty-two percent of the heavy abusers had used amphetamine and amphetamine as a main drug was reported for 48%, cannabis for 17% and opiates for 26% (compared to 15% opiate abusers in 1979). Most of the remaining heavy drug abusers were primary users of alcohol. Polydrug use was the rule — only 23% of the heavy abusers reported using only one drug during the previous year. The most popular second drug for amphetamine abusers was cannabis, whereas heroin abusers used cannabis, amphetamine and benzodiazepines to about the same extent.

First or second generation immigrants constituted 19% of the heavy drug abusers in this study. About half of these came from another Nordic country, the rest from other countries. Of the 576 injecting drug abusers participating in an HIV epidemiological study at the Remand Prison in Stockholm in 1992 there were 50 persons (9%) from a country outside the Nordic countries. Of these 60% used mainly heroin and 40% amphetamine as opposed to the whole population where amphetamine was the main drug for 72% and heroin for 28% (the author's unpublished data).

Import and Trade

According to information from experienced drug abusers, not only the use but also the import and trade with amphetamine is dominated by native Swedes, whereas the trade in heroin is dominated by ethnic minorities, mainly from the Middle East and North Africa. The dominating import routes for amphetamine are from the Netherlands and Poland and also increasingly from other parts of the former Soviet Union. The purity of the amphetamine on the street is about 8%–10%. The amphetamine from the East European countries is considered to be of lower quality than the Dutch amphetamine. The price in the street is around 300 Swedish Crowns ($40 US) per gram compared to around 1000 ($134 US) for heroin. The prices have been remarkably stable since the 1970s, which in effect means that that drugs have become much cheaper due to inflation.

Treatment

Treatment for drug abusers in Sweden has been developed gradually and has been influenced by different ideologies. One issue of debate has been whether treatment should be voluntary or compulsory. Before 1982 treatment for drug abuse was compulsory only for persons under the age of twenty years. Compulsory treatment of adults was legislated only for heavy alcohol abuse. In 1982 the new Social Services Act took effect, which was supplemented the Care of Alcoholics and Drug Abusers (Special Provisions) Act LVM (Ministry of Health and Social Affairs International Secretariat, 1989). The 1982 version of the law allowed two months of compulsory treatment with a possibility of two months prolongation. This was changed in 1989 to six months maximum treatment and the inclusion of abusers of volatile solvents. For the law of compulsory treatment to be applicable the drug abuse must be extensive with an abundance of physical and social complications and the drug abuser must have refused all offers of voluntary treatment. Every case of compulsory treatment is tried in a County Administrative Court.

An evaluation of most of the drug abusers treated under the LVM law during 1986 until mid 1988 was published in 1989 (Fugelstad, 1989). Of the 152 drug abusers studied, 37 used mainly amphetamine, 91 opiates and

24 other drugs (mainly alcohol). Fifty-eight were HIV seropositive (only one of these was an amphetamine abuser). This group was followed until the fall of 1988. By then 21 were dead (14 heroin abusers, one amphetamine abuser and six primary alcohol abusers), 25 had received methadone maintenance treatment, 76 were still actively abusing drugs and 30 were either not found, had moved, were in prison or treated for something other than drug abuse. The proportion in active abuse was higher for heroin abusers (excluding those who had received methadone treatment) than for amphetamine abusers. The poor outcome of the LVM treatment may not reflect so much the quality of the treatment as the very heavy abuse of the persons treated. Besides being life saving in many cases, the most important effect of the LVM law may be that its very existence stimulates many drug abusers to seek and stay with voluntary treatment in order to avoid compulsory treatment.

An average of about 40% of the inmates in Swedish prisons are drug abusers (Krantz *et al.*, 1990). Drug treatment is offered in special drug free wings in many Swedish prisons. Inmates can apply to come to these wings if they accept regular urine tests for drugs, which are taken to ensure that the wings remain drug free. Drug abusing inmates may also be allowed to serve the last part of a long (or the whole of a short) sentence in a treatment unit or family care outside prison.

The official responsibility for the treatment of drug abusers relies on the Municipal Social Welfare Committees. They offer outpatient care and decide about institutional treatment for individual abusers. Drug treatment institutions for adults and young people have been influenced by two rather different models of care (Bergmark *et al.*, 1989). Institutional care developed for adult drug abusers tended to follow the tradition of therapeutic communities, with an emphasis on equality within the staff and between staff and clients, voluntary treatment, open communication and shared responsibility. Institutions for young drug abusers (under 20 years), on the other hand, emphasized training in social norms, education and training of new patterns of behaviour. The relationship between staff and clients was more like a parent/child relationship and the responsibility was on the staff. Treatment was compulsory (Care of Young Persons [Special Provisions] Act LVU). The public debate between proponents of the two types of treatment was very polemic but eventually elements from both models have integrated to some extent. In later years 'twelve step' programmes, in the tradition of Alcoholics Anonymous have been introduced in some institutions.

Common to all treatment interventions is that they do not have separate treatment programmes for abusers of different drugs. Abusers of cannabis, amphetamine, heroin and, sometimes, alcohol, are treated together. In addition to these drug-free treatment units there is a strictly regulated methadone maintenance treatment program for opiate abusers, and specialized treatment units for adult alcoholics and abusers of tranquillizers. There is no special treatment for amphetamine (or cannabis) abusers.

In addition to treatment in institutions there is a network of rural families where drug abusers are offered accommodation with a family for about two years. This form of family care is available both for young and adult drug abusers (Tunving *et al.*, 1993). About 300 drug abusers can be accommodated in this way at a time. The families offer both voluntary and compulsory treatment. This treatment form has not been formally evaluated but has a good reputation. Many heavy drug users prefer family care to institutions.

In 1989 an evaluation of institutionalized treatment of drug abusers was published (Bergmark *et al.*, 1989). From the 1,656 clients enrolled in drug treatment institutions during late 1982 and the whole of 1983, 560 persons from 23 different treatment units were selected and of these 438 were interviewed one year after treatment. Both voluntary treatment (65%) and compulsory treatment were represented. After one year 36% of the 438 interviewed drug abusers reported no use of narcotic drugs at all during the follow up year and an additional 15% had not used narcotic drugs during the last six months of the follow up. In other words 51% or 221 persons had not used narcotic drugs during the last six months. Of these, 163 had not abused other drugs including alcohol. When only socially well functioning persons were included no more than 43 individuals remained. It is important to note that this evaluation only looked at the first year after treatment, which by all standards is a very short follow up. Abusers of amphetamine and heroin were not analyzed separately in this evaluation but the majority of the drug abusers analysed can be presumed to have been abusing amphetamine, since this was the dominating drug in 1982/83, even more so than it is at the present time.

Despite the poor outcome of both voluntary and compulsory drug treatment in terms of total rehabilitation of drug abusers the humanitarian aspects of drug treatment should not be underestimated. It is often life saving and for parents, partners and children of drug abusers, treatment is a temporary relief from their normally very strained life situation. The availability of decent treatment is also important to make the restrictive drug policy acceptable in the eyes of the general public. Without it, police and criminal justice could easily be seen as merely repressive instruments.

Regular Intravenous Amphetamine Abusers

Some characteristics of the present population of regular amphetamine injectors in Stockholm are revealed in a recent study of HIV risk behaviour among 200 incarcerated regular injecting drug abusers at the Remand Prison in Stockholm (Käll, 1995). The population of drug abusers in prison is biased towards older male regular drug abusers. Recreational drug abusers can be expected to be less often arrested by the police and, even if they are arrested, they are less likely to be identified as drug abusers, since they are probably less likely to inject their drugs (urinalysis is not routinely employed with arrested persons). Likewise female drug abusers are arrested less often than male, probably because they, to some extent, are supported with drugs from partners or at least play a more passive role in the criminal activity than the men. Some women, but seemingly very few men, finance their drugs with prostitution, which is not illegal in Sweden.

Of the 200 regular injecting drug abusers interviewed in this study 115 injected mainly amphetamine (41 women and 74 men) and 85 (13 women and 72 men) injected mainly heroin. Amphetamine abusing men constituted about 60% of the drug injectors eligible for the study, but to get comparable populations only a quarter of these were selected. These drug abusers were on the whole living an asocial life, starting their criminal and drug abusing career at an early age. Looking at the men in the study the mean age of the amphetamine abusers was 36 years compared to 30 years for the heroin abusers. The 15 oldest male injecting drug abusers in the study (43–52 years) were all amphetamine abusers, reflecting the fact that the present epidemic started with amphetamine abuse. Fifty percent of the men had working class family backgrounds and 22% had not completed compulsory school (higher, although not statistically significant, for the amphetamine abusers in both these respects). Only 20% had held a job two weeks or more during the last year and only 15% had done military service (which is compulsory for men in Sweden). The amphetamine abusing men had been imprisoned for longer time than the heroin abusers, even when their older age was controlled for, a median of five years of imprisonment for the amphetamine abusers versus one year and four months for the heroin abusers. The reason for this difference has not been investigated, but one possible explanation could be that amphetamine abusers were more often criminal prior to their drug abuse. The median age of injection debut was 17.5, similar for amphetamine and heroin abusing men and the first drug injected was amphetamine for 91% of the amphetamine abusers and 47% of the heroin abusers. Most experienced drug injectors had tried both drugs. The frequency of drug injection was somewhat lower for the amphetamine abusers than the heroin abusers (a mean of 21 versus 25 injections during the last week injecting). Table 1 shows the responses of amphetamine abusers to a question on preferred activity when using amphetamine.

Table 1 shows that about half of the amphetamine abusing men who heavily used amphetamine preferred sexual activity compared with 20% of the women. This preoccupation with sex in the subculture of regular amphetamine abusers was probably even more pronounced in the late 1960s and early 1970s judging from early clinical reports (Rylander, 1969). In the light of the HIV epidemic, where injecting drug abusers constitute one of the main risk groups, this aspect of the drug subculture has gained renewed attention and it was shown in this study that for male amphetamine abusers the preference for sex when on amphetamine was a marker of high HIV injection as well as sexual risk behaviour (Käll *et al.*, 1994). Another aspect of the sexual behaviour of the injecting drug abusers that is important in the

Table 1   Preferred activity while using amphetamine reported by primary amphetamine injectors

Preferred activity	Women* N = 40 (%)	Men N = 74 (%)
Sexual activity	8 (20)	38 (51)
Repairing cars	3 (8)	10 (14)
Repairing anything	4 (10)	3 (4)
Driving	9 (23)	9 (12)
Cleaning the house	5 (13)	0
Sorting things	3 (8)	3 (4)
Socializing in various ways	4 (10)	2 (3)
Stealing or preparing for crimes	1 (3)	6 (8)
Miscellaneous	3 (8)	3 (4)

*no information from one amphetamine abusing woman

light of the HIV epidemic was the prevalence of sexual contact with non-injecting partners (Käll, 1994). In this study 69% of the men and 41% of the women reported at least one non-injecting sex partner during the last three years. Among the men 77% of the heroin abusers versus 61% of the amphetamine abusers reported non-injecting sex partners, but the main reason for this difference was the difference in age and experience with drugs between the two groups. The young men with a short drug injecting history on average had more non-injecting sex partners than older more experienced drug injecting men who more often had injecting sex partners only. The latter however tended more often to be HIV seropositive. This may be one reason why few cases of heterosexual HIV infection from injecting drug abusers to non-injecting partners have been reported in Sweden (20 women and one man in Stockholm county by September 20, 1994 compared to 548 HIV seropositive injecting drug users reported to the Medical Officer of Health).

A different sample of drug abusers was studied recently in Malmö in the south of Sweden (Stenström *et al.*, 1994). Needles and syringes are not freely available for injecting drug abusers in Sweden except in the cities of Malmö and Lund. At the needle exchange site in Malmö a study has been carried out on 930 clients who used the needle exchange from January until mid November 1992. Of these 11% had a regular job, were not known by the social services and had not been in treatment or had any contact with the criminal justice system while in the needle exchange programme (which started in May 1989). This group, called by the researcher the 'social' group, was compared with a group of 'asocial' abusers without a regular job, known to the social services and who had been in drug treatment at some time during their time in the programme. The mean ages for the groups were similar but the asocials had started injecting more than three years earlier than the social abusers. There were more women among the asocials (36%)

than among the socials (17%). There were differences between the two groups in their preferred drug of injection. Amphetamine was the main drug for the socials (77%) but not for the asocials (48%). Heroin as the main drug of choice was reported by 11% of the socials and 26% of the asocials. More of the asocials (26%) used both heroin and amphetamine compared with 12% of the socials. It seems that amphetamine abuse is easier to combine with a normal social life in this sample. This is in sharp contrast to the study from the Remand prison in Stockholm where the amphetamine abusers had spent more time in prison than the heroin abusers, indicating that the Malmö study revealed a population of amphetamine abusers largely overlooked in previous studies. The average age of the amphetamine users in the Malmö study was only slightly lower than in the Remand prison study in Stockholm (35 years versus 36 years in Stockholm), indicating that it was not another generation of abusers. These 'social' abusers may reasonably be expected to have more contacts, including sexual contacts, with non drug using persons, with all the implications of possible spread of HIV.

HIV AND INJECTING DRUG ABUSERS IN SWEDEN

HIV was introduced into the population of injecting drug abusers in Sweden in 1983, beginning among the heroin abusers in Stockholm (Böttiger *et al.*, 1993). There was an initial rapid spread of HIV among heroin abusers and when testing started in the fall of 1984 more than half of the heroin abusers tested were HIV seropositive. About this time there was limited mixing between the heroin and the amphetamine using populations in Stockholm. The spread of HIV seems not to have started until about a year and a half later among the amphetamine abusers, and there was no phase of rapid spread in this group. After the initial establishing phase, the rate of seroconversion has been low among injecting drug abusers in Sweden, about 1% annually, with little difference between amphetamine and heroin abusers. The newly infected drug abusers have typically been older and more experienced with drugs.

The HIV testing of drug abusers has been extensive in Sweden. Among regular drug injectors more than 90% have been tested, many of them several times in spite of the fact that testing is voluntary. All new cases of HIV infection are reported to the Medical Officer of Health in each county in accordance with the Infectious Disease Act. On November 1, 1985 HIV infection was included in this act under the section 'venereal diseases'. Reporting is anonymized, and the reporting doctor has the responsibility to monitor the risk behaviour of those patients. If there is reason to suspect that one of the patients is putting others at risk for HIV infection the patient must be reported with full identity to the Medical Officer of Health, who performs an investigation, which can, if every other effort fails, end up with a suggestion that the patient should be isolated in a hospital. The enforced isolation is decided by a County Administrative Court. In Stockholm, where most of the isolations have been undertaken, 35 HIV seropositive persons have been isolated according to this law by November 22, 1994. Of these, 22 were injecting drug users (18 were Swedish citizens). Eight (one woman and seven men) were amphetamine abusers. They were all charged with concealing their HIV status from sex partners as were one female and two male heroin abusers. Seven heroin abusing women were charged with prostitution (illegal for those who are seropositive) and four heroin abusing men with lending their injection equipment. Many of the isolated drug abusers suffer from severe psychiatric conditions, but among those who do not, the time for isolation seldom exceeded twelve months (the prolongation is tried by the Court after three months and then every sixth month).

One reason for the willingness among Swedish drug injectors to take HIV tests may be that there is a certain amount of peer pressure within the drug abusing subculture to take the test and to be open about one's HIV status. Needles and syringes are not legally available for drug abusers (except for in Malmö and Lund) and since most drug abusers calculate that they may have to borrow somebody else's injection equipment at some time, they want to be sure that the person they borrow from is not HIV seropositive. Similarly, since condom use is not customary, they need to know about their sex partner's HIV status.

The most recent investigations point to a HIV seroprevalence among injecting drug abusers in Stockholm of about 28% among heroin abusers and about 6% among amphetamine abusers (Käll, 1994). There has been some speculation about the reason for this remarkable difference. One reasonable hypothesis is that the two populations are separate in some sense and that HIV started to spread among the heroin abusers before they were aware of the risk of infection, whereas when the infection had broken into the population of amphetamine abusers they were already aware of the risk. The heroin abusers may have used riskier injection practices prior to the awareness of HIV, at least this is what many amphetamine abusers claim. There used to be a certain animosity between the two populations and amphetamine abusers often seemed to consider themselves somewhat above heroin abusers in social status. A typical remark about heroin from amphetamine abusers could be: 'heroin is not a drug it is poison'. In later years this animosity seems to have decreased for some reason, perhaps because many older amphetamine abusers have swiched to heroin. To elucidate these issues, ethnographic studies of the drug cultures would need to be carried out. Unfortunately there has been very little done in this field so far in Sweden.

MORTALITY AND MORBIDITY

Several studies have shown a difference in mortality between amphetamine and heroin abusers, where the mortality for heroin abusers is usually about twice as high (more than 2% annually as opposed to about 1% for amphetamine abusers) (Tunving, 1990). The mortality is somewhat lower for female abusers and higher when there is alcohol abuse and criminality in parallel to drug abuse.

Between 1986 and 1993, 658 drug related deaths have been observed at the Department of Forensic Medicine in Stockholm, where the majority of deaths outside hospitals in Stockholm county are examined (Fugelstad *et al.*, 1994a). In 417 (63%) of these cases morphine was detected (heroin is rapidly broken down to morphine in the body). In 84% of them death occurred soon after injecting (so called over-doses although the actual amount of morphine was typically not impressive). In 147 of the cases amphetamine but no morphine was detected. Only 17 (12%) of these were judged to be death by intoxication, often a combination of amphetamine, alcohol and/or benzodiazepines. Comparing heroin and amphetamine deaths, 40% of amphetamine deaths were from accidents versus 2% of heroin deaths, 20% of amphetamine deaths were from suicide versus 9% of heroin deaths and 14% of amphetamine deaths were murders versus 1% of heroin deaths. Death from organic disease was also more common for amphetamine than heroin abusers (26% versus 4%). Typical causes of death among the amphetamine users were heart disease and stroke (Fugelstad *et al.*, 1994b).

In addition to the risk of disease or death of the drug abuser him- or herself there is the risk for the future generation in terms of perinatal complications of drug abuse. In Sweden there is an ongoing prospective study of 65 children born between 1976 and 1977, whose mothers used amphetamine during pregnancy. At the age of eight years it was found that children exposed to amphetamine during the whole of the pregnancy were more aggressive and had more peer-related social problems than those exposed to amphetamine during the early pregnancy only (Billing *et al.*, 1994).

A well-known complication of amphetamine abuse is amphetamine psychosis (Connell, 1958). Connell in 1958 described the typical clinical picture of this condition as a paranoid reaction with delusions and hallucinations, most often auditory, but sometimes with visual, tactile and olfactory hallucinations. Disorientation, however, is rare in amphetamine psychosis, according to Connell, and most patients recover within a few days of abstinence. In the previously mentioned study of 200 regular drug injectors at the Remand prison in Stockholm, about 80% of the 167 drug abusers who had experience of amphetamine abuse had had at least one episode of both visual and auditory hallucinations as well as at least one paranoid reaction (the author's unpublished data). The most commonly mentioned perceived cause of psychotic episodes was a prolonged period of drug consumption with no sleep for several nights. The typical attitude to psychoses among the amphetamine abusers interviewed was rather casual, and it seems that the more experienced drug abusers teach beginners how to handle psychoses without too much panic and that most psychoses probably never appear at psychiatric emergency wards.

PREVENTION

To deal effectively with drug addiction, preventive efforts are essential. In addition to law enforcement in drug trafficking and abuse, the schools in Sweden are seen to have an important role in educating young people about drugs, and in teaching them to resist peer pressure to experiment with nicotine, alcohol and drugs. The Swedish compulsory school curriculum stipulates that every school creates a plan for tobacco, alcohol and drug instruction. The Police and Municipal Social Services are obliged to assist the schools in this educational task. These kind of 'primary' prevention measures have gained priority over 'harm reduction' strategies in Sweden. The prevailing opinion is that the overriding goal must be to abolish illegal drugs from society and to the extent that harm reduction measures (like, for example, needle exchange services), may compromise this goal, they are not considered desirable.

TRENDS

The injection mark study has indicated a decrease in initiation into drug injection during the 1980s. There are however signals that this trend may be changing. The number of young people accepted at Maria Ungdomsenhet (a ward for young drug abusers in Stockholm) has started to increase after a long period of decrease, and oral abuse of amphetamine has become increasingly popular along with Ecstasy and LSD at certain discos and rave parties for young people (personal communication, S.E. Eriksson, social worker at Maria Ungdomsenhet). The number of young drug abusers (under 20 years) actually injecting drugs is still low, but increasing.

Another important trend may be the gradual shift from amphetamine to heroin abuse noted among the heavy abusers. This is however contradicted by the reports of police confiscations where both amphetamine and heroin have been increasing since 1987, but heroin has stabilized in the '90s whereas amphetamine continues to increase (Swedish National Police Board, 1994). This, as well as the evidence from the Malmö study, may indicate that there is an extensive hidden and recreational abuse of amphetamine which is not yet evident to police and social workers.

The trend in government economic policy at present is to cut down public expenditure in order to reduce the national deficit. For drug abusers this has meant that long term institutional treatment has become much harder to get, which will probably lead to increased death rate and morbidity as well as social misery for the drug abusing population. The fear is also that the increasing unemployment will put larger portions of the young generation at risk for drug abuse.

Sweden and Europe

Sweden's entrance into the European Community is feared to lead to an increased smuggling of drugs into the country when the custom officials can no longer make random checks at the border. With the increased integration within Europe may also come new influences on the existing national drug patterns as well as on policy makers. There is now a new drug liberalization movement in Europe. In November 1990 the cities of Amsterdam, Frankfurt am Main, Hamburg and Zürich issued a document named "European Cities on Drug Policy", the so called Frankfurt Resolution. This resolution states that drug problems in society are primarily due to the illegality of drug consumption, which makes drugs impure and expensive and causes misery, death and acquisitive criminality. Consequently it proposes, among other things, the permission of "'shooting galleries' in which drugs can be consumed under supervision" and that "medically controlled prescriptions of drugs to long-term drug users should be analysed without prejudice and in view of harm reduction". This resolution has now been adopted by 23 cities and municipalities in Europe. The similarity of the arguments of the Frankfurt resolution to the arguments in favour of legal prescription in Sweden in the 1960s is striking. It is therefore not surprising that the first meeting of the opposition to the Frankfurt resolution was held in Stockholm. In April 1994 the document "European Cities Against Drugs", the so called Stockholm Resolution, was issued. In this resolution all proposals to legalize illicit drugs are rejected and a restrictive drugs policy based on the international drugs conventions adopted by the UN is advocated. So far 21 cities and municipalities (among them Berlin, Paris and London and several other capitals) have adopted the Stockholm Resolution.

REFERENCES

Ågren, G., Anderzon, K., Berglund, E. and Dundar, A. (1993) *Narkotika i Stockholm.* Stockholm: Socialtjänsten i Stockholm, FoU-byrån.
Bejerot, N. (1968) *Narkotikafrågan och samhället* (Second ed.). Stockholm: Aldus' Aktuellt.
Bejerot, N. (1970) *Addiction and Society.* Springfield, Ill: Charles C. Thomas.
Bejerot, N. (1975a) *Drug abuse and drug policy.* Copenhagen: Munksgaard.

Bejerot, N. (1975b) *Narkotikamissbruk och narkotikapolitik.* Stockholm: Sober.

Bergmark, A., Björling, B., Grönbladh, L., Olsson, B., Oscarsson, L. and Segraeus, V. (1989) *Klienter i institutionell narkomanvård.* Pedagogiska institutionen, Uppsala Universitet.

Bergvall, B. (1988) *Ingen anledning till oro …* Stockholm: Ordfront.

Billing, L., Eriksson, M., Jonsson, B., Steneroth, G. and Zetterström, R. (1994) The influence of environmental factors on behavioural problems in 8-year-old children exposed to amphetamine during fetal life. *Child Abuse and Neglect,* **18**, pp. 3–9.

Böttiger, M., Biberfeld, G., Janzon, R., Forsgren, M., von Sydow, M., Greillner, L. and Annell, A. (1993) HIV-antibody testings among injecting drug users (IDUs) in the Stockholm area, 1984–91: Information compiled from testing laboratories. *Scandinavian Journal of Infectious Diseases,* **25**, pp. 289–295.

Connell, P.H. (1958) *Amphetamine Psychosis.* London: Oxford University Press.

Fugelstad, A. (1989) *LVM-vård av narkomaner.* Toxikomankliniken, Sabbatsbergs sjukhus. FoU-byrån, Stockholms socialförvaltning.

Fugelstad, A. and Raijs, J. (1994a) *Narkotikarelaterade dödsfall i Stockholm 1986–1993* (Preliminary report). Department of Forensic Medicine.

Fugelstad, A. and Rajs, J. (1994b) Dödsorsaker hos amfetaminmissbrukare i Stockholm 1986–93. *Svenska Läkaresällskapets Riksstämma* in Stockholm (Abstr. MA 10P).

Goldberg, I. (1944) Vänjning och missbruk efter användning av fenopromin-preparat. *Läkartidningen,* **41**, pp. 561–578.

Krantz, L. and Jonsson, U. (1990) *Narkotikaläget, missbrukarna och kriminalvårdens åtgärder* (PSF PM 1990:1). Kriminalvårdsstyrelsen, Forsknings — och utvecklingsgruppen.

Kühlhorn, E. (1994) *Legala och illegala droger i Sverige. Hur hanterar svenskarna alkohol — och andra drogproblem?* Department of Sociology, Stockholm University.

Käll, K. (1994) The risk of HIV infection for noninjecting sex partners of injecting drug users in Stockholm. *AIDS Education and Prevention,* **6**, pp. 351–364.

Käll, K. (1995) *Sexual behaviour of incarcerated intravenous drug users in Stockholm in relation to Human Immunodeficiency Virus (HIV) and Hepatitis B Virus (HBV) transmission.* Karolinska Institute, Department of Clinical Neuroscience, Division of Psychiatry, St. Göran's Hospital, Stockholm, Sweden and the Department of International Health and Social Medicine, Division of Social Medicine, Kronan Health Institute, Sundbyberg, Sweden.

Käll, K. and Nilsonne, Å. (1994) Preference for sex on amphetamine — a marker for HIV risk behaviour among male iv amphetamine users in Stockholm. *AIDS Care,* **7**, pp. 171–188.

Ministry of Health and Social Affairs International Secretariat (1989). *The Care of Alcoholics, Drug Abusers and Abusers of Volatile Solvents (Special Provisions) Act /LVM/.*

Olsson, O., Byqvist, S. and Gomér, G. (1993) *Det tunga narkotikamissbrukets omfattning i Sverige 1992 No. 28.* Centralförbundet för alkohol — och narkotikaupplysning (CAN).

Rylander, G. (1969) Clinical and medico-criminological aspects of addiction to central stimulating drugs. In F. Sjöqvist and M. Tottie (Eds.), *Abuse of Central Stimulants. Symposium arranged by the Swedish committée on international health relations.* Stockholm: Almqvist and Wiksell.

Stenström, N. and Öberg, D. (1994) *Socialt integrerade och utslagna intravenösa* narkotikamissbrukare. *En studie av deltagare i sprutbytesprogrammet vid infektionskliniken, Malmö allmänna sjukhus.* Institutionen för socialt arbete — Socialhögskolan, Stockholms Universitet.

Swedish National Institute of Public Health (1993) *A Restrictive Drug Policy. The Swedish Experience.*

Swedish National Police Board (1994). *Yearly Report from the National Criminal Investigations Service for 1993.*

Tunving, K. (1990) Dödligheten bland narkotikamissbrukare — en översikt. In K. Tunving, B. Olsson, and P. Krantz (Eds.), *Dödligheten bland narkotikamissbrukare i de nordiska länderna* pp. 21–46. (Stockholm, Centralförbundet för Alkohol — och Narkotikaupplysning (CAN)).

Tunving, K. and Nordegren, T. (1993) *Droger A-Ö.* Borås: Natur and Kultur. Ågren, G., Anderzon, K., Berglund, E. and Dundar, A. (1993) *Narkotika i Stockholm.* Stockholm: Socialtjänsten i Stockholm, FoU-byrån. 1'Narcotic drug' in Sweden is any drug scheduled under the Swedish Narcotic Offence Act, which is the domestic Swedish legislation corresponding to the UN 1961 and 1971 Drug Conventions.

Introduction to Section 4:
Germany and the Netherlands

Germany and the Netherlands share a common border but they are very dissimilar in the way they deal with the drugs problem. The Netherlands has been at the forefront of a liberal and pragmatic approach to drug use, particularly the recreational use of cannabis, and achieved some notoriety as a transit nation for trafficking a whole range of drugs. The maritime history of the Dutch with their well developed ports contributes to this. There has been some containment of domestic heroin consumption and injecting, but the policy on cannabis, that allows public consumption in restricted areas, still attracts many visitors from other nations — attention that is not always welcome. Legislative control of amphetamine started in the 1970s and domestic use declined, but manufacture and trafficking to other European nations increased and now stretches even further afield.

One of the target markets for the Netherlands has been Germany, now itself a transit country for supplies of amphetamine and its precursors from Eastern Europe. The approach to drugs in Germany has never been liberal however and the harm reduction model espoused in the Netherlands has not taken root.

The similarity between these two nations lies mostly in the absence of an amphetamine problem until the 'rave' scene with its association with MDMA spread from the United Kingdom. The situation seems similar in several other European countries and there is a new and widespread concern about youthful recreational use of this drug.

12

The Phenomenology of Amphetamine Use in Germany

WOLFGANG HECKMANN

GENERAL TRENDS

Although amphetamines and other stimulants have been available through-out Germany for many years, there has never been an epidemic of 'uppers' or 'speed' in this country. Stimulant use existed during the war and in the first post-war decade, but only to a limited extent. As in many other coun-tries, stimulant use was prevalent in the military system (used by the troops, but neglected by officials) and it was quite common among people involved in the black market after World War II (Amendt, 1993).

Since the mid sixties there has been a youth oriented development of illicit drug use which has changed in nature several times over the years. During the first phase it was mainly the behaviour of artists and 'bohemians' and international youthful fashions that influenced the more academic young to try psychedelic drugs. The purpose was the extension of mind, feelings and emotions. The preferred drugs were cannabis, LSD and other hallucino-gens. Rituals were associated with a contemplative mood and complete physical inactivity (Steckel, 1972).

During the second phase, illegal drugs became popular more generally among less academic adolescents. Drug users gathered together on the streets, in parks and subway stations. The nature of drug use changed to one in which avoidance of reality was the aim and 'downers' were preferred. Although cannabis and LSD were still the most popular, they were not used in the same way. They were no longer used as a celebrated event, but became a daily habit, and experimenting with high doses and mixing 'cocktails' of drugs was common.

A consequence of this trend was that one part of the drug-using subculture developed a pattern of use that focused on classical 'downers' like heroin and other opiates, analgesics and sleeping pills and other pharmaceutical preparations. This was the beginning of a 'hard' drug-use pattern which led to criminal behaviour, destructive lifestyles and deteriorating living conditions. These now dominate public discussion and are the most obvious symptoms of the drug problems among young people.

Although the average young adult in Germany is very familiar with the use of alcohol, only about 20% of them have ever used cannabis. The use of opiates is rare and is estimated at less than 1% of the population for lifetime use. Nevertheless the national disposition up to the end of the eighties was towards the use of legal or illegal 'downers'. Amphetamine did not have a high profile. Only a very small minority of intravenous drug users had ever injected amphetamine or cocaine. The use of crack was known mostly through the media, and was very rare on the streets. Uppers of all kinds, including cocaine were more likely to be used by older people.

Only since the end of the eighties has cocaine begun to be more widespread in western European countries, and has become established to a greater extent in Germany. The epidemic of cocaine use started, predictably, among 'Yuppies' and middle-aged, middle and upper-class people who were mainly involved in (show-) business (Heckmann *et al.*, 1987). Within a few years there were cocaine addicts needing treatment (Stone *et al.*, 1990).

Cocaine crossed the boundaries of social class and became fully integrated into street life from the early nineties. This was the result of Latin American cocaine dealers using aggressive marketing strategies in major western European Countries. The prices on the black market decreased and street sales became an attractive and lucrative proposition for drug dealers. So far, the use of cocaine is not very popular among opiate users, the psychoactive effects are the opposite to those of their favourite drug. But there are some regions, like Frankfurt, where polydrug use (opiates and cocaine) is quite prevalent. The impact of these consumption patterns can be seen on the streets as a visible increase in violence (Heinz, 1993).

Emerging at about the same time were party or designer-drugs. As the decade of the nineties started, the first users of these recreational drugs were recruited into a youth-subculture with only the experience of drugs such as cannabis. The first vehicle of this development were 'house' parties at places outside the established disco venues, where 'house-music' was played and drugs were available. Designer-drugs were well promoted, but in general "acid" was sold. From time to time there was a rumour that PCP ('angel dust') was available too, but no PCP epidemic was observed.

'House-parties' were in vogue for one or two years and were confined to the major cities only.

With the subsequent fashion for 'techno' or 'rave' parties, a completely different subculture with different patterns of drug use was established. When listening to 'techno' music, people dance for many hours and often without concern for serious health problems, like dehydration. Alcohol is not an acceptable part of this scene but soft drinks are used, although they are very expensive. Speed of all kinds is easily available. Those who want to succeed (and to survive) in this party and dance-culture, have to achieve the 'normal' level of performance — and hence need additional power and energy. To get through the weekend from Friday to Monday morning and to dance almost continuously and in a frenetic way is hardly possible without little synthetic helpers.

To perform every weekend in this way leads sooner or later to the use of 'uppers'. This was the route on which young people now embarked in their drug careers. It was characterized by a hitherto unknown pattern of use and driven by an unusual motive — the use of a drug as an agent of active leisure, enabling users to have a good time, and avoiding the physical stresses and strains brought about through dancing for long periods of time. This ideology of the German 'party-family' now formulates the goals of group members which are largely about fantasy, dancing, raging, raving, and identifying and testing one's own creative energies. Drugs are used to reach these goals, and the only problems encountered are incompetent use, wrong timing or dangerous combinations of drugs (Eve and Rave, 1994; Vollbrechtshausen, 1994). This ideology is transmitted by several interest groups and has considerable coverage from the media. The most active group is named "Eve and Rave", characterized by their members as "party-people with long experience in raving". The message of their papers and press releases is a mixture of sociological analysis, new age philosophy and promises of salvation. In short, comparable with Timothy Leary's attitude to hallucinogenic drugs and the affirmative promotion of LSD based on his books (Leary, 1970).

Most 'ravers' have previous experiences with drugs such as cannabis and some of the so-called 'soft' drugs. The temporary and unstable integration of cocaine into the intravenous drug using population is unlikely to occur in a similar way in this culture. However, the use of 'uppers' in some form is likely to be crucial to the development of the German rave scene. The main drugs used in this subculture are amphetamines — even if the drug of choice is Ecstasy. The marketing of drugs is focussing on the designer drugs XTC, Adam and E, but what is sold is seldom genuine since the availability of Ecstasy in Germany is low. Most drugs sold as Ecstasy are in fact amphetamines (Heinz, 1994). Since the need of the ravers is more for the energy-giving component of Ecstasy rather than for the psychedelic effects, most of the users are satisfied.

Another unusual aspect in the German rave culture (comparable only to the Dutch, see Korf and Lettink, 1994) is the occasional infiltration by cocaine into some sub-groups. For example, at the end of parties, when only a core group of people, organizers and their peers are staying.

The impact of German unification on patterns of drug use has been interesting. The raves, house-parties and speed use are not, as most of the other parts of the illicit drug subculture, only a phenomenon in the former Federal Republic of Germany, they have become more and more fashionable in the 'new Bundesländer', that is, the former German Democratic Republic. One of the reasons for this unexpected development is the organization of rave parties for customers from the big cities, such as Berlin, Hamburg and Frankfurt, in old farmhouses and factories out in the countryside. Another reason seems to be that some of the young former GDR citizens are intent on following the newest trend of youth culture in the western democracies. Drug use is no longer taboo in the 'new Bundesländer' but it needs to be affordable. Cannabis is affordable, but it is a drug of an older generation and has less status among the younger generation. Amphetamines are affordable and can take on other forms. In the former GDR it is even easier to sell amphetamines as Ecstasy.

The general trends of drug use and affinity of young people towards drug use in the 'new Bundesländer' are not easy to assess. The early estimates, that all kinds of drugs, which have been available in the western part of Germany for many years would be soon available (and used) in the eastern part, failed. It seems on the contrary, that the general fear among the older and even the younger generation, of trying illegal drugs, is still persisting. Additionally, for those who would be able to afford the expense of costly drugs, other priorities of consuming are set: for example TVs and HiFi sets, Western cars and expensive clothing. In the context of these 'economic imperatives' it is evident that illegal drugs do not have their time yet. There is a growing drugs market and increasing misuse of them — but it is rather limited to cannabis and amphetamines or designer drugs, not including cocaine and heroin. However, the economic development of the former GDR provinces will inevitably be affiliated to the western standard and the climate will be prepared for more costly drugs as well.

The interchangeability of Ecstasy and amphetamine, also of cocaine and legal stimulants has its tradition in the USA. Rapid change among drug users between different stimulants (that seems to have nothing to do with availability) has quite often been reported for New York City (Frank, 1988; Frank and Galea, 1994). But in other regions there are fluctuations in the use of stimulants which are observed in connection with rave parties, be it based on sociological changes for example, crossing the boundaries of social classes in Colorado, (Harrison, 1994), or be it based on changing fashions, for example in San Francisco (Newmeyer, 1994).

SUMMARY

If anything may be concluded about the current drug scene in Germany and predicted for the near future, it is a pattern largely determined by particular demands being met with what can be supplied.

There is a great demand for Ecstasy, generated by the new vogue for raves, and the ideology that underpins it. Minority youth, music and party cultures are the customers. The trend is enhanced by the publicity given to these events in all major magazines and TV programmes. It is fuelled by another campaign for the legalization of cannabis, and also for Ecstasy and cocaine.

On the other hand the current demand is predominantly satisfied by cheaper, affordable uppers than the original: that is, amphetamine. This may eventually lead to a replication of the international trend towards the interchangeability of all kinds of stimulant drugs. If this happens, in Germany the use of amphetamine will have been established almost by default, even though it was never a primary drug of choice.

AVAILABLE DATA

Research on the use of amphetamines in Germany is quite poorly developed. This is not so very different from many other countries throughout the world. The publication of this book draws attention to the lack of information about the nature of amphetamine misuse in many countries of the world and at the same time demonstrates the need for it. Amphetamine is an ubiquitous and easily available drug that comes disguised in many forms.

In the Federal Republic of Germany it is unclear whether amphetamine has established itself in its own specific and restricted subculture, or whether patterns of consumption will emerge that will be comparable to the hard core addiction that is associated with opiates.

Survey Data

Regular surveys on the drug using behaviour of the general population are carried out by the Federal Centre for Health Education in Köln. Recent data (Bundeszentrale für gesundheitliche Aufklärung, 1994, p. 102) on the use of drugs by German youth show the following trend: "Of the 12 to 25 year old in the whole of the Federal Republic, 18% have tried illegal drugs on some occasion or taken them for a time — 21% in the old Federal Länder and 6 percent in the new Federal Länder. This indicator of so-called lifetime drug experience encompasses a whole variety of different substances, ranging from hashish and 'uppers' to 'hard' drugs, such as cocaine and heroin. Hashish is the drug actually taken in most cases, as reported by 96% of those with drug experience. The numbers of cases of hard-drug consumption are correspondingly low, meaning that the results of the drug affinity study cannot be used to make accurate estimates of the lifetime use of cocaine, heroin or other hard drugs."

The data on stimulants are interesting. Only 16% of the age group 12 to 25 years know peers who have tried them. Of the 18% that report drug experiences however, 39% have used uppers as well. This is an increase of between 200% and 300% compared to the eighties (ibid., p. 74).

The number of intravenous drug (opiate) injectors in Berlin has recently been estimated. From two different, carefully controlled surveys, a population of 7,000 injecting drug users is likely to be the more accurate estimate. Among these hard core users more than 20% are experienced in the (mainly non-injecting) use of amphetamines (Kirschner *et al.*, 1994).

From the evidence supplied by local studies in rural regions surrounding the capital, Berlin, it is apparent that up to 25% of the young people have already tried or are motivated to try illegal drugs including amphetamines. Amphetamines (and Ecstasy) are more likely to be used than opiates and cocaine.

Police data

An impressive increase in seizures of amphetamines by police suggests increased use of the drug. In 1993 the seizures of amphetamine tablets increased by 119% over those recorded in 1992 (Bundeskriminalamt, 1993). Also in 1993 a total of 198.6 kg and 425 amphetamine tablets were seized in the country and 15,500 kg of amphetamines, ready for delivery to Germany, were seized outside the country.

Amphetamine is also manufactured in Germany. Twenty two illegal laboratories, 15 of them producing amphetamines, were closed in 1993. More people were apprehended by police for using amphetamine and the number of first offenders increased to 1884, an increase of 15% over 1992. This is in contrast to heroin using first offenders where a decline was recorded from 1992 to 1993. The rise continues and from January to April 1994 an increase of 88.6% of first offenders of amphetamines were reported. The rise in MDMA seizures was even higher with a 300% increase and with a total of 31,459 arrests (Presse-und Informationsamt, 1994).

Socioepidemiological and Ethnological Data

There are research groups in Germany that are involved in epidemiological and socioepidemiological studies of recreational drug use. Some have produced insights into amphetamine use, for example: the use of Guarana (a legal agricultural product with stimulant effects that are stronger than coffee, imported from Latin America) is quite prevalent in the nightclubs of the larger German cities. Some producers of soft and alcoholic drinks have followed this fashion with new products mixed with Guarana and the sales of these costly 'energy drinks' like 'Red Bull', 'Flying Horse' and 'XTC' are increasing (Horx, 1994). The motivation to use Guarana, Ecstasy and cannabis is frequently reported (Rakete *et al.*, 1993). Other data have revealed that amphetamines are popular among truckers, students and managers (Grube *et al.*, 1994).

Drugs are combined with amphetamine by users, for example: with heroin by 26% of heroin users in Berlin (Kirschner *et al.*, 1994), with cocaine and heroin in other metropolitan areas like Frankfurt (Heinz, 1993), with Ecstasy and LSD (Rakete *et al.*, 1995; Saunders, 1994, p. 315). Ecstasy tablets have been found mixed with amphetamines and/or LSD (Traufetter *et al.*, 1995; Müller, 1994; Grube *et al.*, 1994).

An organization of drug users who were interested in the quality of Ecstasy analysed Ecstasy tablets and found they were a mixture of caffeine and quinine or Paracetamol, quinine, caffeine and Ephedrin (Eve and Rave, 1995). The same organization estimated that more than one million persons had used amphetamine or Ecstasy in Germany.

CONCLUSION

Amphetamines are not an intrinsic part of the drug culture of the Federal Republic of Germany. Although there was a period of use of stimulants during World War II and for a time afterwards, misuse was never extensive. The misuse of drugs that developed in various groups of German youth culture tended to focus on 'downers', that is, the opiates for more than twenty years from the late sixties. Only certain members of high stress occupations like truck-driving, prostitution, entertainment and management were attracted to 'uppers', but even here the preferred drugs were cocaine and some legal stimulants.

The contemporary use of amphetamine is a fashion that seems at present to be restricted to young people on the rave and techno-party scene. However, their drug of choice is not pure amphetamine, but the combination of stimulant and hallucinogenic effects that are induced by MDMA. The vagaries of availability of Ecstasy on the black market combined with a limited knowledge about drugs among the customers, has led to the common practice of manufacturing substances in which amphetamine and other drugs such as LSD are sold (and used) as Ecstasy. The widespread use of amphetamine as a hidden ingredient in such 'cocktails' is leading to the rather unexpected and paradoxical consequence — that amphetamine use is developing into an epidemic in Germany despite the fact that, for most users, it is not the first drug of choice.

REFERENCES

Amendt, G. (1993) Sucht — Profit — Sucht. Hamburg.

Bundeskriminalamt (1994) *Rauschgiftjahresbericht 1993*. Wiesbaden.

Bundeszentrale für gesundheitliche Aufklärung (1994) *Die Drogenaffinität Jugendlicher in der Bundesrepublik Deutschland. Wiederholungsbefragung 1993/94*. Köln.

Deutsche Hauptstelle gegen die Suchtgefahren (1994) *Jahrbuch Sucht 95*. Geesthacht.

Eve and Rave (1994) *Selbstverständnis — Perspektive*. Pressematerial. Berlin.

Eve and Rave (1995) *Ecstasy-Pillen. Analysen und die Werte*. Berlin.

Eve and Rave (1993) *Partydrogen: Safer-Use-Info zu: Ecstasy, Speed, LSD, Kokain*. Berlin.

Frank, B. (1988) Current drug use trends in New York City. In: Community Epidemiology Work Group (CEWG) *Epidemiologic Trends in Drug Use*. Maryland National Institute of Health.

Frank, B. and Galea, J. (1994) Current drug use trends in New York City. In: CEWG *Epidemiologic Trends in Drug Use*. Maryland National Institute of Health.

Gesundheitsministerium Brandenburg (1994) *Drogenbericht*. Potsdam.

Grube, L., Märtens, P. and Hoffmann, R. (1994) *Ecstasy — LSD — Speed — eine Information für Eltern, Lehrer, Erzieher*. Hannover.

Harrison, L. (1994) Special Topics: Field notes on "raving" in Colorado. In: CEWG *Epidemiologic Trends in Drug Abuse*. Maryland National Institute of Health.

Heckmann, W. u.a. (1987) *Modedroge Kokain?* Hamm.

Heckmann, W. and Vormann, G. (1980) Zur Geschichte der Therapeutischen Wohngemeinschaften in Deutschland. In: H. Petzold, and G. Vormann, (eds.) *Therapeutische Wohngemeinschaften*. München.

Heckmann, W. (1995) *Der Einfluß sich verändernder Strukturen auf das Suchtverhalten: die Situation in den neuen Bundesländern*. Heidelberg.

Heinz, W. (1993) *Beikonsum von Kokain unter Polamidon-substituierten Opiatabhängigen in Frankfurt. Die Veränderung des politoxikamanen Erscheinungsbildes*. Vortrag. Ärztekammer Hessen. Frankfurt.

Heinz, W. (1994) *Marketing von Amphetaminen als Ecstasy*. Personal Communication.

Horx, M. (1994) Jede Epoche hat den Rausch, den sie verdient. *ZeitMagazin* 50.

Huncke, W. (Hg.) (1981) *Die Drogen-Jugend. Berichte, Analysen und Fakten über die Heroinabhängigkeit Jugendlicher*. Frankfurt: Ullstein.

Kirschner, W., Kunert, M., Grünbeck, P., Markert, S. and Tiemann, F. (1994) *Umfang und Struktur der Population i.v. Drogenabhängiger in Berlin*. Berlin.

Kleiber, D., Soellner, R. and Tossmann, H.P. (1995) *Determinanten unterschiedlicher Konsummuster von Cannabis. Zwischenbericht.* spi. Berlin.

Korf, D.and Lettink, D. (1994) Ecstasy: Trends and Patterns in the Netherlands. In: CEWG *Epidemiologic Trends in Drug Abuse.* Maryland National Institute of Health.

Leary, T. (1970) *Politik Der Ekstase.* Hamburg.

Lintner, E. (1995) *Keine Entwarnung bei Rauschgift!* Bonn: Bundesministerium des Innern.

Müller, L. (1994) *Ecstasy.* Lausanne: SFA/ISPA.

Newmeyer, J. (1994) Drug Abuse in the San Francisco Bay Area, in: CEWG (1994) *Epidemiologic Trends in Drug Abuse.* Maryland National Institute of Health.

Presse- und Informationsamt der Bundesregierung (1994) *Politik gegen Drogen.* Weimar.

Rakete, G., Püschl, M., Flüsmeier, U. and Rabes, M. (1995) *Konsum und Mißbrauch von Ecstasy in Hamburg.* Hamburg.

Saunders, N. and Walder, P. (1994) *Ecstasy.* Zürich.

Senator für Inneres (1995) *Rauschgiftkriminalbericht.* Berlin.

Sphor, B. (in press) *Techno-Party-drogen. Psychologische Aspeckte und therapeutische Erfahrungen.* Berlin.

Steckel, R. (1972) *Bewußtseinserweiternde Drogen.* Berlin.

Stone, N., Fromme, M. and Kagan, D. (1990) *Leistungsdroge Kokain. Szenereport und Ausstiegshilfen.* Basel: Weinheim.

Traufetter, G. and Pilscek, R.F. (1995) *Ecstasy.* Die Woche, **8**, pp. 34.

Vollbrechtshausen, A. (1994) Ecstasy in Deutschland. Partykinder und Technoschwule. In: N. Saunders and P. Walder, (eds.) *Ecstasy.* Zürich.

13

Chasing Ecstasy: Use and Abuse of Amphetamines in the Netherlands

MARGRIET W. van LAAR and INGE P. SPRUIT

INTRODUCTION

In the Netherlands, users of amphetamines have neither been the focus of research during the last decade, nor did they receive special attention from politics and health care services for addicts. This contrasts with the opiate users, who are often associated with serious drug related problems affecting both the individual and society as a whole. Since approximately 75% of the Dutch opiate addicts are estimated to be in contact with official care and treatment agencies, there is a relative wealth of data available about this group. To a certain extent the lack of special attention to amphetamine users reflected a relatively low prevalence of use and a relatively regulated consumption pattern. However, the recent introduction on the Dutch drugs market of 'new' amphetamines, especially Ecstasy, appeared to change this trend. The increasing popularity and use of this drug at 'houseparties' attracted wide attention of the media. In addition, the use of this drug soon became associated with health risks and accidents that could be as serious as death and created a concern for politics and health care authorities. Although the extent to which such adverse health effects occur, under which circumstances and which individuals are most at risk, has not been systematically investigated, such developments require preventive measures.

This chapter addresses the use and misuse of amphetamine and related compounds in the Netherlands. After a short historical overview, epidemiological data will be presented, followed by a characterization of the primary users of amphetamines. Attention will be paid to the quality of the drugs and health consequences that are partly related to the quality issues. Next, preventive actions that typify Dutch drug policy are described. Finally, current trends in illegal drug use as well as predictions on future trends are delineated. The main drugs in question are the stimulant amphetamine (Benzedrine) and several derivatives that are obtained by slight molecular modifications. These include the potent stimulant methamphetamine (Pervitine) as well as drugs with a different spectrum of effects, the hallucinogenic amphetamines. This category contains numerous compounds, the most popular in the Netherlands being methylenedioxymethamphetamine (MDMA or Ecstasy or XTC), followed by methylenedioxyethamphetamine (MDEA) and to a lesser extent methylenedioxyamphetamine (MDA). These compounds are not only chemically related to amphetamine but also to mescaline, a potent hallucinogen. However, they appear to be neither real stimulants nor hallucinogens, although properties of both classes of drugs are observed to different degrees. At a moderate dose they positively affect mood and heighten perception without causing a loss of control or reality. Because these drugs seem to enhance feelings of intimacy and closeness to others they are said to represent a new class of 'entactogens'. MDA is more potent and longer acting than MDMA, and may have some hallucinogenic effects at higher doses. In contrast, MDEA is less potent and shorter acting than MDMA, but its stimulant effects appear to dominate the entactogenic effects. The use of MDMA will be emphasized in this chapter since it plays a major role in the Netherlands. The term amphetamine will be used to refer to both amphetamine and methamphetamine, unless mentioned otherwise.

HISTORY

Compared to opium and cannabis, the use of amphetamine was introduced only recently. First synthesized in 1887, it took some time to reveal its potential therapeutic applications. In 1935, amphetamine was marketed in the Netherlands. The drug was used as inhaler in the treatment of asthma and hay fever, and prescribed for oral use in the treatment of obesity, mild depression, and chronic fatigue.

In the years following the Second World War, Dutch physicians frequently prescribed amphetamine as an aid for weight reduction. Housewives were also given the drug as an 'upper' to counteract the morning hangover sedation, following nocturnal use of a barbiturate or benzodiazepine hypnotic ('downer') (van der Stel, 1992). In this period the amphetamine black market emerged. Several 'professional' groups, such as truck-drivers and workers in the hotel and catering industry, frequently used amphetamines to overcome fatigue during relatively exhausting working conditions. In general, these groups could control their use fairly well. During the sixties (the 'flower-power' period), non-medical use of drugs, such as cannabis, LSD and other psychedelics, was widespread within a particular subculture of intellectuals and well educated, middle-class youth (such as provos and hippies). These drugs symbolised their counter-cultural lifestyle, freedom and resistance against mainstream society's values (Leuw, 1994). Amphetamine, especially injected methamphetamine, soon became popular, however, mainly in the socio-cultural context of the working class.

The consequences of uncontrolled use, such as physical exhaustion, weight loss and even psychosis, soon appeared. The addictive potential of amphetamine and the proliferation of use, prompted the control of this drug under the Dutch Opium Law in 1976. Subsequently, the prices on the black market increased considerably and amphetamine lost much of its popularity. In the early seventies, heroin was introduced on to the Dutch drugs market and heroin addiction soon became the core of the drug problems in the Netherlands (Swierstra, 1994).

In the eighties, the rise of cocaine partly contributed to the decreasing interest of Dutch drug users for amphetamine, although in this period a short-lived rise of amphetamine use was observed among punks and squatters. Currently, the amphetamine scene seems to be dominated by MDMA (and related drugs) that appeared on the Dutch market in 1985. Initially, MDMA was predominantly used in a closed subcultural environment of like minded people in order to enhance certain hedonistic values and personal growth. However, the drug soon entered the 'party world' and became associated with a youth culture that had acid house music and house parties (raves) as symbols (Kaplan *et al.*, 1989). MDMA seemed to fit the spirit of the time, combining the mind-expanding elements of the sixties with the pragmatism of the Dutch eighties. After a lively weekend, this 'light' drug was supposed not to interfere with Monday morning duties at work or at school. In 1988, MDMA was included in the Opium Law but its popularity has not waned since that time. Amphetamine still has a significant role as one of the recreational drugs (whether or not taken intentionally), and there is some evidence for a revival of a separate amphetamine users group.

LEGAL USE

Currently the medicinal use of amphetamine or derivatives in the Netherlands is restricted to only two (psychiatric) conditions. These are the hyperkinetic syndrome in children and narcolepsy. Methylphenidate is the drug of first choice for the hyperkinetic syndrome. This drug is also used in the treatment of narcolepsy if the therapeutic response to tricyclic antidepressants, such as clomipramine, and ephedrine is unsatisfactory (van der Kuy, 1994). With the exception of fenfluramine (not included in the Opium Law), amphetamine and congeners are not now indicated as medicine for obesity because of the rapid development of dependence, the addiction potential and limited efficacy. Because of these few accepted indications, amphetamine abuse as a consequence of medical prescription is unlikely or very small-scaled. In the United States, MDMA was investigated as a 'truth-serum' for military purposes in the fifties. In the seventies and eighties it was used as an aid in psychotherapy until its listing on Schedule I by the Food and Drug Administration in 1985. There has never been a clinical indication for MDMA in the Netherlands.

PREVALENCE OF USE

The current prevalence of the use of amphetamine and MDMA in the *total* population is not exactly known. It is assumed that the use of MDMA has increased during the last years, whereas that of amphetamine is more or less stable, or showed some temporary fluctuations due to the emergence of MDMA on the market. Some field experts try to indicate the extent of MDMA use, revealing estimates of the number of people who used this drug at least once in their life that vary widely from 20,000 to about half a million on a total population of 15 million (Jamin, 1994). Based on non-systematic participant observation it is suggested that 10% to 40% of the 2,000 to 20,000 visitors of house-parties may use MDMA (Kaplan *et al.*, 1989).

Amsterdam Population

Epidemiological data on the use of illegal drugs are only available for the overall Amsterdam population and, at the national level, for Secondary School pupils in regular education. Referring to the former, results of a household survey in 1990 among 4,445 inhabitants of Amsterdam of 12 years and over, revealed that cannabis was the illegal drug used most frequently (Sandwijk, Cohen and Musterd, 1991). The percentage of people who used this drug at least once in their life (life-time prevalence) was 24.1%. 'Recent' use (as last month prevalence) was reported by 6%. Although among addicts heroin still is largely the most used hard drug, in the population survey, cocaine appeared to be the most popular hard drug. The life-time prevalence of use was 5.5%, followed by amphetamine and hallucinogens (both 4.1%) and MDMA (1.3%). 'Recent' use of cocaine or amphetamine was reported by 0.4% of the respondents; only 0.1% had 'recently' used hallucinogens or MDMA. Prevalence rates of amphetamine and MDMA use were about twice as high for men than for women. This is a relatively stable finding, applying to most illegal drugs. The considerable difference between life time and 'recent' use, as well as the low frequency of use by 'recent' drug users, suggests that the pattern of use is experimental and recreational, rather than 'dependent'. In this respect, it must be emphasized that most of the respondents did not belong to the estimated 7,000 hard drug addicts living in the capital city, since their life-style (for example, being homeless) makes them difficult to capture in surveys. The low prevalence of MDMA use should also be interpreted with caution since this drug was introduced in the Netherlands only shortly before the start of the study. Moreover, it is important to realize that the Amsterdam drug situation can not be generalized to other areas of the country (van de Goor and Spruit, 1990). When compared to other cities or geographical areas, a relatively large amount of data on drug use in Amsterdam is available. Although this is obviously related to the size of the drugs problem that is greatest in this metropolitan area, a drawback is that a distorted picture may arise when taking these data as representative for the Netherlands in general.

Drug Addicts

Amphetamine use is also reported to be used by the 21,000–25,000 opiate addicts living in the Netherlands, but its role is limited. Currently, the dominant pattern for opiate addicts is to use various drugs, alcohol, and/or prescription drugs in addition to heroin. According to 1993 registration data of the outpatient addiction institutes, the number of *newly* registered drug clients was 9.238. The majority (68%) of these clients were primarily dependent on opiates, followed by those dependent on cocaine (13%), cannabis (11%), medicines (4%), amphetamines (3%) and other drugs (<1%). More than half (56%) of these drug clients used two or more addictive substances problematically (poly-users). Cocaine was most the most popular co-drug being used by 62% of the poly-users. In contrast, only 4% used amphetamine as co-drug (Stichting IVV, 1993). This pattern of results is generally confirmed in other studies, amphetamine being one of the least preferred drugs among opiate addicts (Driessen, 1992; Hartgers *et al.*, 1991; van Ameijden, van der Hoek and Coutinho, 1994).

Pupils

The most recent data on the prevalence of drug use at a national level are based on the National Youth Health Care survey in 1992 among pupils attending Secondary School (12–18 years). School surveys represent the 12–16 year population rather well, with the exception of pupils in special schools. The 16–18-year-olds are less well represented since the school age ends at 16. The results of this study revealed that illegal drug use, apart from cannabis, was relatively low (de Zwart, Mensink and Kuipers, 1993). MDMA appeared to be the most popular hard drug: 3.3% had used this drug at least once and 1% did so recently. The next most popular drug was amphetamine, followed by cocaine and heroin. Life-time prevalence rates were only 2.1%, 1.5% and 0.7%, respectively. Recent use of these drugs was reported by even less than 1% of the pupils, and no more than 0.2% reported weekly use of these drugs. In general, substance abuse was higher among boys than among girls, and showed an increasing trend with age. Yet the dominant pattern of use was experimental or incidental and most pupils did not move into regular drug use. Generally school or population surveys suggest that intensive use of illegal drugs, with the exception of cannabis, occurs at a very low rate. Stated differently, these surveys are largely studies of non users. In order to increase knowledge of the users of illegal (hard) drugs, specific methods have been developed (Hartnoll, 1992).

Problematic Youth

A high risk group with regard to drug use consists of youngsters who have relatively frequent contact with youth care facilities. They often drop out from regular education, start working at an early age or are unemployed. Experimentation behaviour and recent use of hard drugs appears to be considerably higher among these 'problematic' youngsters than among 'average' pupils. In a recent survey, Korf and van der Steenhoven (1993) showed that about one-third of 105 problematic youngsters (mean age 17.4 years) had ever tried at least one hard drug and 15% did so last month. MDMA was the most popular of these: 23% had experience with the drug and 11% reported recent use. Cocaine, amphetamine and LSD were next popular. Prevalence figures were three to four times higher than those regarding a sample of 679 pupils of comparable ages. Problematic youngsters had also more experience with cannabis and tobacco but they used slightly less alcohol than the pupils. The majority of the respondents from both groups lived in Amsterdam.

USERS AND PATTERNS OF USE

People may use drugs for various reasons, with different frequencies and in very diverse settings. The previous epidemiological studies may contribute to the characterization of the amphetamine and MDMA users. However, more detailed information is available from anecdotal and empirical data derived from nonsystematic field observations (de Loor, 1993; Fromberg and Jansen, 1993; Fromberg et al., 1994), more systematic studies using standardized interviews (Lettink and Tulfer, 1993), and 'ethnographic' research methods (Korf et al., 1991). Korf et al. have applied several data collection techniques such as field observations and interviews with visitors and organizers of houseparties and owners of discotheques, as well as individual and group (in-depth) interviews with Ecstasy users. In some cases a snow-balling method was used to recruit them. It should be noticed that these typologies are by no means exhaustive or mutually exclusive.

Several types of users can be distinguished based on the place, function or pattern of use. Mass use of amphetamine and MDMA appears to be related to the entertainment circuit ('out users'), although subtypes of primary amphetamine users as well as primary MDMA users are found outside this scene.

Home and Home/Out Users

Generally these users were the first to use MDMA since its introduction on the Dutch market. This category resembles the former United States therapeutic and spiritual scene like the 'New Age' movement. MDMA may be used in intimate home settings withdrawn from a wide social context, or in group sessions with friends, to communicate feelings and deepen self-understanding. Some of these users may have a strong affection for nature and use drugs outside their home, but hardly ever at house-parties. On the average these home and home/out users are in their late twenties and they use MDMA less frequently than the out users (see below). They may have experience with other drugs too.

Out Users

These users tend to visit discotheques, houseparties or other places of entertainment where the use of amphetamine and MDMA is functional. Those who predominantly use MDMA are attracted to its euphoric and stimulating effects as well as the sense of solidarity. These may intensify perceptual functions and facilitate dancing and interpersonal communication. The social background of this user group varies widely, and includes relatively highly educated, working people, students, artists and 'yuppies', as well as more deviant less educated, often unemployed youngsters, spending the largest part of the day in cafes and frequently experimenting with other drugs. In between are the moderately educated, fanatic partygoers, who especially appreciate the dancing and social contacts with friends (Korf *et al.*, 1991; de Loor, 1993; Kaplan *et al.*, 1989).

Most of the out users are white, older adolescents and young grown-ups (early twenties) who have in common that they are open to any new experience. The majority also regularly uses tobacco, alcohol and cannabis. They may also have experience of cocaine and amphetamine, and to a lesser extent of psychedelics, such as LSD and mushrooms, and 'poppers' (amylnitrite) (Sandwijk *et al.*, 1991; Korf *et al.*, 1991). These drugs are also reported to be used *simultaneously* with MDMA, either to augment or to control its effects.

Some users first experiment with high doses of MDMA and appear to prefer the more stimulant properties instead of the social effects of this compound. These 'going hard' youngsters may also have tried the more stimulant compound MDEA, often switching over to the much cheaper amphetamine (Fromberg *et al.*, 1994, de Loor, 1993). House-parties and house-music have no dominant role in their lives and drug use outside the 'house-scene' may be more prevalent. A minority of them is found among football supporters, repeatedly displaying aggressive behavior. According to some Dutch amphetamine (ex)users, speed seems to fit less well within the spirit of this era when compared to the seventies or early eighties, but it is still popular among a small users group. They say that "… Ecstasy makes them sluggish and is associated with the anti-political 'house', cocaine is too expensive, decadent and shortacting, LSD carries the risk for flipping, and heroin makes them dull and is too sedative." (Nabben, 1992).

Instrumental Users

As several decades ago, amphetamine may be used to enhance mental performance, for example to perform a job, to stay awake during prolonged driving or to study before an examination. Others may use amphetamine to enhance physical performance in the field of sports. Amphetamine is used by top sportsmen and women as well those who play sports recreationally (for example, racing cyclists). It is, however, the least popular drug among the total 'top 10' of doping agents. The most frequently used performance enhancer is the anabolic steroid Nandralon. Within the category stimulants, amphetamine occupies only a fourth place (Stoele, 1994). In the Netherlands, amphetamines are nevertheless detected in urine samples, especially from sportsmen and women living in the south of the country where the drug is produced in illegal laboratories.

Regular Users

Regular users of amphetamine are found among the addicted polydrug users, as mentioned previously. Both cocaine and amphetamines may be used as 'uppers' combined with the 'downer' heroin, either apart or simultaneously ('speed-balling'). A functional relationship between heroin and cocaine is established in that cocaine is the primary source of pleasure and heroin is the medicine, used to antagonize the adverse stimulant effects of cocaine (Grund, 1993). In a survey of the economy of 'druglife' using a representative sample of hard drugs users in Amsterdam, it was reported that most had a pronounced preference for cocaine, but their financial position might force them to buy speed (Pervitine) as a cheap substitute (Grapendaal, Leuw and Nelen, 1991).

Patterns of Use

The dominant pattern of use of both amphetamine and MDMA is experimental and recreational (Sandwijk *et al.*, 1991; de Zwart *et al.*, 1994). It is suggested that Dutch recreational users take amphetamine mainly by the oral or nasal route, but in fact there are no data available to confirm this. The intravenous injecting of amphetamine is primarily associated with a fundamentally different (dependent) pattern of use found among a minority of heavy polydrug addicts. Doses of amphetamine may vary widely, depending on the quality of the drug and degree of tolerance, resulting in a hundredfold dose difference. High dose use is often limited to a few days ('speed run')

because of the advent of adverse symptoms and rapid development of tolerance to the feelings of well-being and euphoria. Most of the recreational
MDMA users appear to regulate their use. Sometimes an initial period of
frequent use is observed, followed by a decline. The majority stabilize the
frequency of MDMA use at less than once a week, largely at weekends. One
(oral) dose per session, sometimes divided in two doses, is usually sufficient
given its time of action (4–6 hours). A minority devoted to 'going hard' may
take several tablets of MDMA in order to enhance the stimulant effects. The
advent of after-effects, such as fatigue and depressive feelings, that can last
for several days, may contribute to a limitation of its use. The same applies to
the adverse effects of MDMA that appear to overshadow the entactogenic
and calming effects of the drug after frequent dosing.

SOURCES AND QUALITY

The chemicals to produce synthetic drugs like amphetamine, MDMA, MDA
and MDEA are reported to come from Belgium, Germany and recently also
from East-Europe, China, Italy, Denmark and France (Centrale Recherche
Informatiedienst, 1993). In the Netherlands, the production of these drugs
takes place not only for the home market but also for international markets.
In 1993, about 12 drug laboratories were exposed that produced drugs
largely for the British and Scandinavian (Sweden) and also German markets.
According to the Dutch Criminal Intelligence Service of the Ministry of Justice, in 1992 and 1993, a total of 560 kg and 30,846 tablets of amphetamine
were confiscated as well as 776 kg and 2,500,335 tablets of MDA, and 302 kg
and 1,635,677 tablets of MDMA. Enormous quantities of synthetic drugs were
sometimes seized at once, pointing to the activities of highly organized criminal groups who are involved in this business.
  Currently, at the consumers level, prices may vary from fl. 25 (£10) to
fl. 100 (£40) per gram amphetamine and from fl. 20 (£8) to fl. 50 (£20), but
mostly fl. 35 (£14), per 'XTC' pill. However, price and quality of the drugs are
generally not related. The substances sold as amphetamine and particularly
MDMA, may vary widely, both with respect to the types of active ingredients
and to purity levels. This is especially true for samples bought on the street
and at house-parties and for samples obtained from unfamiliar dealers. For
several years what is sold as MDMA has been a variety of substitutes, combination preparations, wide dose ranges and so-called 'look-alikes'. The last
refer to pills that are identical in appearance but contain very different active
substances, often in highly variable concentrations. This phenomenon appears to be a growing problem on the Dutch 'MDMA' market.
  According to some field experts, there is a temporal relationship between
criminalisation of drugs and subsequent repressive actions of the police, and
the pollution of the drugs market, especially that of MDMA (Fromberg *et al.*,

1994; Korf and Verbrack, 1993). When MDMA initially entered the small Dutch market, most tablets were imported from the USA and Spain, or were produced at a small scale by some Dutch non-deviant producers (the 'soft fringe'). Following the introduction of MDMA in the entertainment circuit the demand for this drug increased considerably, not only in the Netherlands but also in the United Kingdom. At the same time, Poland became a major competitor for the 'hard' Dutch amphetamine producers on the international markets after the opening of the borders between East- and West-Europe. These developments first stimulated Dutch amphetamine producers to retail amphetamine as MDMA (the 'look-alikes'), but they soon turned over to the production of MDMA tablets. In 1988, MDMA was brought under control in the Dutch Opium Law, mainly because of international pressure. Some of the 'soft fringe' producers switched to the production of a then legal alternative, MDEA, in order to avoid prosecution. This drug can be described as a 'designer drug'. In 1993, MDEA was also included in the Opium Law. However, the supply did not subsequently wane and this was explained either by the dumping of stores on the market or by the appearance of a new consumer group.

The criminalisation of MDMA appeared to have several consequences, although the available data do not allow the determination of causal relationships. With increasing frequency, producers attempt to avoid prosecution by designing new drugs. 'Bad' drugs may appear on the scene as amateur chemists enter a lucrative market vacated by more experienced manufacturers. In this context the famous handbook "Pihkal" (Shulgin and Shulgin, 1991) is mentioned, in which numerous 'recipes' are described that synthesize 'new' mind-altering drugs, mainly belonging to the class of the hallucinogenic phenethylamines. Moreover, the criminalisation of MDMA combined with the high demand for the drug resulted in an increased number of distributors between producer and consumer. Although this did not significantly affect the prices at the consumers level, it appeared to contribute to the pollution of the MDMA market (Korf and Verbraeck, 1993). One of the new links in this distribution chain is the pill manufacturers. In order to reduce the risk for detection by the police, clandestine laboratories sell their base-powder to 'pill-rollers'. The latter often use the same logos for all pills irrespective of the ingredients, thereby compromising the recognition of drugs by their users. Quality control may also be of low order resulting in impurities and variable doses due to inferior cleaning and mixing. In addition, the relatively high cost of MDMA explains the frequent substitution of less expensive amphetamine. It must be emphasized, however, that the waxing and waning of drugs on the market as well as their quality is not only dependent on their legal status and actions of the police. Other factors, such as prices, availability of chemicals, effects of preventive measures and preferences of the consumers creating for example a small MDA market, may also contribute to their prevalence.

The Drugs Information Monitoring System (DIMS)

The above information is partly derived from the Dutch Drugs Information Monitoring System (DIMS) that was developed in 1992 at the Netherlands Institute for Alcohol and Drugs. This project was set up to provide information on several drugs markets in addition to existing data from addiction agencies, scientific research, police and justice. Up-to-date knowledge is obtained about users who are to some extent hidden to the previously mentioned organisations. The major objectives are the protection of public health by providing relevant information to drugs users as well as to policy makers. Direct interaction with the users as well as the suppliers of drugs is a prerequisite. A nation wide network of informants is set up consisting of drug treatment agencies, social welfare workers and (ex)users. They provide relevant inside information about the markets and also regularly deliver drugs samples for the purpose of monitoring the quality. In co-operation with the Safe House campaign (see under 'prevention') thousands of tablets of MDMA have been identified based on a qualitative coding system and 'acid-test'.[1] Drugs that can not be qualitatively identified are, at a smaller scale, identified by chemical laboratory analyses. It should be noted, however, that the drug samples of the DIMS are neither systematically obtained nor randomly sampled from a 'total' pool of drugs at the consumers level. A selection bias may be introduced by identifying samples that are brought up by the 'network' and by visitors at house-parties who can test their pills on a voluntary basis. Moreover, only a highly selective sample of drugs is analysed quantitatively. Therefore, the representativeness of these samples for 'the' drugs markets can be questioned and some caution should be practised in interpreting the following results in terms of drugs prevalence figures.

In the first half of 1994, qualitative identification of 3945 'MDMA' pills at houseparties revealed that 41% contained MDMA, 33% contained MDEA and 15% consisted mainly of amphetamine. In addition, 6% were identified as yeast, medicines or high doses of caffeine. The remainder contained MDA, MDOH (methylenedioxy-N-hydroxyamphetamine, resembling the actions of MDA) and in a few cases the potent hallucinogen DOB (dimethoxy-bromo-amphetamine) that may act as long as 18–36 hours. Occasionally, tablets were found to contain dangerous compounds like the anaesthetic ketamine or very high concentrations of amphetamine. Laboratory analyses of 254 MDMA samples obtained during the second half year of 1993 revealed several combination preparations

---

[1] The so-called acid test is applied at house-parties and in the field as a first qualitative screening test to determine the contents of 'XTC pills'. A minor amount is scratched from the pill and combined with a drop of the test compound. The colour reaction is an indication of the tested substance: No colour means a fake pill (such as paracetamol), orange points to 'speed' and blue indicates an XTC-like substance. The last can be further identified using a coding system based on 'appearance' (colour, size, logo, weight). Those not identified are sent to the laboratory for a full chemical analysis.

consisting of two compounds. These contained primarily MDMA and MDA, MDMA and MDEA, or MDA with MDEA, sometimes adulterated with caffeine or paracetamol. Usual 'recommended' doses of MDMA and MDEA are about 100 mg and 135 mg per tablet, respectively. The laboratory analyses revealed that most doses of MDMA tablets fell within the range of 30 mg to 180 mg with a peak at 90 mg. However, high doses up to 210 mg were also found. Consistent with its lower potency, doses of MDEA were generally higher than that of MDMA, showing a peak at 120 mg.

The amphetamine market has not been investigated to the same extent as the MDMA market. Analyses of 26 samples sold as amphetamine in the entertainment circuit revealed 14 samples consisting of caffeine and 1 consisting of ephedrine. The remaining samples contained amphetamine in concentrations varying from 1% to 48%. Results from a different study, analyzing 76 samples obtained at several places in Amsterdam, showed that about 20% contained either no active ingredients or lidocaine. Most of the low quality samples were bought at street. The remaining samples contained amphetamine (sulphate) varying from 12% to 100% purity. The analyses also frequently revealed the addition of caffeine (Korf and Verbrack, 1993).

LEGISLATION

In 1976, amphetamine was listed on Schedule 1 of the Dutch Opium Law, together with drugs such as cocaine, heroin and LSD. This schedule contains the so-called hard drugs, i.e. drugs with an unacceptable risk of use. This risk is not only based on the pharmacological properties of the drugs. It also depends on the reasons to use, the characteristics of users and the circumstances of use. Schedule 2 contains the so-called soft drugs (cannabis products like hashish and marihuana). Possession, trade, production, exportation/importation (etc.) and any preparatory act relating to serious drug offenses, are penalized for *all* drugs, except for medical and scientific purposes. In the latter cases, a licence from the Minister of Public Health, Welfare and Sports is required. The maximum punishments for acts and omissions in relation to hard drugs are much harsher than those concerning soft drugs. The Opium Law also distinguishes between suppliers and consumers of illegal drugs. This means that the possession of drugs for one's own use is less severely punished than possession for purposes of trade. These distinctions result in a differentiated system of punishments. For example, the maximum penalty for possession and dealing of soft drugs is 1 month custody and/or a fl. 5,000 fine, and that for importation and exportation of hard drugs is 12 years imprisonment and/or a fl.100,000 fine. The maximum penalties may be increased by one-third when the offence has been committed more than once.

In 1988 MDMA was added to Schedule 1 (hard drugs). However, the motive was not primarily its unacceptable risks for public health but the production networks and exportation to Scandinavia, the USA and the UK. Pressure from international authorities contributed to the prohibition of MDMA. In 1993, MDEA was also listed on schedule 1. In practice, users of MDMA and related drugs are treated with the same 'lenience' as if they were using soft drugs. This means that the detection of trade and production of these drugs have highest priority while the detection of possession of these drugs for personal use have a lower priority. In the latter case, the Public Prosecuter may decide not to prosecute.

ADVERSE HEALTH EFFECTS

The health risks of drugs, including amphetamine and MDMA, are dependent on several factors, including their pharmacological properties, the patterns of use, user characteristics (sensitivity, predisposing factors), circumstances of use and the concomitant use of other drugs. The risks may be related to the acute and subchronic use or to the longterm use of these drugs.

The pharmacological and behavioural effects of amphetamine in both animals and human subjects have been well documented in the international literature, especially in the sixties and seventies. Data regarding the effects of MDMA are comparatively scarce. These mainly concern animal experiments to elucidate its mechanism of action and neurotoxic effects, and studies to classify the drug. The described human (psycho) pharmacological effects primarily rely on anecdotes and retrospective reports of users. Generally, there is no control for confounding variables such as concomitant drug use and quality or dose of the administered drugs. Yet, apart from quantitative differences, a comparable pattern of wanted and unwanted effects is reported in several countries (Peroutka, Newman and Harris, 1988; Solowij, Hall and Lee, 1992; Korf *et al.*, 1991). However, life-threatening adverse reactions appear to be highly bound to the circumstances of use, in particular the Dutch and British 'rave scene'.

Acute and Subchronic Effects

The mechanism of action of amphetamine is mainly by stimulating the release of dopamine (DA), norepinephrine (NE), and to a lesser extent serotonin (5-HT), from nerve terminals as well as by blocking the re-uptake of these transmitters. High doses may also inhibit tyrosine hydroxylase and tryptophan hydroxylase activity, the rate-limiting enzymes of NE and 5-HT synthesis, respectively (King and Ellinwood, 1992). The effects of MDMA are predominantly mediated by the serotonergic system. The drug is shown to block 5-HT re-uptake and to produce a long-lasting inhibition of tryptophan hydroxylase. To a lesser extent, MDMA interacts with DA and NE systems (Rattray, 1991).

Amphetamine and MDMA share several sympathomimetic side-effects such as tachycardia, hypertension, palpitations, dry mouth, tremor, jaw clenching, and sweating. In addition, anxiety and agitation may occur as well as a 'kick-down' phase with fatigue and depression that may last for several days. Higher doses and frequent use of both amphetamine and MDMA are reported to cause anxiety, panic, confusion, insomnia, depression, psychosis and hallucinations. With respect to MDMA, the last symptoms may be related to its metabolic conversion to MDA that is known to have hallucinogenic properties (Lim and Foltz, 1989). LSD-like flashbacks have been described after abuse of MDMA (Korf *et al.*, 1991). Overdose can easily occur because of the varying concentrations of amphetamine (often in powder) and MDMA in tablets.

According to registrations of fieldworkers, the number of visitors to house-parties needing first aid has been relatively low. Up to August 1993, on average fifteen people per houseparty experienced negative psychological or somatic symptoms associated with the use of MDMA (de Loor, 1993). These are manifestations of anxiety caused by overwhelming emotions or by the perception of palpitations and jaw tension, as well as a general malaise, feeling sick and vomiting. The former symptoms appear to be more frequently experienced by women, often combining MDMA with hashish, and the latter symptoms are more common in men, often combining MDMA with alcohol. Users are often afraid that these feelings will not diminish. As with an LSD intoxication, a 'talk down' is sufficient in most cases, that is, reassuring and supporting someone who is on a bad trip or in a frightening intoxicating state. Most of the symptoms wear off within one hour and emergency room admissions occur infrequently. However, recent newspaper reports (September and November, 1994) mentioned a considerable increase in adverse incidents that were associated with the use of high dose amphetamine tablets (sold as MDMA) and unfavourable environmental factors, such as high ambient temperatures.

It must be emphasized that the relationship between adverse effects and the use of MDMA or amphetamine has never been established objectively in these cases. Given the described pollution of the MDMA market, other drugs might as well have produced unwanted effects, such as high doses of caffeine causing nausea, palpitations and vomiting, or multiple doses of MDEA resulting in disorientation, lethargy and even hyperthermia, to mention only a few.

According to the National Poison Information Center, the number of requests for information and assistance with regard to MDMA has risen over the years. In 1993, there were 89 questions related to the possible use of MDMA of which 27 concerned the combination of MDMA with alcohol or stimulating drugs. The reported symptoms were nausea, dizziness, hyperthermia, hypertension, agitation, hallucinations, palpitations and cardiac arrhythmias, occurring primarily in subjects aged between 20 and 30 years (Ministerie van Volksgezondheid, Welzijn en Sport, 1994).

Occasionally the use of amphetamine and especially MDMA is related to severe diseases or even death. Several cases have been described world-wide. The most frequently reported is the hyperthermia syndrome with renal and hepatic failure, rhabdomyolysis, intravascular coagulation and convulsions. This pattern was first described in relation to an amphetamine intoxication (Ginzberg, Hertzman and Schmidt-Nowara, 1970). The use of MDMA by subjects presenting this syndrome has been confirmed by toxicological analyses in most of the internationally reported cases (de Man, 1994). The hyperthermia syndrome is likely to be due to an interaction between the pharmacological properties of the drugs and the circumstances of use such as a high ambient temperature, bad ventilation, insufficient fluid intake and sustained physical activity. The concomitant use of alcohol heightens the chance of dehydration. Other serious conditions related to the use of MDMA (determined by case history) include hepatitis and acute hepatic failure, cardiotoxic effects, cerebrovascular accidents and subarachnoidal bleeding, and psychiatric disorders. In the Netherlands, four cases of hepatotoxicity have been described. Two patients successfully underwent a liver transplantation (de Man, 1994). In addition, one case of acute myocardial infarction following use of MDMA and alcohol was reported (van Brussel, 1991).

In the Netherlands a total of six (previously healthy) young people died at house-parties in 1993 and 1994. It is suggested in newspaper reports that either MDMA, amphetamine or their combined use with cocaine were involved in these cases. However, no results from toxicological analyses are available. The same applies to seven Dutch houseparty visitors who were recently (September 1994) hospitalized and needed treatment at an intensive care unit. They probably suffered an amphetamine intoxication intensified by the previously mentioned hyperthermic factors.

Longterm Effects

Chronic users of amphetamine exhibit only limited sympathomimetic effects due to tolerance, but increasing mental problems and physical deterioration may appear. These include paranoid psychosis, cognitive impairment and malnutrition with an increased susceptibility for diseases. Physical and psychological dependence to amphetamine is reported but abrupt withdrawal produces relatively mild symptoms when compared to the opiate withdrawal syndrome.

Following chronic use of MDMA, Dutch users report an increased susceptibility for cystitis, cold, sore throat, dermatological problems as well as menstrual irregularities (de Loor, 1993; Korf *et al.*, 1991). Some of these may point to negative effects on the immune and hormonal system. The former may also be secondary to physical exhaustion, sweating and temperature changes related to the visiting of house-parties. Physical dependence and withdrawal syndromes as a consequence of MDMA use have not yet been described. However, some users show symptoms of psychological dependence, such as 'craving' to MDMA and feeling empty without the drug. Neurotoxic effects related to the serotonergic system following relatively high doses of MDMA in animals, have been repeatedly described in the literature. These effects received special attention because MDMA is structurally related to both methamphetamine and MDA which have been shown to produce degeneration of DA and 5-HT neurons, respectively. The effects of MDMA are primarily attributed to its S(+) isomer and there is some evidence for the involvement of one of its metabolites. The effects are generally reversible although long lasting reductions in levels of 5-HT, main metabolite 5-HIAA and number of 5-HT re-uptake sites were found in non-human primates (Ricaurte, Martello, Katz and Martello, 1992). However, the results from these animal studies are often disputed with regard to their relevance to the human recreational consumption pattern. Clinical symptoms of serotonergic dysfunctioning could be related to sleep, mood, pain and cognition. Yet, apart from a few studies including sleep and neuroendocrine parameters, these functions have hardly been objectively investigated (Price *et al.*, 1989; Allen, McCann and Ricaurte, 1993). These studies would however also be unlikely to elucidate possible effects in the long run, for example, after twenty years of use.

Potential Hazards

It has been suggested that MDMA may act as a 'gateway drug' to the use of other, more hazardous drugs. As an Amsterdam GP states: "I have seen people who never abused drugs but, after using MDMA for a few times they ingested or sniffed everything they could get: LSD, speed, coke, mushrooms, spacecake, uppers, downers etc., often in high doses" (de Groot, 1994). Currently, there is no strong evidence, however, to verify or reject this MDMA gateway hypothesis. Another potential risk is related to the sexuality enhancing properties of amphetamine and MDMA, resulting in increased (unsafe) sex and transmission of HIV. Although MDMA is said to be more like a 'hugging' drug than an aphrodisiac, some users are convinced of the potential risk to get involved into sexual activities. To be on the safe side, condoms are often provided at house-parties. Risk of HIV transmission related to the injecting of amphetamine appears to be primarily confined to the injecting 'polydrug' users (in the Netherlands about 30% of the addicts) of whom only a minority injects amphetamine too. Hazardous habits in drug use still result predominantly from heroin use in a minority of smaller networks, or from polydrug use in which heroin and cocaine are the more important drugs. Most of these users participate in needle-exchange programmes or participate in other prevention programmes. It is therefore not expected that amphetamine alone has any specific role in the dispersion of AIDS or other blood-blood transmittable diseases.

Problematic Use and Treatment

Relatively few users of amphetamine and MDMA appear to have turned into problematic users. Only 1% of all registered clients in outpatient addiction facilities (Consultation Bureaus for Alcohol and Drugs or CADs) has an amphetamines related problem (Stichting IVV, 1993). The absolute number of amphetamine using clients increased from 133 (<1%) in 1987 to 519 (1%) in 1993. This increase may be attributed to MDMA. The CADs are nonresidential mental health institutions specifically oriented towards addiction problems. They offer a variety of care, treatment and social welfare programmes including psychotherapy, group therapy, material assistance and counselling as well as the supply of methadone. The nature of the assistance (psychological, social or medical) to amphetamines users is not known, however. Predictably, the mere recreational use of amphetamines, the number of users who presented for treatment in inpatient facilities (general psychiatric hospitals, addiction clinics) has been low. In 1992, 23 persons were diagnosed with addiction to psychostimulants (International Classification of Diseases or ICD code 304.4) and 19 with psychostimulant abuse (ICD code 305.7). This is less than 0.5% of the total of hospital/clinic admissions related to drug addiction and abuse. No distinction is made between amphetamine and MDMA users. The major types of treatments offered in these institutions are crisis intervention and detoxification, followed by clinical treatment to overcome the addiction.

In conclusion, what evidence do we have in the Netherlands to help us to estimate the risks from amphetamine misuse, in particular MDMA? To summarize, six deaths have been reported the past two years, as well as four hepatotoxic and one cardiotoxic case. In addition, the number of problematic users is very low but has nearly doubled in the past two years, the number of people getting sick at house-parties is rising, the request for information increases and, from animal experiments, knowledge of several potentially harmful effects is growing. Yet, given the magnitude of the exposition to MDMA, the toxicity appears to be modest. A complicating factor is that we do not know if the reported incidents and health problems are just the tip of the iceberg because generally only the most severe and new clinical cases are described (mainly of the hospitalized patients) and reach the media. Moreover, we are not sure that MDMA has been the (only) drug in question in these cases. Currently, an objective estimate of the risks of MDMA in human (recreational) users seems therefore impossible.

PREVENTION

One of the basic tenets of the Dutch drugs policy is that the reduction of the hazards related to the use of drugs is as important as the prevention of drug use itself. The former is internationally referred to as 'harm reduction' and is based on a pragmatic approach to the drugs problem. It is acknowledged that drugs will be used anyhow, despite their legal status and despite activities directed towards demand reduction. The best strategy therefore is to inform users and potential users in a realistic, non-dramatized, non-judgemental way about the positive and negative aspects of drug use, and try to reduce health risks in this way. Instead of a mass-media approach, this information should be given directly to the users and at the places of use. With regard to MDMA and related substances, it is essential to adjust the 'message' to suit the (youth) culture and to cooperate with intermediates, such as the organizers of house-parties or owners of discotheques.

The Dutch initiative, the 'Safe House' campaign developed by the Drug Consultation Bureau A. de Loor, integrates all these elements and is characterized by an outreach approach. The name 'Safe House' refers to the safe use of drugs and to safe sex in relation to house parties. In response to requests by the organizers, campaign workers place a Safe House information desk at house-parties where information (personal advice, flyers) and condoms are available. Visitors can also make use of the pill testing facility described before. In addition, Safe House professionals support the First Aid workers in dealing with drug related medical and psychological problems.

The previously described Drugs Information Monitoring System (DIMS), works in close relationship with the Drug Consultation Bureau. Harm reduction is one of the main objectives of this project. One of the 'instruments' in realizing this objective is the up-to-date monitoring of the drugs markets by means of quality control of drugs samples delivered by a nationwide network. Feedback on the results from drugs analyses is given to the participants in the system to allow immediate preventive actions if necessary. In the past years, these comprised the supply of information to the users, such as the distribution of flyers with a warning message that followed on the detection of chlorpromazine in MDMA samples or very high dose MDEA/MDA pills. In some cases, a public news campaign directed at the producers was set up in order to persuade them to withold their pills from being marketed and to adjust the doses (Jansen and Fromberg, 1993; Fromberg and Jansen, 1993).

In addition, several local authorities have developed regulations with regard to the organization of house-parties. For example, organizers of house-parties have to make sure that there are several facilities, such as sufficient ventilation, chill-out rooms, a First Aid staff, enough water or soft drinks and information. These have turned out to be essential. Yet local authorities are increasingly prohibiting large-scale house-parties because they fear local problems, disturbance of Public Order and drug related incidents (Bos, 1995).

At a national level, politicians show an increasing concern for the public health consequences of XTC use. In the note 'policy on Ecstasy' of the Ministry of Public Health, Welfare and Sports several policy plans are defined (Ministerie van Volksgezondheid, Welzijn en Sport, 1994). First, a better understanding and estimation of the health risks of MDMA and related compounds is required. In this respect, a comprehensive inventory will be made of the pharmacological effects and medical consequences of these drugs. This will result in the design of a research project directed to investigate the (neuro)toxicological and pharmacological effects of the respective drugs. In addition, an education campaign on the risks of MDMA and related compounds will be developed. The outpatient drug agencies and municipal health agencies will be more involved with these preventive activities. Third, the development of local regulations with regard to public order and safety at house-parties will be stimulated and worked out at a national level. Criteria will be defined with regard to the organization of house-parties (minimum age, number of visitors per square meter etc.) and a protocol will be developed to improve assistance to Ecstasy victims. Finally, drug use in the entertainment circuit will be monitored and a central registration point for all MDMA related incidents will be established. Recently, three working groups have been established to work out these plans.

CURRENT AND ANTICIPATED TRENDS IN DRUG USE

Trends in illegal drug use in the general population are hard to establish in the Netherlands because there is no tradition (that means, governmental support) of periodical and systematic data collection on this topic. This applies particularly to trends in the prevalence of use of relatively new drugs such as Ecstasy or cocaine, that are more difficult to determine than trends in the use of drugs that have a longer history of use such as cannabis. At a national level, school surveys have been conducted with some regularity in the past. However, these do not reliably include the higher age groups (>16) in which the development of (more) problematic patterns of drug use may take place. Occasionally, surveys are conducted at a regional or local level. These obviously generate useful data but often do not allow the monitoring of trends. Data are also hard to compare because of differences in methodologies. Moreover, prevalence figures from certain geographical areas, specific subcultures or age groups can not be generalized to other populations. This adds to common problems in interpreting epidemiological data on illegal drug use from surveys due to, for example, sampling bias, under — and overreporting and non-response.

Indicators of problematic drug use, such as the number of registered clients, treatment demand and deaths, should be interpreted with caution too. The same applies to criminal justice data such as the number of drug arrests and amount of seized drugs. These data may indicate trends in drug preferences or, more important, trace priorities and developments in drug control and the effect of drug control on the illicit drugs market (Korf, 1992). In this respect, some developments can be traced back to the former cabinet (1991–1994), showing influences of the Christian Democrats on Dutch drug policy that resulted in a more repressive approach and more stringent prosecution policy, especially with regard to drug trafficking. This appeared from a number of measures such as an increase in police activities and the formation of specialized criminal investigation teams. Moreover, changes in legislation broadened the scope for the detection and prosecution of drug offences and made it possible to seize illicit gains from drug trafficking, to curb the laundering of money and to use, for example, sophisticated telephone tapping equipment (Ministry of Welfare, Health and Cultural Affairs and Ministry of Justice, 1994). Valid estimates of the number of Dutch drug users based on drug seizure data become even more complicated because the Netherlands has a role as drug transit-country too. Synthetic drugs produced and seized in the Netherlands also may be destined for the markets abroad. Therefore, the general increase in quantities of seized synthetic drugs over the past years, as reported by the Dutch Criminal Intelligence Service (Centrale Recherche Informatiedienst, 1993) have only limited value with regard to national drug consumption. Yet, while recognizing the reported limitations, pieces of information may be placed together in an attempt to describe some trends in drug use.

Today, cannabis is the most prevalent illegal drug in the Netherlands. It is estimated that about 600,000 people use this drug regularly. National school surveys showed a three-fold increase of life-time and 'recent' use of cannabis among Dutch pupils from 1984 to 1992. The increased availability of cannabis in coffeeshops[2], increased hemp cultivation and changes in Western European youth culture have been implicated when accounting for this trend (Kuipers, 1993). However, the significance of these factors remains to be established. Next to cannabis the popularity of cocaine appears to be growing, but hard evidence is lacking. The suggested increase in cocaine use is based on a considerable rise in seized quantities of the drug and on registration data from outpatient addiction agencies. The latter show an increasing number of clients with primary cocaine problems as well as an increase in drugs (mainly opiate) clients using cocaine as secondary drug (Stichting IVV, 1993). Both types of indicators are, however, unreliable as estimates for the prevalence of cocaine use in the general population. Apart from opiate addicts, there is evidence that cocaine is used in several other social networks that are largely unknown to addiction treatment services. These include adolescents and young adults (outgoing trendys), criminals, prostitutes, professionals and (other) recreational non-deviant users (Bieleman, Bosma and Swierstra, 1990; Cohen, 1989). Crack, the ready to use smokable 'rock' form of cocaine, is rarely seen in the Netherlands.

In the late eighties and nineties, the most remarkable change from earlier decades has been the introduction of MDMA. Among young people this drug is currently the most popular, and heroin the least popular hard drug. Although the use of both MDMA and amphetamine is most visible in the entertainment circuit, its 'hidden' use outside this scene also appears to be

---

[2] Café-like shops in the Netherlands where one can buy cannabis products such as marihuana and hashish. The sale of these soft drugs is 'tolerated' when owners of these shops conform to certain official regulations.

prevalent. Several years ago it was shown that MDMA did not create a new market but seemed to be integrated in the repertoire of drugs from those people having experience with other (illegal) drugs (Sandwijk, 1991; Korf *et al.*, 1991). It is not known to what extent this statement is relevant today.

In the past years a great variety of drugs has been observed for recreational use. On the one hand these are psychedelics such as MDA, MDOH, LSD and mushrooms, and on the other hand the more stimulant compounds such as amphetamine and MDEA (de Loor, 1993; Fromberg *et al.*, 1994). This trend towards variety may suit the current 'multiple choice generation' that is confronted with numerous life-styles, types of education, music and drugs. As a consequence people may experiment frequently to determine their preferences. Observational data reveal that some drug users change to more 'healthy' alternative stimulant or psychedelic drugs such as qat, guarana, psylocyben, peyote cactus etc. The use of these 'ecodrugs' is still confined to a small users group (the 'psychonauts') and they seem to be more popular in countries where soft drugs are difficult to obtain. Most of these drugs can be bought in specific (New Age) shops in the Netherlands.

The Future

The use of MDMA appears to be more than a short-term fad and it is expected that the specific effects of this drug will continue to attract new users. However, there are also several reasons why people may limit or stop using this drug, such as the negative publicity concerning its health effects and the advent of adverse after-effects following use. In predicting the spread of MDMA use, Kaplan *et al.* (1989) suggest that this drug may have a functional relationship with cocaine because its use is observed in the same 'groups' of (largely non-deviant) users. The authors also speculate that MDMA, from a pharmacological viewpoint, may partly function as a substitute for cocaine. MDMA may be preferable because it lacks the aggressive impulses that accompany cocaine use and it is considerably cheaper. Their 1989 prediction that MDMA will probably occupy a place on the illegal market appears to have come true, but there is currently no evidence that it serves as a desirable substitute for drugs of more unacceptable risk. This should be determined by carefully designed studies repeated over time. In addition, the acceptability of the risks of this drug still remains to be established. Nevertheless, as a consequence of the criminalisation of MDMA, field experts fear and also observe that the use of amphetamine is increasing. Since the abuse potential of amphetamine appears to be high, lacking the self-regulating or self-limiting mechanisms associated with the use of MDMA, this might compromise public health. There are, however, no hard data to confirm the increased use of amphetamine.

With regard to the 'designer drugs', it appears that the race between drugs designers and legislative control is not yet finished. Those who have a chemical/analytical education and appropriate chemicals at their disposal may continue producing new drugs and try to reach an appropriate consumers market. Recently (November 1994), two new designer drugs ('2CB' and 'FLEA') were detected by the police in Amsterdam. According to the Ministry of Public Health, Welfare and Sports, these compounds are meant to change the functioning of a bodily organ and can therefore be regarded as unregistered medicines. Therefore it is being considered to bring all drugs of the class of phenylethylamines (MDMA and derivatives) under legislative control in future. According to some field experts such a decision would decrease the pollution of the MDMA market since the issue of prosecution would be no longer a drive for producers to synthesize new drugs of this class.

Inevitably there are many factors that can affect patterns of drug use and the result of their interplay is hard to predict. Statements on future developments are highly hypothetical and unreliable. Ideally they should be based on results from studies using the currently popular 'scenario' methodology. These studies make a careful analysis of the effects of several possible drug policy strategies and allow predictions of developments of aspects of the drug problem, such as the number of users and degree of criminality. At present, however, predicting drug use is something which the Dutch call 'koffiedik kijken' (reading tea leaves).

REFERENCES

Allen, R.P., McCann, U.D. and Ricaurte, G.A. (1993) Persistent effects of 3,4-methylenedioxymethamphetamine (MDMA, Ecstasy) on human sleep, *Sleep*, **16**, pp. 560–564.

van Ameijden, E.J.C., van den Hoek, J.A.R. and Coutinho, R.A. (1994) Injecting risk behavior among drug users in Amsterdam, 1986 to 1992, and its relationship to AIDS prevention programs. *American Journal of Public Health*, **84**(2), pp. 275–281.

Bieleman, B., Bosma, J.J. and Swierstra, K. (1990) Cocaïne: van mythe tot probleem, *Tijdschrift voor Alcohol en Drugs*, **16**, pp. 11–16.

Bos, I. (1995) De houseparty, in steeds meer gemeenten verboden, *Binnenlands Bestuur*, **2**, pp. 20–22.

Van Brussel, G.H.A. (1991) XTC, een nieuwe softdrug, *Nederlands Tijdschrift voor Geneeskunde*, **135**(44), pp. 2062–2063.

Centrale Recherche Informatiedienst (CRI) (1994) *Jaarverslag 1993*, Den Haag.

Cohen, P. (1989) *Cocaine use in Amsterdam in non-deviant subcultures*. Amsterdam: Instituut voor Sociale Geografie.

Driessen, F.M.H.M. (1992) *Methadoncliënten in Nederland* Rijswijk/Utrecht: Ministerie van WVC/Bureau Driessen.

Fromberg, E. and Jansen, F. (1993) *DIMS: Het drug informatie en monitoring systeem. September 1992-juni 1993.* Utrecht: Nederlands Instituut voor Alcohol en Drugs.

Fromberg, E. and Jansen, F., de Loor, A. and Matser, H. (1994) *De XTC-markt, juli 1993-juli 1994* Utrecht: Nederlands Instituut voor Alcohol en Drugs.

Ginzberg, M.D., Hertzman, M. and Schmidt-Nowara, W.W. (1970) Amphetamine intoxication with coagulopathy, hyperthermia and reversible renal failure, *Annals of Internal Medicine*, **73**, pp. 81–81.

van de Goor, L.A.M. and Spruit, I.P. (1990a) *Inventarisatie van prevalentiestudies naar alcohol- en drugsproblematiek in Nederland: Samenvatting.* Utrecht: Nederlands Instituut voor Alcohol en Drugs.

Grapendaal, M., Leuw, E. and Nelen, J.M. (1991) *De economie van het drugsbestaan: criminaliteit als expressie van levensstijl en loopbaan.* Arnhem: Gouda Quint.

de Groot, H. (1994) Misvattingen over XTC-gebruik, *Het Parool*, october 24.

Grund, J.P.C. (1993) *Drug use as a social ritual. Functionality, symbolism and determinants of self-regulation.* Rotterdam: Instituut voor Verslavingsonderzoek.

Hartgers, C., van den Hoek, J.A.R., Krijnen, P., van Brussel, G.H.A. and Coutinho, R.A. (1991) Changes over time in heroin and cocaine use among injecting drug users in Amsterdam, The Netherlands, 1985–1989, *British Journal of Addiction*, **86**, pp. 1091–1097.

Hartnoll, R. (1992) *Overview of existing research methods. Proceedings Illegal drug use: research methods for hidden populations.* Rotterdam: Netherlands Institute for Alcohol and Drugs and Municipal Health Service.

Jamin, J. (1994) Out of their minds, *Jellinek Quarterly*, **1**(3), pp. 1–2.

Jansen, F. and Fromberg, E. (1993) Analyse van de drugmarkten, *Algemeen Politieblad*, **14**, pp. 22–23.

Kaplan, C.D., Grund, J.P., Dzoljic, M.R. and Barendregt, C. (1989) *Ecstasy in Europe: reflections on the epidemiology of MDMA.* Rotterdam: Instituut voor Verslavingsonderzoek.

Korf, D., Blanken, P. and Nabben, T. (1991) *Een nieuwe wonderpil?: verspreiding, effecten en risico's van ecstasygebruik in Amsterdam,* Jellinekreeks, 1. Amsterdam: Jellinekcentrum.

Korf, D., (1992) *Administrative data on criminal justice: the validity of drug seizures as indicators for trends in drug use. Proceedings Illegal drug use: research methods for hidden populations.* Rotterdam: Netherlands Institute for Alcohol and Drugs and Municipal Health Service.

Korf, D. and Verbraeck, H. (1993) *Dealers en dienders.* Amsterdam: Criminologisch Instituut "Bonger".

Korf, D. and van der Steenhoven, P. (1994) *Antenne 1993. Trends in alcohol, tabak, drugs en gokken bij jonge Amsterdammers,* Jellinekreeks, 2. Amsterdam: Jellinekcentrum.

Kuipers, S.B.M., Mensink, C. and de Zwart, W.M. (1993) *Jeugd en riskant gedrag. Roken, drinken, druggebruik en gokken onder scholieren vanaf tien jaar.* Utrecht: Nederlands Instituut voor Alcohol en Drugs.

van der Kuy, A. (1994) *Farmacotherapeutisch kompas 1994*: medisch farmaceutische voorlichting Amstelveen: Ziekenfondsraad.

Lettink, D. and Tulfer, N. (1993) *"Dak eraf". Een onderzoek naar het ecstacy-gebruik van ervaren consumenten.* Amsterdam: IADA Jellinekcentrum.

Leuw, E. (1994) Initial construction and development of the official Dutch drug policy. In: E. Leuw and I.H. Marshall, (eds.) *Between prohibition and legalization. The Dutch experiment in drug policy.* Amsterdam: Kugler Publications.

Lim, H.K. and Foltz, R.L. (1989) Identification of metabolites of 3,4-(methylenedioxy) methamphetamine in human urine, *Chemical Research in Toxicology*, **2**, pp. 142–143.

de Loor A. (1993) *De risico's van XTC-gebruik.* Amsterdam: Adviesburo Drugs August de Loor.

De Man, R.A., Wilson, J.H.P. and Tjen, H.S.L.M. (1993) Acuut lever-falen door methyleendioxymetamfetamine (Ecstasy), *Nederlands Tijdschrift voor Geneeskunde*, **137**(14), pp. 727–729.

De Man, R.A. (1994) Morbiditeit en sterfte als gevolg van ecstacygebruik, *Nederlands Tijdschrift voor Geneeskunde*, **10**, 138(37), pp. 1850–1855.

Ministerie van Volksgezondheid, Welzijn en Sport. Tweede Kamer der Staten-Generaal. *Nota Beleid inzake XTC.* Vergaderjaar 1993–1994, 23, 760, nr. 1. Den Haag, 1994.

Ministry of Welfare, Health and Cultural Affairs and Ministry of Justice. The drug policy in the Netherlands, February 1994.

Nabben, T. (1992) Het synthetisch gevoel van speed. *Amsterdams Drug Tijdschrift*, **1**, pp. 3–5.

Peroutka, S.J., Newman, H. and Harris, H. (1988) Subjective effects of 3,4-Methylenedioxymethamphetamine in recreational users, *Neuropsychopharmacology*, **1**(4), pp. 273–277.

Price, L.H., Ricaurte, G.A., Krystal, J.H. and Heniger, G.R. (1989) Neuroendocrine and mood responses to intravenous l-tryptophan in 3,4-methylenedioxymetamfetamine (MDMA) users, *Archives of General Psychiatry*, **46**, pp. 20–22.

Rattray, M. (1991) Ecstasy: towards an understanding of the biochemical basis of the actions of MDMA, *Essays in biochemistry*, **26**, pp. 77–87.

Ricaurte, G.A., Martello, A.I., Katz, J.L. and Martello, M.B. (1992) Lasting effects of 3,4-methylenedioxynmethamphetamine (MDMA) on central serotonergic neurons in non-human primates: neurochemical observations, *Journal of Pharmacology and Experimental Therapeutics*, **261**, pp. 616–622.

Sandwijk, J.P., Cohen, P.D.A. and Musterd, S. (1991) *Licit and illicit drug use in Amsterdam.* University of Amsterdam.

Shulgin, A. and Shulgin, A. (1992) *Pihkal. A chemical love story*. Berkeley: Transform Press.

Solowij, N., Hall, W. and Lee, N. (1992) Recreational MDMA use in Sydney: a profile of Ecstasy users and their experiences with the drug, *British Journal of Addiction*, **87**(8), pp. 1161–1172.

van der Stel, J.C. (1992) Druggebruik en preventiebeleid: een caleidoscopisch overzicht, in: Buisman, W.R. and van der Stel, J.C. (eds.) *Drugspreventie, achtergronden, praktijk en toekomst*. Houten.

Stichting Informatievoorziening Verslavingszorg (IVV) (1993), *LADIS 1992*. Utrecht: Stichting IVV.

Stoele, F.W.J. (1994) Doping, cijfers en trivia. In: E.N. Vrijman and R. Weers, (eds.) *Doping controle stap voor stap; een handleiding*. Papendal: Arnhem; Nederlands Centrum voor Dopingvraagstukken.

Swierstra, K. (1994) The development of contemporary drug problems, in: E. Leuw and I.H. Marshall (eds.) *Between prohibition and legalization. The Dutch experiment in drug policy*. Amsterdam: Kugler Publications.

de Zwart, W.M., Mensink, C. and Kuipers, S.B.M. (1994) *Key data. Smoking, drinking, drug use and gambling among pupils aged 10 years and older*. Utrecht: Netherlands Institute on Alcohol and Drugs.

Introduction to Section 5: Summary

The two final chapters attempt to summarise and interpret the patterns of amphetamine misuse in the nations represented in this book. Advances in technology and communication systems along with rapidly accelerating social change in many parts of the world has increased the complexity of the interplay of factors at a global level. Attempting to predict, and prepare for, future patterns has made a difficult task seemingly impossible. The fallibilities of trend-watching have been exposed before. The prediction that crack-cocaine would be widespread in Europe by the late 1980s, based on the evidence that drug cartels saw the unexploited market there as a solution to the problem of saturation in the United States proved unfounded. There has been a growth in the prevalence of this drug in Europe, and it may yet increase in momentum, but it is still extremely low and now seems likely to be overtaken by the growth of other markets.

Pietschmann provides a valuable summary of the economic forces that drive the illicit amphetamine markets and puts forward a model that may help us understand why they are expanding. There seem to be links associating law enforcement strategies, suppliers' profits and market fluctuations. Profit margins for manufacturers and traffickers, and street prices of the amphetamines are important determinants of the level and extent of misuse that is encountered in communities. His warnings about the increased profitability of amphetamine-type stimulants are consistent with recent observations of world patterns in drug trafficking and herald a major change for which we are at present unprepared.

Looking across the data from the seven nations contributing to this book, some commonalities and contrasts are apparent, and the aim in the last chapter is to expose underlying factors that facilitate or impede the abuse of the amphetamines. No claim is made for an exhaustive coverage of all that may be relevant however.

14

Economic Forces Driving Manufacture, Trafficking and Consumption of Amphetamine-type Stimulants

THOMAS PIETSCHMANN

INTRODUCTION

Economic factors play an important role in determining the direction and speed of expansion of the manufacturing, trafficking and consumption of amphetamine-type stimulants. In this chapter, which draws heavily on the results of a global review on amphetamine-type stimulants (UNDCP, 1995a:1), it will be shown that economic incentives for the expansion of both supply and demand for amphetamine-type stimulants are very strong, even exceeding those for heroin or cocaine. Though economic incentives cannot fully explain or predict developments in clandestine drug markets, they are, nevertheless, key factors influencing the behaviour of the main actors concerned and have thus to be taken seriously. The following analysis will begin with a short presentation of the conceptual/theoretical framework, identifying the main economic incentives and discussing their functioning mechanism. This discussion will be followed by a more detailed presentation of empirical findings.

The main economic incentives for expansion are high profits, comparatively low levels of expected *risk* and relatively low prices. Table 1 provides a more detailed overview of the main economic factors driving/restricting manufacturing, trafficking and consumption of amphetamine-type stimulants.

The table should serve as a frame of reference for the subsequent discussion. The economic incentives, which are considered crucial and will be analyzed in more detail in this chapter, have been underlined. The table shows that expected profits, limited by the perceived level of risks, can be

Table 1:	**Main Economic Factors Determining Expansion of Amphetamine-type Stimulants Markets**

A)   Manufacturing level

Incentives: **Manufacturing profits:**
　　　　　* Gross profit margins:
　　　　　* Volume of manufacture
　　　　　* Fixed costs
　　　　　* Human resources (necessary know-how)
Disincentives: **Risks:**
　　　　　* Risks of detection
　　　　　* Risks related to the manufacturing process (e.g. explosion, accidents)
　　　　　* Risk of non-availability of supply of precursors/chemicals

B)   Trafficking level

Incentives: **Trafficking profits:**
　　　　　* Gross profit margins:
　　　　　* Number of trafficking steps between wholesale and retail level
　　　　　* Volume of transactions
Disincentives: **Risks:**
　　　　　* Risks of detection;
　　　　　* Relation with distribution networks for other drugs (e.g. level of violence)
　　　　　* Reliability of supply

C)   Consumption level

Incentives: **Low opportunity costs**
　　　　　* Low prices compared to other drugs
　　　　　* "Performance" of substance
　　　　　* Easy availability
　　　　　* Other incentives (image, peer group attitudes, etc.)
Disincentives: **Risks**
　　　　　* Risks of detection
　　　　　* Health risks

regarded as the main driving force at both the manufacturing and the trafficking level. Although there are many factors influencing profits, the main factors in illicit drug markets are the gross profit margins (difference between output and input prices) and the actual volume of manufacture/trafficking. The volume, as will be argued in this chapter, is determined by decisions taken simultaneously on both the supply and the demand side. Although it will be argued in this chapter that high profit margins and resulting high profitability ratios are indicators to predict market expansion, it should be mentioned that such a correlation only holds true as long as retail prices are relatively low and do not act as a deterrent for the sale of the end-products. As will be shown, this is the case with (most) amphetamine-type stimulants.

The table also shows that various other factors may determine the expansion of manufacturing/trafficking, such as necessary human resources to organize production, availability of precursors, necessary investment for laboratory equipment, etc. All these factors are important. However, they will eventually in one form or another enter into the economic calculus, affecting either the profit or the risk perceptions and thus will influence via expected profits/perceived risks the outcome of the decision making processes of the actors involved. Thus, expected profits and perceived risk can be assumed to be the key factors driving manufacture and trafficking of amphetamine-type stimulants.

Economic incentives for consumers are important as well (Becker and Murphy, 1988; Schiray, 1992; Stevenson, 1994). Even though consumer preferences are more complex and other factors such as image, fashion, peer pressure, etc., are of significance too, the price level of any specific drug as compared to other substances with similar pharmacological properties is an important determinant for consumer behaviour. Research results suggest that cross-price elasticities among drugs with similar pharmacological properties are relatively high (Klee, 1992; Miron, 1992). These findings are also in line with findings that poly drug abuse is globally on the rise, suggesting that drug consumers are increasingly inclined to shift between various substances, thus enabling economic factors to play an ever more important role in these decision making processes.

A FRAMEWORK FOR THE ANALYSIS OF MARKETS FOR AMPHETAMINE-TYPE STIMULANTS

The functioning mechanism and interplay of incentives in the clandestine amphetamine-type markets will be analyzed in more detail in this section to provide an answer to the question of why these incentives have emerged in the first place and how they can be expected to influence the growth of amphetamine-type stimulants markets in the future. This analysis will start with a presentation of a basic theoretical framework for the analysis of the clandestine markets for amphetamine type stimulants which will subsequently allow us to put empirical results into better perspective and assist in their interpretation. The interplay of the economic incentives above can be best demonstrated, if illegal drug markets are modelled, by (downward moving) demand and (upward moving) supply curves, with the interception of the two curves representing the 'natural' price/quantity equilibrium. Though empirical data are difficult to obtain and there may be some disagreement concerning the exact location and the precise shapes of these curves, there should not be any doubt that the general market model with downward sloping demand curves and upward sloping supply curves also applies to illicit drug markets (Wagstaff and Maynard, 1988), including the clandestine markets of the amphetamine-type stimulants. This means that, contrary to general belief, the general phenomenon of 'price elasticity' (i.e., of markets reacting to price signals) also exists in illicit drug markets (Silverman, Spruill and Levine, 1975; Moore, 1990; Niskanen, 1992; UNDCP, 1995b; CASA, 1995, Hardinghaus, 1995).

Higher prices, *ceteris paribus*, tend to result in lower demand for drugs (Wagstaff and Maynard, 1988; Goldstein and Kalant, 1990; Kleber, 1994). Particularly recreational users tend to reduce or may give up consumption while new consumers will keep consumption at a minimum level or may be deterred from entering the market in the first place. Heavy drug addicts may initially take recourse to increasing their crime activities (Miron, 1992; Niskanen, 1992) to overcome the financial restraints (Pearson, 1991; Grinspoon and Bakalar, 1994). However, even the possibilities to generate on a regular basis ever larger funds through criminal activities are not unlimited. Ever more urgent needs to generate quickly large funds tend to reduce the level of precautions taken, thus increasing the likelihood of detection. By increasing the level of risks for manufacturers and traffickers, law enforcement efforts are successful in driving up prices from their original price/ quantity market equilibrium (Fazey and Sevenson, 1990), and thus effectively contribute to a reduction of demand (Wagstaff and Maynard, 1988). Moreover, as a result of the legal status of drugs that makes consumers in most countries potentially subject to legal prosecution, law enforcement tends to prevent a number of potential consumers from entering the market and from experimenting with drugs (Thies and Register, 1993), which — in economic terms — corresponds to an inward (left-ward) shift of the demand curve, i.e., to a smaller level of consumption at any given price level. Although some consumers may have special preferences and may be attracted by the illegality status of drugs, these people tend to be outnumbered by those prevented from entering drug markets.

To sum up, from an economic perspective law enforcement efforts shift both the supply and the demand curve to the left. As the impact is stronger on the supply side, the shift of the supply curve tends to be of larger importance than the shift in the demand curve. The resulting post-intervention market equilibrium will be characterized by higher prices and smaller numbers of consumers compared to any 'pre-intervention' market equilibrium (Wagstaff and Maynard, 1988).

Unfortunately, however, this emerging 'post-intervention' market equilibrium fails to be stable in the long-run. As an unintended side-effect, law enforcement that targets manufacture, trafficking and consumption of drugs tends to contribute towards a substantial increase in profit margins (Block, 1993; Reinarman, 1994). Though the increased profit margins represent, to a large extent, simply a 'risk premium', i.e., a compensation for the additional risks taken by manufacturers and drug traffickers (Thoumi, 1994), the expectations of extremely high profits, nevertheless, tend to remain a strong incentive for manufacturing and trafficking to expand again from any given 'post-intervention' market equilibrium level (Choiseul-Praslin, 1991; Schiray, 1992). This is particularly the case whenever the perceived risk/profit equilibrium differs strongly among various groups in society and/or whenever new, (often) marginalized groups are emerging and willing to take the risks for the given profit potential, thus shifting the (risk premium including) supply curve again to the right, leading to a market expansion ('supply push'). The theoretical limit for this process of market expansion is the location of the original (pre-intervention) supply curve. As drug traffickers would not be willing to run the risk of prison without having chances to reap higher profits than to be expected in other fields of business activities, it means that in practice any market expansion will still fall short of the pre-intervention equilibrium situation. However, expectations and subsequent realization of high profits do not only fuel market expansion by channelling funds into drug manufacturing activities, but — and this may be perhaps an equally important danger — may lead to increased marketing efforts, particularly by improving the operations of the distribution networks, thus actively contributing to a rise in the level of demand. Research has shown that improved (i.e. reliable/regular) availability of illegal drugs is indeed an important factor for market growth (Goldstein and Kalant, 1990; CASA, 1995; Reuband, 1995). In short, high profits for any specific drug can be expected to lead to a market expansion from any given 'post-intervention' market equilibrium by eventually shifting both the supply and the demand curve to the right, offsetting again some of the original gains obtained through law enforcement.

The 'risk factor' has already been mentioned several times. In addition to the scenario discussed above of a lower profit/risk equilibrium for some groups living at the margin of society, the risk factor — or better the lack of risks — seems to play a potentially very dangerous role in the case of amphetamine-type stimulants. There are strong indications that prices of amphetamine-type stimulants, though in general cheaper than cocaine prices, may have still 'benefitted' from high cocaine prices and have been kept 'artificially' high. Prices of amphetamine-type stimulants are in most countries currently above the to be expected 'post-intervention' market equilibrium price. The actual risk premium — which should not be higher than that for cocaine or heroin — suggests that the actual supply curve may be at a lower level than one would expect from the current price levels. This leaves amphetamine-type stimulants manufacturing and trafficking with windfall profits which go beyond risk compensation and thus offer ample incentives for further expansion in the future. In other words, as it can be assumed that the risks associated with manufacture and trafficking of amphetamine-type stimulants are definitely not larger than those associated with cocaine or heroin where several borders have to be crossed and law enforcement authorities have developed skills in detection, higher profitability of amphetamine-type stimulants, as compared to cocaine or heroin, cannot be explained by the existence of any higher risk factor. It is particularly this additional profitability of amphetamine-type stimulants that goes beyond that of heroin or cocaine, which represents a special danger for fueling further expansion in the future.

EMPIRICAL RESULTS

Based on the considerations discussed in the previous section, the following analysis will compare 'profitability' (indicator for the economic incentives on the supply-side) and 'prices' (indicator for the economic incentives on the demand-side) of amphetamine-type stimulants (amphetamine, methamphetamine, methcathinone and ring-substituted amphetamine-derivatives such as the substances of the ecstasy group, i.e., MDMA, MDA, MDEA, etc.) with those of the other two main drugs of global concern, cocaine and heroin. It will be argued that the higher the profitability and the lower the price of any specific drug, the larger is the likelihood for further expansion.

Detailed profit and loss accounts of operators in clandestine drug markets are, of course, not available. As a proxy (see Table 2), the difference between output prices (i.e., prevailing wholesale prices for the manufacturing level; retail prices for the trafficking level) and input prices (i.e., raw material prices for the manufacturing level; wholesale prices for the trafficking level) have been used. This difference, which in economic theory constitutes the 'value added' of economic activities, was termed for the purposes of this paper as 'gross profits'. As the main indicator for 'profitability', gross profits as a percent of input costs (raw material prices; wholesale prices) were calculated. The relative price level was used as indicator for the incentives on the demand side.

Based on the concept of 'value added', some general observations can be made from the very outset. Since amphetamine-type stimulants are typically manufactured in the country of final consumption (or in a neighbouring country), the overall 'value-added' to be reaped in the (consumer) country/ region in question is higher than for illicit plant-based drugs where the value-added in consumer countries is *de facto* limited to trafficking activities. Only minor manufacturing processes, such as transformation from cocaine hydrochloride into crack-cocaine, take place in the country of final consumption. Previous analyses of plant-based drugs have shown that 'only' half (Europe) to about two thirds (USA) of the retail price represents the value-added (mostly a risk premium) generated in the countries of final consumption (UNDCP, 1995). By contrast, in case of amphetamine-type stimulants almost all of the total retail price remains as 'value-added' in the county (or region) of final consumption.

Supply

The following tables, based on US data (1991–1994 averages), illustrates the enormous profit potential of amphetamine-type stimulants. Profitability of amphetamine-type stimulants is particularly high at the manufacturing level (see Table 3). This is true for methcathinone, methamphetamine and even more so

---

Table 2   Concepts used: Profitability/Opportunity Costs

i)   Supply side:

Economic concept to make profits comparable and guide investors in their investment decision:

"Profitability"

In finance/accounting defined as: Profits / Equity

Proxies used: **Gross profit margins / weight units**
                                     Gross profit margins / costs of main inputs

The following analysis on economic incentives will concentrate on the supply side on the following elements:

-       at the manufacturing level:
        *   **gross profits** (wholesale prices less manufacturing costs) **per weight units**;
        *   **gross profit margins in percent of manufacturing costs**

-       at the trafficking level:
        *   **gross profits** (retail prices less wholesale prices) **per weight units**;
        *   **gross profit margins in percent of wholesale prices**

ii)   **Demand side:**

Parameter used: **retail prices**

*   development of retail prices of amphetamine-type stimulants over a period of time (time series data)
*   comparison of retail prices of amphetamine-type stimulants with those of other drugs, notably cocaine.

---

for the more knowledge intensive — and thus less easy to manufacture — ring-substituted amphetamines such as MDMA (Ecstasy). Given the far higher input prices for crack/cocaine, data show that profitability of the manufacture of crack/cocaine, by contrast, is comparatively low. The calculations revealed that (i) gross profits per weight units are significantly (two to three times) higher than for crack/cocaine; (ii) with profitability similar, but methcathinone manufacturing technology even simpler than for methamphetamine manufacture, the potential dangers for expansion of methcathinone might be even larger; (iii) the critical factor for profitability and thus for the incentive to expand manufacture, is the price of the precursor (ephedrine/pseudoephedrine in the case of methamphetamine/methcathinone); costs for other chemicals are almost negligible.

A higher profitability of amphetamine-type stimulants in the USA at the trafficking level is less clearly identifiable. However, if variations in purity between the wholesale and retail level are included in calculations, the

Table 3: Manufacturing level: gross profit comparisons in USA, based on 1991-1994 averages					
	MDMA	**METH-AMPHETAMINE**	**METH-CATHINONE**	**CRACK COCAINE**	**HEROIN**
Raw material costs (in USA)	$0.3* - $0.6*	$0.3* - $2.0**	$0.3* - $2.0**	$15***	****
Whole-sale price for 1 g (street purity)*****	$60 - $100	$10.2 - $50.6	$25 - $40	$10.8 - $40.5	$50 - $250
GROSS PROFITS AT <u>MANU</u>-FACTURING LEVEL — Per kg	$59,000 - $99,000	$8,000 - $50,000	$23,000 - $39,700	up to $26,000	-
Average per kg	$79,000	$30,000	$31,000	$13,000	-
In % of expenditure for raw material	9,900% - 33,200%	400% - 17,000%	1,100% - 13,000%	up to 180%	-
Average profitability	17,800%	2,600%	2,700%	90%	-

*   Prices, if access to precursors from licit sources is given.

DEA reports for 1995 suggest that prices for illicit ephedrine have gone up strongly to $2.3-$5 per gram. Licit ephedrine was available at around $0.15 per gram in the 1991-1994 period. Overall input prices for methamphetamine/methcathinone may have thus increased to $2.6-$5.6 per gram in 1995. Even at this price level manufacturing costs for methamphetamine/methcathinone manufacture are significantly lower those for the manufacture of crack/cocaine.

**   Price based on (licit) ephedrine tablets.

***   Initial purchases of some US$ 15,000 worth of cocaine HCl are needed for conversion into 1 kg of crack cocaine.

****   Heroin is in general not manufactured in the USA

*****   Prices for MDMA are for 1994 only.

Sources: UNDCP, ARQ Data; Merck and various other chemical catalogues; Andrews, K.M. (1995), Ephedra's Role As a Precursor in the Clandestine Manufacture of Methamphetamine, *Journal of Forensic Sciences*, 40 (4), pp.551-560; DEA (1994), Illegal Drug Price/Purity Report, January 1991-June 1994; Shulgin A. and Shulgin (1992), *Pihkal - A Chemical Love Story*, Transform press, Berkeley.

analysis of available data suggests that trafficking of methamphetamine may be slightly more profitable than that of crack/cocaine and significantly more profitable than the trafficking of heroin (see Table 4 and Figures 1–2.)

Calculations of gross manufacturing and gross trafficking profits combined suggest that in the USA, methamphetamine and MDMA generate higher gross profits per kilogram than crack/cocaine. When calculations are based on the gross profits of *pure* substances, the higher profitability of methamphetamine and MDMA is even more pronounced. Calculations of total gross profitability (total gross profits from both manufacturing and trafficking as a percent of initial costs of raw materials) suggest that MDMA may be the economically most attractive substance to manufacture and distribute, followed by methamphetamine and methcathinone (see Table 5). Although the profitability of crack/cocaine is high as well, calculations suggest that it is at a significantly lower level than that of the amphetamine-type stimulants.

Heroin still generates the largest gross profits per kilogram of pure substance. However, the necessary input costs for traffickers in the USA are

Table 4: Trafficking level: gross profit comparisons in USA, based on 1991-1994 averages						
		MDMA	**METH-AMPHETAMINE**	**METH-CATHINONE**	**CRACK COCAINE**	**HEROIN**
Whole-sale price for 1 g (street purity)*****		$60 - $100	$10.2 - $50.6	$25 - $40	$10.8 - $40.5	$50 - $250
Retail price for 1 g (street purity)*****		$80 - $250	$42.5 - $162.5	$75 - $120	$21.3 - $181.3	$65 - $540
Average purity wholesale level		-	92%	-	84%	82%
Average purity retail level		-	53%	-	63%	45%
GROSS PROFITS AT (DOMESTIC) TRAFFICKING LEVEL unadjusted for changes in purities	Average per kg (street purity)	$85,000	$22,100	$65,000	$75,600	$148,800
	Average in % of wholesale prices	100%	240%	200%	300%	100%
adjusted for change in purities	Average per kg pure substance	n.a.	$160,400	n.a.	$130,100	$483,000
	Average in % of wholesale prices	n.a.	485%	n.a.	430%	260%

***** Prices for MDMA are for 1994 only.

Sources: UNDCP, ARQ Data; DEA (1994), Illegal Drug Price/Purity Report, January 1991-June 1994.

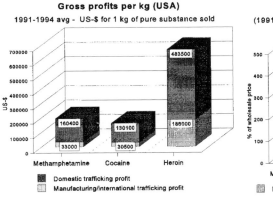

Gross profits per kg (USA)
1991-1994 avg - US-$ for 1 kg of pure substance sold

Domestic trafficking profit
Manufacturing/international trafficking profit

Figure 1
Source: UNDCP ARQ Data; DEA, Illegal Drug Price/Purity Report; Communication by DEA, 7 November 1995.

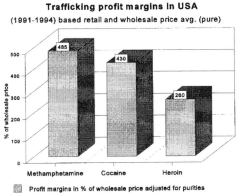

Trafficking profit margins in USA
(1991-1994) based retail and wholesale price avg. (pure)

Profit margins in % of wholesale price adjusted for purities

Figure 2
Source: UNDCP ARQ Data; DEA, Illegal Drug Price/Purity Report; Communication by DEA, 7 November 1995.

considerable. Thus, when higher input costs are taken into account, the net profitability of heroin appears to be a small fraction of that for the amphetamine-type stimulants.

Table 5:	Manufacturing and trafficking level combined: gross profit comparisons in USA, based on 1991-1994 averages				
		MDMA	**METH-AMPHETAMINE**	**METH-CATHINONE**	**CRACK COCAINE**	**HEROIN**
TOTAL GROSS PROFITS (unadjusted for change in purity)	Average per kg (street purity)	$164,000	$102,000	$96,000	$89,000	$149,000
TOTAL GROSS PROFITS adjusted for change in purity	Average per kg (pure substance)	($164,000)	$190,000	($96,000)	$143,000	$483,000
OVERALL GROSS PROFITABILITY	Average total gross profits in % of prices of raw materials acquired in USA	36.000%	16.5000%	8.300%	950%	(260%)* *gross profits (pure substance) in percent of wholesale price (adjusted for purity)

Sources: UNDCP, ARQ Data; Merck and various other chemical catalogues; Andrews, K.M. (1995), Ephedra's Role As a Precursor in the Clandestine Manufacture of Methamphetamine, *Journal of Forensic Sciences*, 40 (4), pp.551-560; DEA (1994), *Illegal Drug Price/Purity Report*, January 1991-June 1994; Shulgin A. and Shulgin (1992), *Pihkal - A Chemical Love Story*, Transform press, Berkeley.

Despite rapidly rising prices for the precursors required to manufacture amphetamine-type stimulants in the USA in 1994/1995, the effect of successful law enforcement efforts on overall gross profitability ratios have not yet been enough to remove the incentives that drive the expansion of the illicit manufacture and trade. Overall gross profitability seems to have fallen from a few million percent (1991–1994) to several thousand percent (1995), a considerable reduction but not one which eliminates the considerable profit opportunities in the illicit market.

Very high profitability of manufacturing (Adelaars, 1992) of amphetamine-type stimulants and a higher profitability of trafficking of amphetamine-type stimulants than of cocaine or heroin has also been confirmed in a number of other countries, including the UK, Germany and the Nordic countries as well as most countries in the Far East region (see Figures 3–6).

Significantly higher profitability ratios for methamphetamine trafficking than in the USA, Europe and most other countries in the Far East region have been found to prevail in Japan and the Republic of Korea (see Figure 7), which seems to reflect strong law enforcement efforts in these countries, driving up the risk premium.

Demand

There are also economic incentives on the demand side. Among a number of parameters influencing the final decision on consumption, such as availability, image of a certain drug, pharmacological properties, side-effects, etc., economic considerations do play a role as well. Economic incentives on the demand side become particularly relevant when there is an alternative

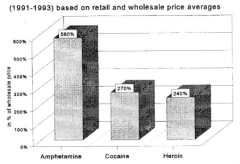

Trafficking profit margins in UK
(1991-1993) based on retail and wholesale price averages

Unadjusted for change in purities.

Figure 3
Source: UNDCP ARQ Data.

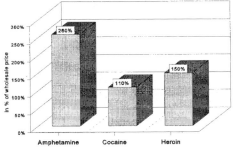

Trafficking profit margins in Norway
(1991-1994) based on retail and wholesale price averages*

*Unadjusted for change in purities.

Figure 4
Source: UNDCP ARQ Data.

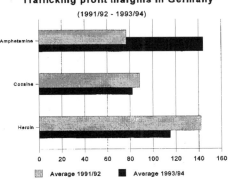

Trafficking profit margins in Germany*
(1991/92 - 1993/94)

* Unadjusted for changes in purity

Figure 5
Source: UNDCP ARQ Data.

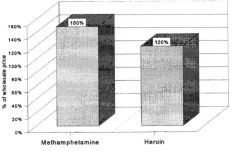

Trafficking profit margins in Thailand
(1991-1992) based on retail and wholesale price averages*

* Unadjusted for changes in purity.

Figure 6
Source: UNDCP ARQ Data.

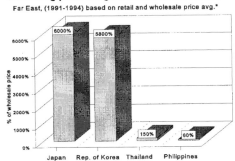

Trafficking profit margins of methamphetamine
Far East, (1991-1994) based on retail and wholesale price avg.*

*Unadjusted for changes in purity.

Figure 7
Source: UNDCP ARQ Data.

substance available which provides a consumer with similar pharmacological effects at lower prices. Thus cross-price elasticities among substances with similar pharmacological properties, such as among the various amphetamine-type stimulants and between amphetamine-type stimulants and cocaine, can be expected to be high.

This is an important issue, as a review of prices confirmed that prices of amphetamine-type stimulants in most countries are lower than cocaine prices. This is particularly true for the Far East region, Australia (ABCI, 1994) and Europe (see Figures 8–11). There has also been a slight decline of prices of amphetamine-type stimulants since the early 1990s (Council of Europe, 1995).

Data for the USA give a less clear picture at first sight. In contrast to Europe or the Far East, prices per given weight units (street purities) in the USA have been at about the same level as cocaine prices over the last decade. Methamphetamine prices have slightly grown in nominal terms (see Figure 12); in

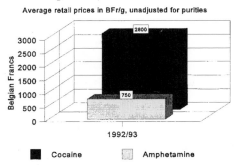

Figure 8
Source: UNDCP ARQ Data.

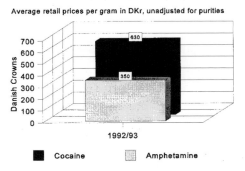

Figure 9
Source: UNDCP ARQ Data.

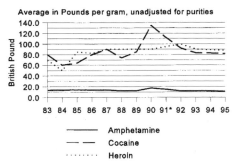

Figure 10
Source: UNDCP ARQ Data; National Criminal Intelligence Service, Nexus, Jan. 1996.

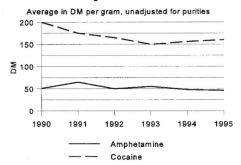

Figure 11
Source: UNDCP ARQ Data; BKA.

USA: Retail Prices

Average per gram, in $, unadjusted for purities

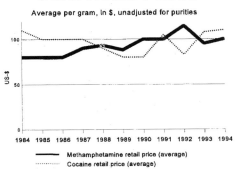

Figure 12
Source: UNDCP ARQ Data. DEA (1994), Illegal Drug Price/Purity Report; DEA (1987), The Illicit Drug Situation in the United States and Canada, 1984–1986 — Special Report, DEA (1985), DEA Quarterly Intelligence Trends, 12, (2).

USA: Retail Prices

Average per gram, in $, adjusted for purities

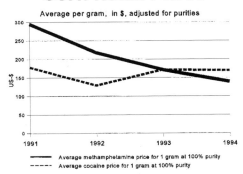

Figure 13
Source: UNDCP ARQ Data; DEA (1994), Illegal Drug Price/Purity Report; Communication from DEA, 7 November 1995.

real terms they stagnated. However, the picture changes once the price comparison is based on pure substances. Then data suggest that until the early 1990s methamphetamine had been significantly more expensive than cocaine; since then, however, fast increasing purity levels have led to strong *de-facto* price falls of methamphetamine. By 1994 methamphetamine prices were clearly below those of cocaine (see Figure 13). Thus, economic incentives for abusers clearly shifted from cocaine to methamphetmaine.

The lower prices of amphetamine-type stimulants in most countries and the *de-facto* fall of retail prices of methamphetamine in the USA may help to explains the fast rising attractiveness of these substances in the 1990s. They confirm the notion that amphetamine-type stimulants — from an economic point of view — have become highly 'competitive' in the illicit drug markets of the 1990s.

SUMMARY AND CONCLUSION

Though all quantitative data describing illicit markets are subject to wide margins of error, the above analysis of clandestine drug markets from both a supply-side and a demand-side perspective, seems to provide sufficient evidence to conclude that economic incentives for a further expansion of both manufacturing, trafficking and consumption of amphetamine-type stimulants are considerable.

Clandestine manufacture and trafficking of amphetamine-type stimulants are financially highly lucrative activities and tend to be even more profitable than cocaine or heroin. This holds true for the manufacturing phase, and, at least partly, also for the trafficking phase. This is even more surprising, as the risks associated with manufacture and trafficking are not larger than those associated with heroin or cocaine. At the same time prices for amphetamine-type stimulants, as compared to other drugs, are relatively low in most countries, which is an economic incentive for consumers to turn to these substances.

Given such strong economic incentives, it seems to be only a question of time until more clandestine manufacturers and traffickers will be tempted to enter and exploit this lucrative market. Intelligence information suggests that this is already happening (NNICC, 1995). Although this may lead to a further decline in retail prices and thus in profit margins, the market as a whole can be expected to expand, both through new consumers attracted by lower prices, and a large number of existing drug consumers who may be tempted to switch from cocaine to cheaper amphetamine-type stimulants.

This scenario of fast expanding markets for amphetamine-type stimulants might, however, still be prevented from taking place if efforts on the demand side (improved information and prevention efforts, improved availability of treatment facilities to allow intervention at an early phase, etc.) were to succeed in prompting an inward (left-ward) shift in the demand curve, and if concerted efforts to strengthen national and international control systems of precursors were to lead — as economic theory predicts — to further strong price rises of illicit precursors, shifting the supply curve (to the left), and thereby limiting at least the extremely attractive economic incentives in this field.

REFERENCES

Adelaars, A. (1992) quoted in Saunders, N. (1994) *Ecstasy,* (German version of *'E for Ecstasy'*) Verlag Ricco Bilger, Zürich, p. 137.

Australian Bureau of Criminal Intelligence (ABCI), (1995) *Australian Illicit Drug Report 1994*, p. 46.

Becker, G. & Murphy, K. (1988) A theory of rational Addiction, *Journal of Political Economy*, pp. 675–700.

Block, W. (1993) Drug prohibition: A legal and economic analysis, *Journal of Business Ethics*, pp. 689–700.

Center on Addiction and Substance Abuse at Columbia University (CASA) (1995) *Legalization: Panacea or Pandora's Box*, White Paper #1.

Choiseul-Praslin, C.H. (1991) *La Drogue, une Economie Dynamisee par la Repression*, Presses du CNRS.

Council of Europe (1995) Group de Cooperation en Matiere de Lutte contre l'Abus et le Trafic Illicite des Stupéfiants (Groupe Pompidou), *Reseau Multi-Villes du Groupe Pompidou*, Strasbourg, P-PG/Epig (94/12 rev. 2), p. 3.

Fazey, C.S.J. & Stevenson, R.C. (1990) *The Social and Economic Costs of Drug Abuse in the U.K. and the Netherlands*, (Report prepared for the Commission of the European Communities), London, p. 12.

Goldstein, A. & Kalant, H. (1990) Drug Policy: Striking the Right Balance, *Science*, 249, pp. 1513–1521.

Grinspoon, M.L. & Bakalar, J.B. (1994) The war on drugs — a peace proposal, *The New England Journal of Medicine*, 330, pp. 357–360.

Kleber, H.D., Our current approach to drug abuse — progress, problems, proposals, *The New England Journal of Medicine*, 330, February 3, pp. 361–365.

Klee, H. (1992) A new target for behavioural research — amphetamine misuse. *British Journal of Addiction* 87(3) pp. 439–446.

Miron, J. (1992) Economists and Drug Policy, *Carnegie-Rochester Conference Series on Public Policy 36*, pp. 249–260.

Moore, M. (1990) Supply reduction and drug law enforcement, *Drugs and Crime*, Crime and Justice: An Annual Review of Research, 13, pp. 109–158.

Moore, M. (1992) Drugs: getting a fix on the problem and the solution, In Rod. L. Evans and I.M. Berent, (eds.) *Drug Legalization For and Against*, pp. 123–155.

Niskanan, W.A. (1992) Economists and drug policy, *Carnegie-Rochster Conference Series on Public Policy 36* (North-Holland), pp. 223–248.

The National Narcotics Intelligence Consumers Committee (NNICC) (1995), *The NNICC Report 1994, The Supply of Illicit Drugs to the United States* (DEA-95051), p. 71.

Pearson, G. (1991) Drug Control Policies in Britain, *Crime and Justice: a Review of Research*, 134, pp. 167–277.

Rainerman, C. (1994) Temperance ideology and sociological denial: prohibitionism in drug policy discourse, *The International Journal of Drug Policy*, 5, pp. 123–130.

Reuband, K.H. (1995) Addiction research in Europe: an overview; drug use and drug policy in Western Europe — Epidemiological findings in a comparative perspective, *European Addiction Research*, 1, pp. 32–41.

Schiray, M. (1992) Economie de la Droge: Construction d'un Champ de Recherche, in Ehrenberg, *A. Penser la Drogue — Penser les Drogues*, Paris, Edition Descartes, pp. 155–174.

Silverman, L., Spruill, N. & Levine, D. (1975) *Urban Crime and Heroin Availability*, Center for Naval Analysis: Public Research Institute Report 75-1, Washington D.C.

Stevenson, R. (1994) Harm reduction and optimal prescribing of illegal drugs, *Contemporary Economic Policy*, XII, July, pp. 101–108.

Thies, C.F. & Register, C.A. (1993) Decriminalization of marijuana and the demand for alcohol, marijuana and cocaine, *The Social Science Journal*, 30, No. 4, pp. 385–399.

Thoumi, F. (1994) *Economía Política y Narcotráfico,* Bogata: Tercer Mundo Editores.

UNDCP (1995a) *Amphetamine-Type Stimulants — A Global Review,* December 1995 (to be published).

UNDCP (1995b) *Economic and Social Consequences of Drug Abuse and Illicit Trafficking: An Interim Report,* E/CN.7/1995/3.

Wagstaff, A. & Maynard, A., (1988) *Economic Aspects of the Illicit Drug Market and Drug Enforcement Policies in the United Kingdom,* (Home Office Research Study 95), pp. 32 ff.

15

Patterns of Amphetamine Misuse in Seven Nations: Factors Affecting Growth and Decline

HILARY KLEE

Internationally the attention paid to the amphetamines has been scant. With the exception of Japan and Sweden, other drugs have claimed centre stage and monopolised the resources allocated to drug control and treatment. Research data and prevalence estimates for cannabis, heroin and cocaine are deficient in many respects, but information about amphetamine is even more limited and partial. This book makes a start on rectifying this, and the contributors have welcomed the opportunity to offer views of the situation in their countries at a time when international concern, stimulated by market growth, is increasing.

In trying to identify factors that affect the growth and decline of the use of amphetamines, the approach adopted in this chapter follows the well-established demarcation between the control of supply and reduction of demand. The novelty lies in trying to make sense of the interactions between the factors that are identified and the patterns that emerge as a result. It is possible that some of the observations will be common to all drugs. However, the specific form they take here will claim relevance only for amphetamine use.

SUPPLY CONTROL

Availability

It is generally acknowledged that one of the most influential factors governing the use of a particular illicit drug is its availability. This observation drives the efforts by governments towards drug control through interventions in prescribing practices, drug production, penetration of dealer networks, and through seizures and arrests. Perfect control of supply eradicates the illicit market for that drug. However, the belief that effective control at an international level is possible has gradually been eroded by costly and so far largely unsuccessful strategies by governments even when acting together (see Hartnoll, 1989 for an account of the international context of drug use). There is now greater emphasis on addressing issues associated with the demand for drugs, in particular with aspects of prevention such as education and harm reduction.

The availability of synthetic drugs such as the amphetamines and their derivatives is subject to a different set of constraints from those of natural and organic drugs such as cocaine, cannabis and heroin. The production of the amphetamines is potentially fairly easy since the formulae are simple and can be widely disseminated to interested parties unimpeded by national and regional boundaries, a consumer group expanded most recently by 'Internet'. Provided appropriate chemical precursors are available, rudimentary laboratories can be constructed almost anywhere. As a result, production can be close to the point of sale, thus limiting the opportunities for detection and interventions in transit. An interesting account of the manufacture of methamphetamine in the US (Irvine and Chin, 1991) describes the use of a range of premises such as motel rooms, horse-trailers and house-boats, which are either temporary or easily moved to evade detection.

The United Nations International Drug Control Programme (UNDCP), becoming aware of the lack of information about the amphetamines, has now instituted a two year global review of amphetamine type stimulants and their precursors. The problem of amphetamine misuse and control is acknowledged to have been overshadowed by the concern with opiates, cocaine and cannabis and, in commenting on the growth in the market, the report states that "… amphetamine-type stimulants are becoming a major concern for international drug control. Simple and flexible manufacturing techniques, easily available starting materials, high profit margins for producers and low prices for consumers — all offer considerable potential for an expansion of illicit markets" (UNDCP, 1995). An analysis of the gross profitability of amphetamine and methamphetamine suggests that these drugs are more profitable than the main competing stimulant, cocaine, in Europe and the USA (see Chapter 14). The economic incentives for expansion are, therefore, considerable.

The nature of the market is rather different for plant-based drugs. The high level dealer in an organic drug that is indigenous only to specific regions, faces problems associated with its cultivation, harvesting, processing, and bulk transportation across borders. This requires an exceptionally high degree of organisation and control over large numbers of people often distributed widely across nations as well as within them. Ruggiero and South (1995) describe how participants in international drug markets form a hierarchy with several levels, the top levels usually embedding drug imports and distribution within legitimate businesses. To overcome the difficulties of control of large scale illegal enterprises there is recourse to bribery, blackmail and various types of corruption of government employees as well as savage violence, which has been so graphically described with reference to cocaine by the media for many years.

This is not to say that amphetamines are not transported over long distances. When local facilities are undeveloped or not competitive, or have been subject to effective law enforcement, amphetamine manufacturing bases spring up in other regions. In the early 1970s after the first epidemic in Japan, increasingly restrictive law enforcement brought about a decline in local production and this was taken over by Taiwan and South Korea (Cho, 1991; Suwaki, 1991). From being both a producer and consumer, Japan has become largely a consumer, its manufacturing role taken over readily by criminal entrepreneurs in less well-policed neighbouring countries who are keen to get into this very lucrative market. The Netherlands and east European nations, particularly Poland, supply the Nordic countries. Australia, although it has a significant manufacturing capability, gets a proportion of its supplies from Europe. Most of Hawaii's 'ice' comes from Asian Pacific areas. These patterns may change of course if new national or international policies improve detection and arrests.

Control of the availability of amphetamine seems to involve predicting who might replace existing suppliers and then devising strategies that will deter their entry into the market. Keeping one step ahead relies on good intelligence and resources. If demand is still high and financial gains large, the threat of apprehension will be seen as a risk worth taking by opportunists waiting on the sidelines.

Intervening in Production

Interventions in the supply of synthetic drugs occur at any stage of the process from producer to consumer. Whereas fields of poppies, coca or cannabis plants may be spotted and destroyed, a similar intervention with synthetic drugs involves detecting and disabling the clandestine laboratories that produce them. However, when local production feeds a major part of the market, these laboratories can be numerous, small, mobile and elusive. A more effective policy may be one that involves an intervention at an earlier stage that limits access to the ingredients (precursors) used in amphetamine manufacture. However, just as laboratory production can move to more hospitable areas, so can the trade in precursors. The effects can be unpredictable in other ways too. Hando and Hall note that precursor control in 1992 led to lower purity levels, a decline also noted in the UK at about the same time and probably for the same reasons. Prices remained stable however, demand was hardly affected and lowered purity may have been partially responsible in the UK for a rise in injecting which involves procedures for filtering the powder in order to remove additives.

Ephedrine is the precursor most often used today and there are a number of countries exporting this substance. There are many legitimate uses for ephedrine and it is subject to extensive world trade, but information about imports and exports is limited making the detection of diversions on to the illicit market difficult. Although recent increases in seizures of ephedrine have been reported by the US, Mexico and Korea, other nations do not always include it in their reports to the United Nations International Narcotics Control Board (INCB). It is difficult to intercept diversions from licit channels since the passage from producer to consumer may be through one or more transit nations and companies. The route into the US via Mexico, with consequences for the pattern of drug use in Southern California, is noted by Miller (Chapter 6) in this volume. Traffickers have sophisticated ways of avoiding the import controls of target countries, even those of the US, with its stringent surveillance systems, and a popular way is for shipments to follow a tortuous path through countries with poor monitoring systems, falsifying documentation on the way. For this reason the INCB, following a 'series of large-scale diversions and attempted diversions of ephedrine' is encouraging governments to strengthen existing controls and improve communication between manufacturing and importing countries (INCB, 1995). It is thought that tightening of international control through co-ordinated action by all UN member governments could make a significant impact on such trade.

Ephedrine is not the only precursor to have been used in the manufacture of amphetamines however, and the technical expertise of chemists and the innovativeness that is evident in developing 'designer' derivatives, such as described by van Laar and Spruit in Chapter 13, suggest that what would be accomplished by effective control of ephedrine would be delays in supplies rather than their disappearance. There are likely to be many experimental shifts between substitute precursors that will ensure a continuing supply of amphetamine-type stimulants that will maintain the market. Many of these substances will not be subject to international control, making effective policing and rapid responses very difficult.

An example is the Ephedra plant (from which ephedrine is derived synthetically). Crude extracts are contained in a large number of dietary additives, herbal medicines and 'energy' drinks which are rarely controlled. In addition, there has been an increase in the use of a very simple process using dried plant material to produce home-made methcathinone, a substance with more potent psychoactive effects than methamphetamine. Widely known in Russia, where it is made regularly for personal use in about ten minutes in many thousands of kitchens, the drug was 'discovered' in the '90s in the US and became popular in some states very rapidly. A similarly disturbing situation exists with respect to access to the precursors of Ecstasy which include oils and plant material rich in safrole. This is a component of many soaps and perfumes that are widely available.

Changing Patterns of Availability

Drug use patterns are subject to continuous flux that is due to some extent to the changing availability of particular drugs within and between nations. Polydrug use is the norm in most countries that have established illicit markets, and the repertoire from which a consumer is able to choose continues to increase. There are several factors that influence shifting patterns of use. Pearson (1991) has described the diffusion of heroin in the UK and US and the factors that facilitated and impeded its spread. Natural barriers such as mountain ranges and water are, perhaps, obvious, but more unpredictable and sometimes fortuitous links between groups in distant communities can also play a role. The current spread of methamphetamine in the US from the West Coast to certain areas inland is attributed in part to the easy access provided by particular interstate highways. The border with Mexico, a manufacturing and transit country, has facilitated sustained methamphetamine use in cities close to it — San Diego, Los Angeles, San Francisco and, more recently, Phoenix, Arizona. (For an account of drug use in this border area see Harrison and Kennedy, 1996.) The proximity of North America to the Colombian coca producers ensures access to a very large market in the US for drug cartels. Access is eased through these links and will therefore influence the reliability of supplies and price, but their absence does not preclude the adoption of a drug anywhere in the world if demand is high.

A useful distinction is that between availability and accessibility, a distinction used in psychology when considering how memory works. A memory trace may be laid down in the brain, and is therefore potentially available, but it can be temporarily, or even permanently inaccessible for various reasons. (The only ultimate proof of existence is when it is retrieved or can be shown to affect behaviour in some way.) It is a distinction that can be applied to aspects of overt behaviour, for example, the availability of sterile injecting equipment may be necessary for a reduction in needle sharing to take place, but injectors may not use the facilities provided because access is difficult — exchanges are too far away, not on the route to or from the dealer, or not open when needed. Drugs may be available in a society, but they may be relatively difficult to access for a given individual — dealers may be involved who are not trusted or they may belong to a different subcultural group, or they may be found in areas that the buyer fears to enter. Heightened police surveillance on the streets is another impediment to access, and an alternative drug may become popular because it is easier to obtain without risk. In polydrug markets such shifts are common when there is a 'drought' of the preferred drug on the streets. It follows that barriers to access will have an ultimate effect on availability and supply. The factors that promote accessibility comprise any aspect of formal or informal control that fails to provide barriers to obtaining the drug: public and official ignorance, acceptance or disregard; local and uninhibited distribution.

The Sufficiency of Accessibility for Predicting Consumption

In the early days of amphetamine use in Europe, the US and Japan, when pills and inhalants were available over the counter, access was easy and they were sold in their millions. Legislation that limited access to the drug through prescriptions created black markets that tended at first to be fed mainly by diversions through over-prescribing and thefts from factories and pharmacies. This was insufficient to meet the demand, and methods of small scale illicit production took over the markets.

Post second world war, perhaps the most dramatic impact of accessibility was in Japan when the illicit market was flooded with unused war-time supplies. The other nation that took to amphetamine as a preferred drug very early was Sweden. It was like many other nations in that a widespread network of legal distribution was already established and many people had been introduced to the drug. There did not seem to be a higher degree of availability there than elsewhere in Europe. Sweden and Japan are often cited as examples, almost curiosities, of amphetamine-oriented cultures and it is tempting to look for correspondences between them in order to find the reason for this and perhaps learn from it. With a smaller population that is highly concentrated in a few major cities, Sweden's drug problem is more contained. Its geographical location in Northern Europe is less central than Japan, which is surrounded by developing nations, some with limited law enforcement capabilities, that are, despite efforts on their part, breeding grounds for enterprising drug producers and dealers. The prospects for continuing problems in Japan are high. However Sweden would also claim to be affected by countries close to its borders. The Netherlands and Denmark have more liberal drugs policies and Sweden tends to adopt a highly critical and fortress-like stance towards them. Whether this can be maintained may depend on the exploitation of increased freedom of movement in areas of Europe further east. Sweden is a target market for Polish manufacturers, who are now making MDMA for west European markets.

Sweden and Japan share both a prediliction for amphetamine over other drugs and a strongly punitive approach to law enforcement — drugs are criminalised and treatment compulsory. Despite the tough policy there is no shortage of amphetamine in either nation. Demand for it has to be high to justify such risks. It has been suggested (Olsson, 1996, personal communication) that the pre-occupation with amphetamine is connected in Sweden with the problem of alcohol. A common practice there is heavy weekend drinking, despite official disapproval and limited sales outlets. State monopoly of retail sales of strong beer and spirits, prices kept high to keep demand low, stores closed at weekends all contribute to a policy that aims to hold consumption down. By contrast, Japan's history is one of tolerance towards alcohol. Male drinking is part of a culture that seems to demonstrate its masculinity and bonding through alcohol. This is common to many cultures in Europe. What is interesting here is the comparatively liberal attitude to alcohol compared to illicit drugs. Alcohol can be purchased from vending machines in the street outside stores. The fear is not of adolescents buying beer, but sniffing solvents (a major problem of this age group also seen in Taiwan) or injecting methamphetamine. In Sweden all inebriation is comprehensively condemned.

Using amphetamine and alcohol together is common, some groups, notably bikers, are known for it. However, this tends to be just one combination of drugs in the context of a larger repertoire, or a strategy used by social drinkers to delay inebriation. In Russia the anti-alcohol laws now verge on prohibition and there has been a major increase in use of methcathinone since the '80s. The nature of the relationship between amphetamine and alcohol in different cultures may vary and is worth much closer scrutiny.

To return to the point that increasing availability does not necessarily mean increasing consumption, a case that seems to support the view is that of the Netherlands which is a producer and major supplier of amphetamine. Despite large quantities readily available, the drug is not seen as a problem there. Of course, what is regarded as a problem in one country may be easily tolerated in another. According to van Laar and Spruit (Chapter 13), it is amphetamine derivatives such as MDMA that have become popular in the Netherlands, as in Germany, on the dance scene. There is some indication of greater use of amphetamine sulphate in parts of the south where it is manufactured, but a generally low prevalence confirms the view that access is only a small part of the answer. Hartnoll (1989) deals with this issue with reference to drug use in general. Availability and accessibility are important but need to be evaluated in the context of other factors. It is also paradoxical that Denmark, the Netherlands' immediate neighbour, and rather similar in adopting a pragmatic approach (some critics would say overly liberal) to drug misuse, seems to have developed an amphetamine problem among its young people (Jepsen, 1989).

DRIVING THE DEMAND: IMAGES, MODELS AND SELF-PERCEPTIONS

The Transition from Licit to Illicit Use

It could be argued that the transition of amphetamine from an acceptable, widely used and applauded, medically approved therapeutic drug to an unacceptable harmful illegal drug has never been achieved in the minds of the general public. Understandably attitudes are difficult to change when people are not convinced by official reasons for a change in policy. What results is likely to be, at best, grudging compliance rather than conviction. The prevailing view in most countries, more than a century after amphetamine was first synthesized, is that it is relatively harmless, controllable and not to be thought of in the same way as heroin. This is despite its illegal status and occasional evidence of casualties. It seems that the authorities are not believed or perhaps the advantages of using the drug outweigh the costs, particularly if those costs are low in terms of health, social and economic consequences. Strict and punitive law enforcement inevitably increases those costs and reduces its attractiveness to more people, but there remain large numbers, not otherwise criminally oriented, who are prepared to take the risk.

The past and current status of forms of amphetamine as licit medication offers a rationale to use it. In certain forms amphetamine is still prescribed in many countries and retains its status as a medicine. Berridge (1988) provides an interesting account of the development of ideological and practical barriers between legitimate medical and illegitimate non-medical use of drugs, notably opium, in nineteenth century Europe. We seem to face a similar problem with amphetamine — but the properties of this drug make the erection of such barriers difficult since there is confirmation from people's own experience or observation of benign effects. Evidence of serious damage to health is rare in view of the prevalence of use and can be dismissed as the result of incompetence by the user or endemic pre-disposition. This is easily contrasted with the damage caused to individuals and society by heroin and crack-cocaine. In addition, if kept under control, all the psychoactive effects are socially acceptable — good mood, sociability, energy and confidence — attributes that are not only highly valued in contemporary society but contribute to a sense of self-worth through feedback from positive interpersonal relationships. As a corollary to these observations — if it is widely regarded as relatively harmless then the credibility and motives of official views become suspect, particularly to the young, and they may be challenged.

Images

The image of a drug is an important factor in its marketability. There are several instances in history. In the 1840s the stimulant used by bohemians and the avant garde in Paris was coffee — and they were criticized for it at a time when opium was widely used and not subject to much concern. The use of opium in literary circles in the UK was highlighted in Thomas De Quincey's *Confessions of an Opium Eater* in 1821 (Lindop, 1981). According to Berridge (1984) it was only when the working classes were believed to be using the drug that it was condemned and efforts made to control it. Fears that they may be using it recreationally and for pleasure provoked moral outrage particularly when it was associated with infant doping (to keep children quiet). Berridge makes the point that the real function was medication in the context of low standards of health care at that time.

A similar pattern of a deteriorating image occurred in the US where ethnicity combined with social class to draw the fire of the moral majority. Immigrant Chinese, already accused of taking work from American citizens, were associated with 'opium dens' and were an easy target. The Harrison Narcotic Act in 1914 made possession of heroin illegal, users were placed outside the law and, as criminals, were now shunned by doctors and social workers. Treatment for addicts effectively disappeared with drug criminalisation.

Cocaine followed a similar track, having been enthused over by Freud for its therapeutic properties, it was taken up at the turn of the century by actors, actresses and their clientele among the rich upper-classes in London. This seemed to persist through the first world war to become the symbol of status in the 'Roaring Twenties' when it was used by a larger group of trendy 'jet-setters' and media stars. Before the start of the slide into the Thirties recession, the frenetic club scene kept it alive. Female actresses and dancers were particularly susceptible, wanting to remain lively through the night. The death of one very popular actress was followed by hysterical press coverage which stimulated public concern, parliamentary questions and a search for a legislative solution. The European cocaine market did not expand significantly however and cocaine retained its image as a luxury drug for the rich and famous. This was in contrast to the image of 'crack' cocaine that developed much later in the US which is now associated wholly with criminality and violence. The original status of other forms of cocaine may have been preserved as a result of the distinction.

There are other drugs that started with a reputation for exclusivity but only stayed popular with the pioneering user group while it remained so. Lysergic acid (LSD), synthesised in the '40s was used at first for psychological research in the US but the range of subjects in experiments gradually widened to include the 'intelligentsia' and alternative sub-cultures in the '50s. Interest was strengthened by publicity about various writers' views of the drug. Academics pronounced on the benefits of its mind-expanding properties and therapeutic value, but Timothy Leary, having advised American youth to 'turn on, tune in and drop out', was ultimately dismissed from his university post. Once LSD had been widely adopted in the mid '60s, it was thoroughly exploited commercially, became subject to rampant press coverage, was associated with violence and then started to decline. Attention turned elsewhere and it now draws little comment as part of the repertoire of available drugs.

Although synthesized earlier, MDMA only emerged in the '70s. Its relative MDA had been tried and tested on the Haight-Ashbury scene in San Francisco in the '60s (for a more extended account see Beck and Rosenbaum, 1994). Like amphetamine and LSD it started out with medical approval when used by therapists to create greater 'openness of emotional expression' (Shulgin, 1990) among their patients. It gradually acquired a recreational market and the opportunity for commercialisation was soon identified. The drug was given the name of Ecstasy and it was being aggressively promoted by the beginning of the '80s among the young and upwardly mobile (yuppies). It then became known for its value when dancing, the government became alarmed, the media were in full pursuit and pressure for control could not be ignored. A rearguard action by psychiatrists failed to rescue it from criminalization in 1988 and Ecstasy became an illicit drug used by various sub-cultures, including large numbers of 'ravers' in a movement that started in the UK and has continued to spread in Europe and the US since. The Ecstasy phenomenon is the latest development in the history of amphetamine and one that continues the close association with music that started in the '60s.

Amphetamine can claim a unique place in medical and social history. It was a drug used for many years in Europe and the US and officially approved as a 'cure' for a wide range of health problems. Distribution to troops in the second world war to improve their performance gave it legitimation and advertised its attractions to people associated with the war effort. Subsequently, for Japan, suffering the throes of post-war depression and loss of confidence, its effects were particularly potent. It also resonated with the ethos of aggressive consumerism and material success that Japan shared with the US. This perhaps contributed to its continued use by American troops for some years after European nations tightened up control.

In its new role as an illicit drug, the image of amphetamine was initially constructed with reference to glamorous sub-cultures that challenged the norms of conventional society — musicians, artists and poets living a 'bohemian' lifestyle. In the '60s resurgence in Europe and the US, music again played a part (Shapiro, 1988) and the images were of youthful rebellion. More disturbing images developed, but initially the psychoactive effects were attractive to many people and it could be concealed by the young since it was not easily identifiable by others as drug related. In societies in which heroin is the standard for 'junkie' stereotypes, the image is of personal neglect, criminal tendencies and violence. The controlled or occasional amphetamine user can assume a low profile and escape the attention of the authorities.

Becoming visible

The dangers of uncontrolled use and the physical and mental changes that can occur are not apparent to the recreational user and the temptation to consume greater amounts of amphetamine, and administer the drug more frequently, is strong, particularly if prices are very low. However, while the image remains untarnished it appears to be tolerated and even ignored by governments, particularly if they are preoccupied with other drugs. Continued use tends to lead to abuse, harmful effects on health, and disruption of social order. The authorities then become aware of the need for action and public opinion, often mobilized by media attention, can then change rapidly.

Hedonism vs self-medication

The image of amphetamine has wide appeal. Many people use amphetamine-type substances simply to enjoy themselves. However, a significant minority have self-medicating personal inadequacies, depression, tiredness, obesity and the stress of environmental pressures (see Chapter 3). These are symptoms that are commonly treated by doctors with fluoxetine (Prozac) and other drugs, and independent self-medication can be partially justified. Among the self-medicators are those with potentially serious mental disorders that are revealed when amphetamine is abused. It is evident that this is not simply a recreational drug — it is highly functional in a variety of ways and will therefore have additional appeal — people not only feel good, they perform better too. Added to this is the knowledge that there are others who are also attracted to the drug whose opinions are valued, or whose lifestyle is glamorous or who belong to a desirable reference group.

Role Models

The identification with people who are admired or envied, and the construction of idealised images to be used as guides for behaviour is very common, if not universal, among the young seeking to establish their own identity. Role models have played a significant part in attracting people to illicit drugs, including amphetamine. The early models of amphetamine users, before the introduction of the accessible and rapid visual communication channel of television, were the 'avant garde' and bohemian groups in the sophisticated atmosphere of European and American cities. Their alternative lifestyles endowed the drug with a particular risqué image — however in the '40s and early '50s their impact was limited.

The Sixties The 'Swinging Sixties', as they were known in the UK, heralded a new age. It was a time of unprecedented and rapid social change in most developed nations as young people found economic freedom, and developments in communication technology started their exponential rise towards the diversified forms of mass media we know today. The young felt they could safely rebel against parents and their conventions. Counter-culture role models emerged and rebellious teenagers appeared as stars in plays and films. Perhaps even more important, popular music, born in the '50s, became the focus of adolescent lifestyles.

'Pop' idols became major formative influences. The role models in the UK were all the more powerful because they were young and working class, just like their fans. Groups like the Beatles and the Rolling Stones were exported to the US, and American bands were seen on international tours. The record industry boomed and different styles of music became associated with a series of deviant youth sub-cultures. Drugs were a part of the image and different cultures (hippies, mods, rockers and punks) were linked with different drugs, mostly cannabis, LSD and amphetamines. In the UK the Drugs (Prevention of Misuse) Act of 1964 focused on LSD and amphetamine. Teff

(1975) argues that the act was mainly aimed at amphetamine because of the use of Drinamyl (purple hearts) by the young, because of the popularity of anorectics among women and because of the large-scale bloody confrontations between mods and rockers at respectable holiday resorts.

Pop stars were known to take drugs. Amphetamine was popular with them because it provided the energy to perform all night and survive periods on tour. Drugs were mentioned in songs, and not always cryptically. This persists today — a group recently received an award in the UK on the basis of a song called 'Sorted for E's (Ecstasy) and Whizz (amphetamine)' which, although it caused controversy, resisted attempts to get it banned on the grounds that it described the 'down' side of stimulants. This is irrelevant in terms of its impact, since the critical issue is the fans' need for shared experiences with their idols, not moral messages or health warnings. Fringe cultures such as bikers, particularly Hell's Angels in the US, became associated with amphetamine at this time — and a level of deviance that had been just tolerable to the older generation threatened to become unambiguously criminal as drug use grew and drug-dealing and violence were reported in the media.

Into The Nineties   Role models have changed since the sixties although those for the young always display the feature of rebelliousness — a voice that will articulate the transition to independent thought and living and away from parental dependence and beliefs. The positive attributes of amphetamine do not change but their value to specific groups may. Contemporary society has values that are rather different to those operating thirty or forty years ago — the world has changed and youth expectations have changed too. With economic recession affecting a large proportion of the world, an enterprise culture with emphasis on personal achievement and upward social mobility is widespread. To succeed is to survive. The young are now better informed, perhaps more cynical and less likely to follow slavishly individual role models — though they are still important to the very young who are newly inducted into the music scene.

The need to achieve is strong but, since opportunities are restricted where unemployment is high, success is often beyond the control of the individual. There are many non-achievers seeking to fill their lives with consoling activities that will preserve self-esteem and rescue them from depression. The antithesis to the philosophy of material gain, aggressive competition and selfishness was perhaps inevitable and can be seen in a variety of forms. Just as 'flower power' caught the imagination of hippies and was manifest in their passive, tolerant and non-violent lifestyles in the Sixties, there are those who want a 'caring society'. One British sociologist (Redhead, 1990) has noted what he describes as a trend towards 'pop humanism' in the UK that is associated with the use of MDMA — a drug that induces interpersonal warmth. This trend is understandable in a generation that has been called in the UK the 'lost generation' — those who have failed to find work, have then become the long term unemployed who have never worked, and have given up hope of finding work. To preserve self-esteem one strategy is to deny that material success matters. An alternative strategy is to induce a psychoactive state that offers the user a self-image of success and well-being, and this is easy to achieve with amphetamine. The difference for consumers now is that the value of the drug has so much more significance than it has had in the past.

For recreational use and hedonistic effects, MDMA is the drug chosen by millions of young people. From its origins in therapy in the US it is now associated with the 'rave' culture which was born in Britain in the late '80s, and which has now spread to Europe and back to the US. There was a period of strong '60s nostalgia in which fashions in clothes and music were revived, but the music scene had changed radically in the UK and continues to do so. From Acid House music, which is something of a hybrid incorporating hard-edged Detroit 'Techno' hypnotic dance-beats and Chicago soul harmonies — experimentation with new synthesizing equipment has led to diversification in sounds and fragmentation of styles.

Some House music tries to re-create through sound and visual effects the experience of psychedelic experience, as it did in the '60s, but now it is expressed in trance-like dancing. Ecstasy helps enhance the mood of unity and sensuality in settings that bring thousands of young people together in close proximity in visually disorienting laser shows and repetitive lighting sequences. Dancing carries on for hours boosted by the energy-giving effects of Ecstasy or amphetamine. It was inevitable that there would be casualties with hundreds of thousands of the young pill-popping across Europe and the US every weekend. A number of deaths over the years, mostly from dehydration, have driven the tabloid media into a moralizing but barely articulate frenzy. They choose not to make some obvious comparisons with the high rate of casualties from alcohol excess, or that as a proportion of the total number of users the morbidity rate is extremely small.

MEDIA IMAGES

The visible effects of media intervention have regularly punctuated events in the course of drug abuse history. Their role in the popularisation of drugs is ambiguous. On the one hand they play an important part in drawing attention to the dangers of a drug and alerting the public, but at the same time such coverage advertises it. This reduces the overall deterrence value of the message since there are many who will become curious and some will then try the drug. If media attention is followed by government action then the perception of harm gains credibility in the minds of the public and subsequent law enforcement interventions are likely to get greater support. This is important since the opinions of the citizens who live with drug use in their midst act as a major preventive mechanism. Communities that are drug sophisticated but law abiding are potential sources of information and support for prevention and enforcement agencies and this is known to users and makes their lives more difficult. It is hard for agents of law enforcement to achieve results without the co-operation of the general public.

The media facilitate the effects of role models and mediate change in public attitudes to drugs largely through alarmist language and dire predictions. They are very powerful since drugs are a growing problem apparently without a solution and appear to constitute a public danger and threat to family health and structure. Worried parents and unsuccessful police actions are effective goads towards political action.

CRIME, MEDIA AND PUBLIC ATTENTION

Crime

The growth in amphetamine use in Japan and the US was closely connected to criminal syndicates that ultimately controlled trafficking. Criminal activity by amphetamine misusers is noted in Sweden, Australia, the Netherlands and the UK. The street price of the drug seems to bear no obvious relationship with the prevalence of property crime by amphetamine users (Klee and Morris, 1994a). A heroin or cocaine habit is very expensive and robbing to pay for drugs is understandable, but many low dose amphetamine users commit such crimes, though more for the 'buzz' and without the sense of desperation reported by heroin or crack addicts. They do not even have the excuse that they are 'driven' to crime to feed their habit. From being a drug with fairly harmless and even positive social effects, there have been points in the history of amphetamine epidemics at which the image of the drug has changed radically. The reference groups associated with amphetamine acquire a reputation for crime and violence. Most recently, the AIDS pandemic has added a disturbing association with injecting risks, which are, of course, not limited to heroin or cocaine (see Chapter 9). Amphetamine is now included on agenda for HIV-preventive interventions.

Media and Public Response

It is in the context of a deteriorating image that particularly dramatic drug-related events have been seized on in a sensationalistic way by the media, seeking to sell copy through inducing alarm and indignation in readers. The early Swedish experimentation with amphetamine prescribing as a form of treatment for addicts ended with the death of a young girl. It caused a public outcry and led to the termination of the programme, marking a change towards a more punitive drugs policy. Public condemnation has been a strong spur to government action in other places too. In Japan, the deaths in 1954 and 1981 of victims of people under the influence of methamphetamine brought about more stringent law enforcement and changes in public attitude that contributed to the end of the first epidemic and may have had some effect on amphetamine use in the second.

'Speed freaks' and bikers on the US west coast became notorious in the sixties through national and international press coverage. In Australia more recently, major lorry crashes have revealed drivers' habitual use of amphetamine to stay awake — a phenomenon that is ubiquitous wherever the drug is used and has been documented regularly over several decades. They caused a public outcry and have helped increase pressure for action. A vigorous policy of control and education is now in progress there. Deaths of young Ecstasy users in the UK and Germany have also been in the news, and harrowing appeals from their parents for the young not to take Ecstasy help to increase general anxiety.

These images do not fit with the concept of successful, socially integrated people enjoying recreational use of a fairly harmless drug. They may help to build drug resistance in the public but their effects on user-groups are uncertain.

Effects on Control and Demand

It is difficult to determine what is important and influential here. When a public outcry presses governments into law enforcement action, these two factors are confounded in their effects. However, enforcement measures would be less effective on their own, they need reciprocal and complementary changes in demand. Hostile public attitudes may help a decline in demand if such majority attitudes are considered relevant by the target group. If the users are marginalised and alienated, they will be part of a sub-culture with norms and values at odds with the larger community, they will be detached from majority norms and their discordant behaviour will be accepted if not acceptable. The drug market is likely to remain unaffected unless the users are still a part of the community and susceptible to its influence, or perhaps direct pressure or action from the community obstructs dealing and disrupts consumption patterns.

LAW ENFORCEMENT — ITS ROLE AND LIMITATIONS

More aggressive law enforcement does seem to effect a decline in use though this may only be temporary. Japan's supplies diminished after policing was stepped up after the first epidemic, the price of amphetamine rose, demand dropped with adverse public opinion and improved economic growth, and it took time before the market re-organised itself. Police success seemed to have an effect in Sweden too where a decline in use was noticeable after the apprehension of only one major dealer. Action against criminal elements on the US west coast was also associated with a decline, although this was not without negative effects as Morgan and Beck (Chapter 7) point out, since the distribution networks governed by 'bikers' gave way to smaller concerns which were more numerous and diffuse and were more difficult to control. The maintaining of control solely through seizures and arrests seems destined to be unsuccessful.

The approaches to the control of amphetamine and methamphetamine abuse adopted by Sweden and Japan are instructive. At first sight it seems that, irrespective of demand factors, a strongly punitive policy aimed at curtailing trafficking, possession and use can work. Nevertheless, in both nations amphetamine was adopted as the drug of choice. A closer look reveals other factors that may have been important.

There seems to have been little competition with other illicit drugs — while other countries became embroiled in problems with heroin (or cocaine in the US), Sweden and Japan did not appear to suffer in the same way — though there was a period in the late fifties in Japan when enforcement of the Stimulant Control Law turned dealers' attention to heroin. Official attention was not diverted away for too long and methamphetamine re-established itself a few years later.

The general approval of amphetamine in Japan after the war is likely to have been fuelled by the needs of a population demoralised and yet faced with the enormous task of re-building their economy and self-esteem at the same time. It must have been difficult to abandon this drug during the first epidemic. Suwaki and colleagues' description of this in Chapter 10 suggests that strict law enforcement combined with public concern brought about a decline in consumption. We are told that the decrease in amphetamine use also coincided with economic recovery. This too is likely to be a critical factor since a buoyant economy would normally indicate high employment and a confident workforce. There would be less need for stimulants to improve mood and fill the tedious and unproductive hours of large numbers of people. Stringent law enforcement may have been a major factor in its decline, but it also may have become less useful to the populace as the fruits of their hard work appeared, living standards improved and the future looked bright. There would be less need for self-medication.

Sweden's problems have traditionally been attributed by them to the more liberal drugs policies in neighbouring countries. Their reaction was similar to that in Japan — the gradual escalation of punitive legislation and policing. The apparent containment of the drug problem at a relatively low level may be the straighforward consequence of this, but there have been other factors too that may have contributed, notably the small size of the illicit drug-using population and the unremitting attack on the evils of intoxication — with any drug (but most particularly alcohol) through education and treatment.

THE REALITY OF AMPHETAMINE EPIDEMICS

The ebb and flow of amphetamine abuse in communities over the last half century seems to follow a pattern — of discovery by a new generation of users, adoption by role models, more widespread penetration, the development of markets, association with deviant or criminal subcultures, over-use and abuse, increasing social and health problems, deterioration of the image, increased law enforcement supported by public approval and the media and a consequent decline in demand — which removes its economic attractions to suppliers. The residual market seems to remain dormant however, only to revive after some years. A contribution to these revivals could be complacency followed by neglect on the part of authorities that have forgotten the intrinsic functional value of this drug to a wide variety of people across different social and occupational strata.

Amnesia and Rediscovery

Some groups are more susceptible than others (see Chapters 3 and 7) to the attractions of a long-acting stimulant. More generally, it is a common observation that those living in conditions of deprivation, unemployment, poverty and other stressors are vulnerable to various forms of drug abuse. Wealthy societies in which the welfare of all its inhabitants is high priority should not see severe drug problems. Though some countries may have experienced such times in the past, this ideal is now rare. For the individuals and societies not so well cared for, the controlled use of a stimulant can seem a panacea for all ills and the functional aspects allow its use to escape notice and therefore censure. The anti-depressant effects of amphetamine are similar enough to a variety of prescribed substances to allow users either to see themselves as no different from those who present as patients to their doctors, or permit recreational or occasional use without fear of danger. The good mood, confidence, energy and alertness are conspicuous benefits, and without strong evidence of the negative aspects they dominate. The negative side of amphetamine is easily forgotten when the media fall quiet, law enforcement relaxes and the problem declines and/or drops out of view, but the positive aspects remain at first hand to attract a new generation of users.

The Progression of an Epidemic: Who are the Players?

By definition, a drug epidemic involves the rapid uptake of the drug by increasing numbers of people. The starting point is a group of users with characteristics that the 'followers' find agreeable and with whom they can identify. It is suggested (Chapters 5 and 10) that the cyclic nature of epidemics is due to the nucleus of users who have persisted in the face of general decline to act not only as a repository of information but as the fuel that keeps the market alive. The market remains dormant until the memories of harmful effects recede and a new generation becomes interested in the positive psychoactive effects. It then takes perhaps relatively few experimenters to sample the drug and extoll its virtues in order to be taken up by others who are disposed to try it, perhaps for the reasons given above, perhaps because they are curious, want to join in, or express defiance. This seems to be accelerated if the role models are anti-establishment and this is advertised by the media. In societies with few resources; inadequate law enforcement capabilities; limited field intelligence; distractions from other social problems or political instability, the economic opportunities are then exploited by criminal elements. The use of amphetamine then increases, with casualties among users and the public, there is concern and condemnation that precipitates action, the drug acquires a bad reputation, law enforcement tightens and use among the less dedicated declines. A residue of converts persists to 'seed' another generation and the cycle is complete.

If this has been the nature (perhaps over-simplified) of past epidemics, will it be the same in the future? Can we learn from history and even risk being a little complacent that another epidemic would burn itself out?

FUTURE USE: EPIDEMICS, CONTROL AND DEMAND

The conditions that, on past form, are conducive to an epidemic are likely to be repeatable — a number of existing users, raw materials and easy production, a period of social change, uncertain future and challenge to prevailing values, marginalised and alienated groups, ignorance, minimal drugs education, patchy international communications and under-resourced or inexperienced law enforcement — but there will be differences too. Some of them seem likely to produce an epidemic will take a rather different form, and one that is more global and diffuse. The opportunities for production now include variations in precursor materials with new and so far unknown suppliers in Eastern Europe, Russia, South-West Asia and China, areas that have been subject to great social change in the last decade and have yet to establish their place in world affairs. Developing countries such as Taiwan, Malaysia and the Philippines that still have low wages and highly competitive pricing are attracting investment and experiencing rapid growth, while most of Europe and the Americas languish and continue to cut public spending in an effort to balance the books. The world patterns of political and economic health are changing and new international power structures are being formed. In such a time the opportunities for exploitation of illicit drugs will increase unless there is some agreement on the advisability for all concerned of their containment. Communications and universally-agreed procedures on international trade are still in an early state of development, and although there are continuing efforts by the UNDCP, the possibilities for exploitation, given the amphetamines' profitability and level of demand, are unlikely to overlooked by criminals in most countries.

New Problems of Control

Another development is the chemical inventiveness that is now available to design many new amphetamine-type substances. Legal control is too slow a process in a such a quickly changing and flexible market, and strict enforcement of the law is made more difficult and more expensive. Internationally agreed control of precursors and substances that are listed in generic forms, if regularly updated and monitored may help but it will take some time for less well developed countries to acquire the administrative infrastructure to apply them effectively.

Multiple choice of other drugs in the illicit market is a factor that affects the market performance of any one of them. Transitions to other drugs are possible when there is a street drought of the preferred drug, or prices rise or purity drops. If local law enforcement agencies have one or two drugs as their main concern, the rest are relatively popular by default. Amphetamine and methamphetamine, or a traditional stimulant, are much cheaper in most countries than cocaine, and comparison of relative costs can make a decision more likely in their favour. Their relatively long-lasting effects can be seen as more cost effective too. It is also a useful ingredient in a polydrug repertoire when the preferred drug is an opiate. In markets with restricted preferences such as Sweden and Japan the options are more limited, law enforcement more focused and preoccupation by the public is not diverted away. A common form of rationalising a piece of aberrant or deviant behaviour is to compare it favourably with a widely condemned alternative and for this reason the impact of prevention and control interventions may be greater in a more monopolistic drug market.

Demand

A drug's image is influential in attracting new consumers. In the case of amphetamine these are mostly young people who are increasingly likely to encounter the drug through the dance scene. Friendliness and sustained energy to keep dancing, with the added bonus of confidence, ensures it a market. The demand for amphetamine, paradoxically, may increase if damage attributed to Ecstasy use continues to appear in the headlines. Deaths are sufficiently rare, and ambiguous in terms of causation to be discounted as irrelevant by many 'ravers' but may be powerful enough to recommend transfer to a similar drug thought to be more predictable. In the UK the price of MDMA is off-putting to the impoverished young who make it an occasional 'treat' and use amphetamine sulphate and LSD together in an attempt to mimic the combined stimulant and hallucinogenic effect of Ecstasy. Amphetamine as well as Ecstasy is seen as a benificent drug, rather like cannabis, that has none of the bad reputation of 'harder' drugs. In the Netherlands and Germany, as in the UK, it is frequently substituted by dealers for Ecstasy, and Heckmann in Chapter 12 speaks of epidemic use almost by default.

The image of amphetamine takes on a more serious and sinister aspect if one considers user groups other than young party-goers. A theme repeated through these chapters is a connection with unemployment, marginalised groups and alienation. The social context of these accounts are societies that are competitive and materialistic, where achievement is applauded and the rewards are on display for those who can afford them. Non-achievers are susceptible to the charms of a drug that will soften perceptions of personal failure and damaged self-esteem, particularly if they feel helpless and incapable of effecting a change. The greatest danger of an epidemic outbreak of amphetamine in such societies is when it does not yet have a bad reputation. Currently heroin and crack-cocaine are regarded as more dangerous to the individual and to society — amphetamine tends to be more prosaic and less problematic and its low public profile allows for insidious growth among the large number of people struggling to adapt to the stress of failing economies and the resulting social divisions. The meteoric rise in the popularity of Prozac, the medical answer to pressure, insecurity and depression, is testament to the potential consumer group for a benign stimulant to enable the workers to function and non-workers not to mind so much. Stress affects the employed as well as the unemployed in societies experiencing economic recession, and licit or illicit medication with drugs is the standard response. The range of effects produced by amphetamine means that a wide variety of needs can be met: — sustained energy for dancers and shift workers; extended alertness for long-distance drivers; motivation for people with boring jobs; confidence for the socially awkward and troops in combat. The sociability it generates brings positive responses from others as does weight control in societies where a slim appearance is valued. Add to this a good mood, and the market seems potentially vast, only limited by the fear of detection and dependence.

PREVENTION AND HARM REDUCTION

With such an alluring combination of hedonistic, therapeutic and socially reinforcing effects what could possibly deter the potential user? One could start with education, but there is an argument that says there are dangers in drawing attention to the use of a drug unless one can be sure that the infomation will not lead to an interest in trying it. The attraction of amphetamine is such that it may be seen as worth the risk by the young and curious. In societies in which use is already increasing there is little choice but to educate potential risk groups about the dangers. However, perhaps more than most other drugs, such as heroin or crack-cocaine which have a negative public image, the preventive messages have to be very carefully communicated. The target audience characteristics have to be known.

There are many reasons for using amphetamine-type stimulants and prevention strategies should be related to them — thus self-medicators will need different messages to those aimed at young dancers out for a good time. But perhaps there are aspects that are common to both. Some idea about deterrents emerges if, having experienced the effects of the drug, amphetamine users are asked whether they wanted, or had wanted to stop, and why. Analyses of such data from young amphetamine users (Klee and Morris, 1994b) suggested that what turned them off was the experience, or prospect, of behaviour that was socially unacceptable to their peers — aggression, deep depression, and paranoia, particularly if this bordered on psychosis. These were likely to invoke judgements from others that they had mental problems — which is particularly stigmatizing to the young. It was 'abnormal' behaviour and psychological changes, not the physical symptoms of palpitations, headaches, poor circulation, 'bad hits' and so on, that were associated with seeking help or thinking about it. The consequences of abuse for mental health and social relations should be emphasized when communicating with young people, more than dangers to physical health which, in fact, have some appeal to young 'macho' males.

Social isolation for an adolescent is a potent force, particularly if the reasons for using the drug have included its socially facilitating properties. If social withdrawal develops with regular use of amphetamine, it could act as a deterrent. Along with this goes the 'junkie' image that is the antithesis of the one the young user has in mind. Such a progression would be similar to the deteriorating lifestyle of a 'smack-head' (heroin addict). Convincing novitiates that this could happen to them is the main problem of course. Many experienced users live through these states, regain control and continue to use. The culture may be sophisticated enough to recognize that hallucinations, paranoia and irritability are part of the experience hence to be tolerated and, if possible, guarded against. Just as the actions induced by alcohol can be excused by others up to a point, so too can those arising from amphetamine. Even then, permanent damage to important relationships can occur if the user persists despite warnings. A current study of amphetamine users in treatment (Klee *et al.*, 1995) has shown that the influence of a partner's ultimatum is strong, along with fear for children. Unfortunately there are also some partner's who are quite happy and even prefer the persona induced by amphetamine.

Amphetamine is a beguiling but also a frustrating drug — it does not consistently deliver the state that it promises. The hedonic effect if injected is likened to an orgasmic state but it is short-lived and declines in intensity with increasing tolerance. Most experienced injectors say that they have never recaptured the sensual force of the first experience. People self-medicating with the drug for depression can find that this worsens when withdrawing, and they easily fall into the trap of continuous dosing in order to avoid it.

Those who are lured by its sociable nature and come to depend on it as a social facilitator can find themselves suspicious of friends, assume that they are the target of malicious gossip and start to become withdrawn and isolated. A highly functional energy boost becomes a disabling state of mental overdrive with continuous dosing — what starts out as a capacity to cope efficiently with different tasks develops into a state of high distractibility and confusion as attention switches rapidly from one job to another, the previous one left unfinished. A useful tendency to be thorough in cleaning, home decoration and so on can become obsessive and actions are repeated ad nauseam until interest switches elsewhere. Morgan and Beck (Chapter 7) highlight what they term the 'paradoxical' effects of continued use of amphetamine. Sadly, the ideal image of the drug persists even then and users struggle to get back to a degree of control that will re-instate the original effects that were so valued. There is a double frustration for those whose use increased because of dissatisfaction with their social status. The antidote to the aimlessness, isolation and demoralisation of unemployment is now seen as superficial if not illusory — the original problems still remain and the user may be in no better position to deal with them.

Social research into substance abuse has consistently identified some potent protective factors such as religious beliefs and family stability — but the list of risk factors is, unfortunately, much longer. They include endemic factors of stimulus-seeking and poor coping skills, social background, particularly the care received during childhood and parental drug use, and situational factors such as peer influence. The profile of the vulnerable has been known for some time, yet we seem a long way from using the information appropriately to formulate effective prevention messages. There are gaps however that need filling. Research on the effects of media reporting of news on drugs would help to identify those elements of communications that encourage rather than dissuade people from using drugs. For health messages to have impact, the 'down' side has to be convincing and recognised as personally relevant — not dismissed as something that happens to foolish and inexperienced people.

It is also important to target the level of drug use with specific messages. This is where the concept of prevention merges into harm reduction. Primary prevention (from non-use to use of a drug) is only one of several stages in a drug-using career — interventions are needed that aim for later stages too in order to arrest further development. Current thinking suggests an approach that — 'would offer a combination of strategies consistent with the needs and developmental level of the individual while sequencing these interventions to be appropriate to each stage of drug abuse behaviour' (Bukoski, 1991). Thus progressions from 'soft' to 'hard' drugs, from using amphetamine alone to using it with various 'downers', from oral administration to injecting need to be addressed (see Klee and Reid, 1995).

In some countries, including the UK, there is little public awareness of amphetamine, patchy drugs education in schools and a focus on heroin. The authorities seem to ignore amphetamine, and in the absence of warning messages, it is convenient for the young to assume that it is safe.

Prevention is a long-term strategy and involves many aspects of interventions that may pay no quick dividends but are investments in the future. The development of community participation is one, and can spontaneously occur in situations of high anxiety and low official action. Despite their low cost these initiatives are mostly grossly underfunded by governments, who tend to prefer punitive law enforcement despite the social and educational benefits of using informal mechanisms of control that are tailor-made for local needs. These choices concerning strategy raise the issue of priorities in resourcing.

QUESTIONS ABOUT PRIORITIES

Public opinion and media attitudes about drugs range across a spectrum of views and it is the more vociferous that often attract attention. Drug use is an issue with a high profile and a low threshold for public alarm, and priorities have to be set by governments in the face of great pressure. There have been noticeable biases. For example, the allocation of resources in many countries has tended to favour legislation and law enforcement at the expense of education and treatment and to favour drugs that, though comparatively rarely used, are seen as the more damaging to health and public order. The political pay-offs in funding treatment are low in comparison to the more visible police actions and media campaigns.

To some extent this arises from different attitudes to drugs — whether abuse is to be regarded as mainly a medical or criminal problem. The crime associated with drug use is a strong influence towards repressive measures — the public have little sympathy for those who threaten their lives and property. It makes harm reduction policies difficult to introduce and sustain, and statements about abstinence, though they may be uninformed, unrealistic and uncompromising at times, are the ones that take root. Nevertheless the apparent incapacity of governments to slow the epidemic of illicit drug use increases pressure towards new strategies. The research data base on the customers is small and needs attention. We need to know much more about the users. Research on the beliefs, norms and values of the target groups, and how the use of the amphetamines is controlled by social forces within groups would be particularly valuable. Informal methods of social control are key elements in changing patterns of drug use and there has been little research so far that can inform policy.

CONCLUSION

There are issues to be resolved if the predicted trend towards another epidemic is to be thwarted. The most long-standing and intractable of these is a resolution of the differing viewpoints, within and between nations, on substance control — particularly with respect to the relationship between traditional licit drugs like alcohol and recreational drugs like cannabis. The issue would best be resolved on logical and not emotional or historical grounds in order to be credible. Ideally, relative risks to the individual and to society of different drugs should be calculated objectively. Comprehensive agreement about what are fair and reasonable constraints on use is remote however. Unfortunately, accepting nicotine and alcohol excess while condemning occasional use of cannabis or MDMA damages the credibility of the forces of law and order in the eyes of young people. There are other perceived anachronisms in attitudes towards drugs and it is easy to cite differences between nations as evidence of inconsistency by the 'experts'. The contemporary drug scene is confusing in several ways. Traditional evaluations of drugs of abuse, distinguished on a continuum from 'soft' to 'hard', are less clearly applied to the prescribed pharmaceuticals now widely sold on the illicit market. Received wisdom from official sources is no longer trusted and the legitimacy of the legal classification of drugs has become a matter for individual judgement. A good case study is Prozac, now appearing on the illicit market, which is prescribed for anxiety, loss of confidence and depression — symptoms for which people take amphetamine. The complex mix of vested interests, moral arguments and health warnings about drugs is confusing without competent, credible, consistent and authoritative guidance.

To the young the agents of law and order appear to have feet of clay — not only are they incapable of out-thinking the dealers, they frequently find the law unenforceable. Changes in drug patterns may or may not be influenced by their actions. The heroin market seems to be declining and there are signs that cocaine may follow. If this could be attributed directly to government policy that has aimed to control supply, one could draw greater comfort from their demise. A belief in the effectiveness of such strategies is difficult to sustain however. It is more likely that the economics of an enterprise market, overflowing with business and technical expertise and high level chemical and communication technology, are driving a change towards cheap synthetic stimulants.

Inconsistency combined with unsuccessful law enforcement undermines police authority and makes it easy to challenge. A policy based on the belief that if an offending drug can be removed then the problem will go away is likely to fail in the long term unless tactics that are wholly repressive are used. The problem needs to be addressed at a much more fundamental level if the solution is to be acceptable on humanitarian grounds and not produce further alienation. Why do people take the risk of using a drug that may lead to exposure, arrest, fines or even imprisonment?

Medically prescribed psychoactive drugs that change mental states are generally approved because they will improve the psychological and perhaps the physical and social health of the patient too. Acceptance of the recreational use of a psychoactive substance is more unpredictable and varies at individual, national and international levels. Alcohol is a major problem in many countries yet tends to be tolerated if under licensing control. To deny access to it in most nations would be regarded as an infringement of personal freedom. It is a substance widely abused and therefore dangerous but supply is controlled — there are standards and licences that can be checked by the authorities. People can drink themselves quietly to death, but that is regarded as their choice provided they do not infringe the rights of their fellow citizens by damaging them or stealing from them.

The argument for alcohol restraint may have gone unheard in several nations but a change of control status is unlikely — there are too many vested economic interests. In the UK, despite well-known problems of alcohol-related violence, there is a trend in government thinking towards a more relaxed approach. Recommended maximum weekly levels have been increased recently. However, the 'battle' with other drugs with little therapeutic application like MDMA (US therapists might disagree) may still be won. Understandably, the growing attraction of the amphetamines and related synthetic stimulants that is associated with widespread law-breaking at all levels has alarmed the international community. Legalisation is generally seen as a dangerous option but there is a clear need to devise a strategy that will contain amphetamine abuse rapidly, preferably without having to deal with uncomfortable and complicated questions that are difficult to answer. Answering difficult questions, however, may be necessary before success is achieved.

Meanwhile, what is clear from an examination of the trends in amphetamine use is that a cooperative international endeavour to devise a balanced approach is needed before the next phase of drug history overwhelms us. Control of supply is the traditional reactive measure but this becomes more difficult as demand increases. It is now important to focus much more on the reasons for the demand and why the law is being ignored. Repressive handling of the self-medicating tendencies of confused, threatened and demoralised communities is certainly not the answer in the long term. Neither is blanket disapproval of what the young see as harmless activities. Easy and rapid access to rewarding mental states can be obtained almost everywhere, licitly or illicitly, and this is now a fact of life. Some realistic decisions have to be made that acknowledge basic human vulnerabilities to hedonism while curbing the damage from exploitation and excesses. Perhaps more importantly, ways have to be found that replace temporary changes to well-being with more powerful social devices by which more long-lasting positive change can be achieved.

POSTSCRIPT

Factors that appear to be associated with the rise and fall in the use of the amphetamines have been summarised in the following tables. Although the lists are long they may not be comprehensive — but they do comprise concepts that seem to be important influences on supply and demand. They illustrate the interactional and cumulative nature of such influences to the patterns of amphetamine abuse. Estimating their relative importance is futile since such weighting will depend on the presence or absence of other factors. No particular relevance should be attached, therefore, to the ordering.

FACTORS THAT FACILITATE THE USE OF THE AMPHETAMINES

FACILITATING SUPPLY	FACILITATING DEMAND
Over prescribing	Accessibility
Established dealer networks	Role models and reference groups
Poor crime control	Socially acceptable
Disparate national control policies	Reputation as controllable/harmless
Poor training of police, customs and excise	Media references to positive models
Political instability	Media coverage of positive lifestyle
Local laboratories	Low price
Ease of manufacture	Low morale, high stress
Access to precursors	Unemployment
Low price of precursors	Functional
Technical/chemical inventiveness	Need for achievement
Technical expertise	Poor understanding of effects
Poor international co-operation	Alienation of sub-cultures
Incentives for traffickers: fixed costs high volume easy transit high profits	Few other drugs
Government preoccupation with other drugs	Other drugs dangerous/inaccessible
Poor official information base	No government strategy for prevention/education

FACTORS THAT IMPEDE THE USE OF THE AMPHETAMINES

IMPEDING SUPPLY	IMPEDING DEMAND
Risk of detection	Low accessibility
Unreliable distribution	Negative image — people, events, crime
Limited distribution networks	High price
Expert, vigilant surveillance	Low purity
Punitive sanctions	Fear of additives
Community involvement	Reputation as harmful
Poor access to precursors	Dysfunction — mental and social
High cost of precursors	Sub-cultural preference for alternative
High production costs	Strong religious beliefs or cultural norms
High transportation costs	Highly negative media coverage
International cooperation	Community involvement
	Credible educational campaigns
	Risk of detection

REFERENCES

Beck, J. and Rosenbaum, M. (1994) *Pursuit of Ecstasy*. New York: State University of New York Press.

Berridge, V. (1984) Drugs and social policy the establishment of drug control in Britain, 1900–1930. *British Journal of Addiction,* **79**, pp. 17–29.

Berridge, V. (1988) The origins of the English drug 'scene' 1890–1930. *Medical History,* **32**, pp. 51–64.

Bukoski, W.J. (1991) A definition of drug abuse prevention research. In: L. Donohew, H. Sypher and W.J. Bukoski (eds.), *Persuasive Communication and Drug Abuse Prevention*. Hillsdale NJ: Lawrence Erlbaum.

Cho, B. (1991) Trends and patterns of methamphetamine abuse in the republic of Korea. In: M.A. Miller and N.J. Kozel (eds.) *Methamphetamine Abuse: Epidemiologic Issues and Implications*. NIDA Research Monograph 115. Rockville MD: US Dept. Health and Human Services.

Harrison, L.D. and Kennedy, N.J. (1996) Drug use in the high intensity drug trafficking area of the US Southwest border, *Addiction,* **91**(1), pp. 47–62.

Hartnoll, R. (1989) The International Context. In: S. MacGregor (ed.) *Drugs and British Society*. London: Routledge.

INCB (1995) Precursors and chemicals frequently used in the illicit manufacture of narcotic drugs and psychotropic substances. U.N. International Narcotics Control Board Report.

Irvine, G. and Chin, L. (1991) The environmental impact and adverse health effects of the clandestine manufacture of methamphetamine. In: M.A. Miller and N.J. Kozel (eds.) *Methamphetamine Abuse: Epidemiologic Issues and Implications.* NIDA Research Monograph 115. Rockville MD: US Dept. Health and Human Services.

Jepson, J. (1989) Drug policies in Denmark. In: H. Albrecht and A. van Kalmthout (eds.) *Drug Policies in Western Europe.* Freiburg: Max Planck Institut.

Klee, H. and Morris, J. (1994a) Crime and drug misuse: Economic and psychological aspects of the criminal activity of heroin and amphetamine injectors. *Addiction Research,* **1**(4), pp. 377–86.

Klee, H. and Morris, J. (1994b) Factors that lead young amphetamine misusers to seek help: implications for drug prevention and harm reduction. *Drugs: Education, Prevention and Policy,* **1**(3), pp. 289–297.

Klee, H., Morris, J., Carnwath, T. and Merrill, J. (1995) *Amphetamine misuse and treatment: An exploration of individual and policy impediments to effective service delivery.* Interim Report to Department of Health, United Kingdom.

Klee, H. and Reid, P. (1995) *Amphetamine Misusing Groups: A feasibility study of the use of peer group leaders for drug prevention work among their associates.* Paper 3. London: Home Office Drugs Prevention Initiative.

Lindop, G. (1981) *The opium eater: a life of Thomas De Quincey.* London: Dent.

Olssen, B. (1996) Personal communication, UNDCP Expert Meeting on Amphetamine-Type Stimulants, Vienna.

Pearson, G. (1991) The local nature of drug problems. In: T. Bennett (ed.) *Drug Misuse in Local Communities: Perspectives across Europe.* London: The Police Federation.

Redhead, S. (1990) *The end of the century party: Youth and pop towards 2000.* Manchester UK: Manchester University Press.

Ruggerio, V. and South, N. (1995) *Eurodrugs: Drug use markets and trafficking in Europe.* London: UCL Press.

Shapiro, H. (1988) *Waiting for the Man: The Story of Drugs and Popular Music.* UK: Mandarin.

Shulgin, A. (1990) History of MDMA. In: S.J. Peroutka (ed.) *Ecstasy: The Clinical, Pharmacological and Neurotoxic Effects of the Drug MDMA.* US: Kluwar Academic Publishers.

Suwaki, H. (1991) Methamphetamine abuse in Japan. In: M.A. Miller and N.J. Kozel *Methamphetamine Abuse: Epidemiologic Issues and Implica-*

tions. NIDA Research Monograph 115. Rockville MD: US Dept. Health and Human Services.

Teff, H. (1975) *Drugs, Society and the Law.* UK: Saxon House.

UNDCP, (1996) Amphetamine-Type Stimulants: A Global Review. Discussion paper for the U.N. International Drugs Control Programme, Expert Meeting, Vienna.

Index

After a reference, f = figure, n = note, and t = table.